ARTIFICIAL INTELLIGENCE IN MEDICINE

Kerry Atkinson and Jim Severino

About this book

All figures used in this book are in the public domain or are acknowledged according to their creator’s request. All the text was written by the authors.

Other books by Kerry Atkinson

Medical books

1. Graft-versus-Host Disease. Editors, S Burakoff, H J Deeg, J Ferrara, K Atkinson. Marcel Dekker Inc, New York, 1990.
2. Clinical Bone Marrow Transplantation. First edition. Editor, K Atkinson. Cambridge University Press, Cambridge UK, 1994.
3. The BMT Data Book: A Manual for Bone Marrow and Blood Stem Cell Transplantation. K. Atkinson, Cambridge University Press, Cambridge UK, 1998.
4. Clinical Bone Marrow and Blood Stem Cell Transplantation. Second Edition. Editor, K. Atkinson. Cambridge University Press, Cambridge UK, 2000.
5. Clinical Bone Marrow and Blood Stem Cell Transplantation. Third Edition. Eds, K. Atkinson, R Champlin, J Ritz, M Brenner, P Ljungman and W Fibbe. Cambridge University Press, Cambridge UK, 2004.
6. The BMT Data Book. Second edition. R Munker, HM Lazarus and K. Atkinson, Cambridge University Press, Cambridge UK, 2009.
7. The BMT Data Book: Including Cellular Therapy. Third edition. R Munker, C Hildebrandt, HM Lazarus and K. Atkinson, Cambridge University Press, Cambridge UK. 2013.
8. Hematopoietic Cell Transplants: Concepts, Controversies and Future Directions. Eds HM Lazarus, RP Gale, A Keating, A Bacigalupo, R Munker, K Atkinson, A Syed. Cambridge University Press, Cambridge, UK. 2017.
9. The Biology and Therapeutic Application of Mesenchymal Cells. Ed. K Atkinson. Wiley/Blackwell. 2017
10. Revolutionizing Tropical Medicine. Eds. K Atkinson and D Mabey. Wiley/Blackwell Publishers Inc. 2019.
11. Asthma: Targeted Biological Treatments 2020. Kindle Direct Publishing, 2020. e-book and paperback
12. Atopic Dermatitis: Targeted Biological Treatments 2020. Kindle Direct Publishing, 2020. e-book and paperback
13. Psoriasis: Targeted Biological Treatments 2020. Kindle Direct Publishing, 2020. e-book and paperback
14. Crohn's disease and ulcerative colitis: Targeted Biological Treatments 2020. Kindle Direct Publishing, 2020. e-book and paperback

15. Rheumatoid arthritis, Juvenile Idiopathic Arthritis, Ankylosing spondylitis, Psoriatic Arthritis and Gout: Targeted Biological Treatments 2020. Kindle Direct Publishing, 2020. e-book and paperback
16. Small Cell Lung Cancer: Targeted Biological Treatments 2020. Kindle Direct Publishing, 2020. e-book and paperback
17. Chronic Myeloid Leukemia: Targeted Biological Treatments 2020. Kindle Direct Publishing, 2020. e-book and paperback
18. Melanoma: Targeted Biological Treatments 2020, Kindle Direct Publishing 2020. e-book and paperback
19. Dementia - A Caregiver's Guide. Kindle Direct Publishing 2020. e-book
20. Breast Cancer: Targeted Biological Treatments 2021. Kindle Direct Publishing 2021. e-book and paperback
21. Non-melanoma Skin Cancers: Targeted Biological and Specifically Designed Therapeutic agents. 2022. Kindle Direct Publishing 2021. e-book and paperback
22. Hodgkin Lymphoma: Targeted Biological Treatments. 2022. Kindle Direct Publishing 2022. e-book and paperback
23. Chimeric Antigen Receptor (CAR) T Cells: The second Revolution in Cellular Therapy. 2022. Kindle Direct Publishing 2022. e-book and paperback
24. Acute lymphoblastic leukemia: targeted immune therapeutic agents. Kindle Direct Publishing 2023. e-book and paperback

Natural history/conservation books

25. Bird facts for everyone. K Atkinson. Outskirts Press Inc., Denver, USA. 2014
26. Birds, Birds, Birds. Kindle Direct Publishing 2020. e-book and paperback
27. A Field Guide to the Wild Habitats of Sydney Australia. Kindle Direct Publishing 2021. e-book and paperback
28. Conserving New Zealand's Endangered Species. Kindle Direct Publishing 2021. e-book and paperback
29. Conserving Australia's Endangered Species. Kindle Direct Publishing 2021. e-book and paperback
30. Nature's Wonders: Britain and Ireland. Kindle Direct Publishing 2021. e-book and paperback.

31. Nature's Wonders: Spain and Bulgaria. Kindle Direct Publishing 2022. e-book and paperback.
32. Nature's Wonders: France's Camargue, the Swiss National Park and Portugal. Kindle Direct Publishing 2022. e-book and paperback.
33. Nature's Wonders: Cuba. Kindle Direct Publishing 2022. e-book and paperback.
34. Nature's Wonders: Japan in Winter Kindle Direct Publishing 2022. e-book and paperback.
35. Nature's Wonders: India. Kindle Direct Publishing 2022. e-book and paperback.
36. Nature's Wonders: Tanzania. Kindle Direct Publishing 2022. e-book and paperback.
37. The Silk Road: Uzbekistan and Kazakhstan – A Book in the Nature's Wonders Series. 2022. Kindle Direct Publishing 2022. e-book and paperback.
38. Madagascar – Land of Lemurs and Chameleons: a book in the Nature's Wonders series 2023. Kindle Direct Publishing 2022. e-book and paperback.
39. South Africa - Kalahari to the Cape - a book in the Nature's Wonders series. Kindle Direct Publishing 2022. e-book and paperback
40. Nature's Wonders – Finland - land of owls and lakes. Kindle Direct Publishing 2023. e-book and paperback
41. Nature's Wonders – Ethiopia. Kindle Direct Publishing 2023. e-book and paperback
42. Nature's Wonders – Kakadu National Park and Central Australia. Kindle Direct Publishing 2023. e-book and paperback
43. Nature's Wonders – Lord Howe Island. Kindle Direct Publishing 2023. e-book and paperback

Other books

44. Paintings 2019 – 2021. Kindle Direct Publishing 2021. e-book and paperback.
45. Ferrari Road Cars. Kindle Direct Publishing 2022. e-book and paperback.
46. Paintings II. 2022. Kindle Direct Publishing 2022. e-book and paperback.
47. Samuel Beckett and Bob Dylan – living in a Shakespearean era. Kindle Direct Publishing 2022. e-book and paperback.
48. Paintings and sculptures 2023. Kindle Direct Publishing 2023. e-book and paperback.

49. Ten influential European paintings. Kindle Direct Publishing 2023. e-book and paperback

TABLE OF CONTENTS

Authors' preface

Key events in the 20th Century include the two World Wars, the development of nuclear weapons and their use on Hiroshima and Nagasaki, the invention of the jet engine which led to mass global travel, and the invention of the internet and search engines allowing access to information on practically everything, as long as you have a computer or a smartphone, and an internet provider. Learning to use the internet takes about 1 minute and you do not need to know anything about the computer science underlying it.

Another major event spanning the 20th and 21st Centuries is the development and application of artificial intelligence.

Artificial intelligence is the use of large data bases to solve complex problems.

The concept was born in 1956 and The Journal of Artificial Intelligence was first published in 1993. In 2024 The New England Journal of Medicine started to publish a separate sister journal called NEJM AI.

Like all technical sciences AI involves a large number of jargon terms. The meaning of many of these is not immediately straightforward to most medical practitioners but are so essential to understanding AI and how it works that we have included a glossary of terms used in machine learning and in AI at the beginning of this book (Chapter 1), rather than at the end of it.

Progress on the use of AI got a major boost in 2022 when ChatGPT (Chat Generative Pre-trained Transformer) was released using open (ie freely available) software. Chat GPT is a chatbot developed by the software company OpenAI. (A chatbot is a software application or web interface that is designed to mimic human conversation through text or voice interactions). Modern chatbots are typically online and use generative artificial intelligence systems that are capable of maintaining a conversation with a user in natural language and simulating the way a human would behave as a conversational partner. Such chatbots often use deep learning and natural language processing, but simpler chatbots have existed for decades). Based on a large language model, users of ChatGPT can refine and steer a conversation towards a desired length, format, style, level of detail, and language. Successive prompts and replies, known as prompt engineering, are considered at each conversation stage as a context. By January 2023 it had become what was then the fastest-growing consumer software application in history, gaining over 100 million users and contributing to OpenAI's valuation growing to $29 billion. Other major technology companies working in AI include Microsoft, Alphabet (Google's parent company), Meta (the parent company of Facebook and Instagram) and Amazon.

A word about the brain of mammals, specifically the neocortex, which is the most recent part of the mammalian brain to evolve, is appropriate here, since this is what AI is trying to mimic: the mammalian neocortex is a remarkably complex organ. It is composed by six layers of neurons and appears to be a distinguishing feature of mammals. It covers the whole of the brain and is responsible for connecting each part of the brain with every other part of the brain. It contains many neuronal cell types, oligodendrocytes, and glia, together accounting for over 10 billion cells in the human brain, that form perhaps 10^{13} - 10^{15} intricate connections (synapses) with other regions of the central nervous system. In its human form the neocortex exists at its most complex and evolved state. It is the region of the brain responsible for sensation, action, cognition, and consciousness.

AI is a complex science involving computer science, electrical engineering, mechanical engineering, mathematics, statistics, robotics, biology and linguistics. There are still many things that machines cannot do, such as understanding the nuances of language, common-sense reasoning, and learning a new skill from just one or two examples. AI software will need to master tasks like these if it is to get close to the multifaceted, adaptable, and creative intelligence of humans.

The impact of AI on human activity will be huge, none more so than in medical diagnosis and treatment. AI is now ubiquitous. It is at the core of Google, Alexa, Siri, Cortana, Facebook, Tesla, Watson and AlphaGo. A search on Google showed 105 million entries and counting. Google Trends shows a growing demand for this search term consistent with the exponential rise of deep learning.

As well as medicine, cellular biology and molecular biology, doctors will need to understand the use of AI and will likely incorporate it into their practice.

Chapter 1. Terms used in machine learning and artificial intelligence

Artificial intelligence

AI, sometimes called machine intelligence, is intelligence demonstrated by machines, in contrast to the natural intelligence displayed by humans and other animals. In computer science AI research is defined as the study of "intelligent agents", meaning any device that perceives its environment and takes actions that maximize its chance of successfully achieving its goals. Colloquially, the term "artificial intelligence" is applied when a machine mimics "cognitive" functions that humans associate with other human minds, such as learning and problem solving. The traditional problems (or goals) of AI research include reasoning, knowledge representation, planning, learning, natural language processing, perception and the ability to move and manipulate objects. General intelligence is among the field's long-term goals. Approaches include statistical methods, computational intelligence, and traditional symbolic AI. Many tools are used in AI, including versions of search and mathematical optimization, artificial neural networks, and methods based on statistics, probability and economics. The AI field draws upon computer science, mathematics, psychology, linguistics, philosophy, to mention only a few.

There is no established unifying theory or paradigm that guides AI research. A few of the most long standing questions that have remained unanswered include this: should artificial intelligence simulate natural intelligence by studying psychology or neurobiology?

Machine learning (ML) is a subfield of artificial intelligence (AI) in which computer programs learn automatically from experience without explicit programming instructions. This learning by machines can be supervised, semi-supervised, or unsupervised. In supervised setup, the machine is fed with datasets of problems with the answers. Machines (ie, computers) learn to pick up the correct answer through trial and error. In unsupervised learning, machines analyze input data with no defined answer. The semi-supervised is a hybrid approach that involves both labelled and unlabelled data.

Artificial neural network

Artificial neural networks are flexible mathematical models that use multiple algorithms to identify complex nonlinear relationships within large datasets (analytics). Information enters the artificial neural network through the input layer, which is then fed through the multiple layers of algorithmic processes. These processes are applied according to the weights learned in the machine learning processes. Finally, the processed data come out of the output layer. Artificial neural networks help the machine for deep learning.

Active learning

The computer can only obtain training labels for a limited set of instances, and it also has to optimize its choice of objects for which to label. When used interactively, these can be presented to the user for labelling.

Affective computing - see social intelligence below.

Agent architectures and cognitive architectures

Researchers have designed systems to build intelligent systems out of interacting intelligent agents in a multi-agent system. A hierarchical control system provides a bridge between sub-symbolic AI at its lowest, reactive levels and traditional symbolic AI at its highest levels, where relaxed time constraints permit planning and world modelling. Some cognitive architectures are custom-built to solve a narrow problem; others, such as SOAR (security orchestration, automation and response), are designed to mimic human cognition and to provide insight into general intelligence. Modern extensions of SOAR are hybrid intelligent systems that include both symbolic and sub-symbolic components. SOAR is a software solution that enables security teams to integrate and coordinate separate tools into streamlined threat response workflows. In large organizations, security operations centers (SOCs) rely on numerous tools to track and respond to cyberthreats.

Algorithm

AI revolves around the use of algorithms. An algorithm is a set of unambiguous instructions that a mechanical computer can execute. In mathematics and computer science, an algorithm is an unambiguous specification of how to solve a class of problems. Algorithms can perform calculations, data processing and automated reasoning tasks. An algorithm can be expressed within a finite amount of space and time and in a well-defined formal language for calculating a function. Starting from an initial state and initial input, the instructions describe a computation that, when executed, proceeds through a finite number of well-defined successive states, eventually producing "output" and terminating at a final ending state; some algorithms, known as randomized algorithms, incorporate random input. A complex algorithm is often built on top of other, simpler, algorithms.

Algorithms can be tree-like or in graphic form:

Tree-like algorithm:

Root node = starting point for processing

Branch node = support other branches or leaves

Leaf node = ending point of tree

Graph-like algorithm: unlike binary tree-like agorithms, a graph-like algorithm has a multitude of connections and can connect in any direction.

Domain

The domains in AI include machine learning, deep learning, natural language processing, computer vision, and data science. AI planning typically involves input to a domain model. Such planners are called domain-independent in order to emphasis the fact that they can solve planning problems from a wide range of domains. Examples of the use of such domains are block stacking, logistics, workflow management, and robot task planning. Hence a single domain-independent planner can be used to solve planning problems in all these various domains.

Domains in ML include supervised learning, unsupervised learning, semi-supervised learning, and reinforcement learning.

An artificial neural network (ANN) learning algorithm, usually called "neural network" (NN), is a learning algorithm that is inspired by biological neural networks. Computations are structured in terms of an interconnected group of artificial neurons, processing information using a connectionist approach to computation. Modern neural networks are non-linear statistical data modelling tools. They are usually used to model complex relationships between inputs and outputs, to find patterns in data, or to capture the statistical structure in an unknown joint probability distribution between observed variables.

Ant colony optimization (ACO)

In computer science and operations research, the ant colony optimization algorithm (ACO) is a probabilistic technique for solving computational problems which can be reduced to finding good paths through graphs. Artificial ants stand for multi-agent methods inspired by the behaviour of real ants. The pheromone-based communication of biological ants is often the predominant paradigm used. Combinations of artificial ants and local search algorithms have become a method of choice for numerous optimization tasks such as vehicle routing and internet routing.

Anti-logic or scruffy AI

Scruffy AI ("scruffies") uses any number of different algorithms and methods to achieve intelligent behavior. Scruffies rely on incremental testing to verify their programs and scruffy programming requires large amounts of hand coding or knowledge engineering. Proponents of scruffies have argued that general intelligence can only be implemented by solving a large number of essentially unrelated problems, and that there is no magic bullet that will allow programs to develop general intelligence autonomously.

Artificial general intelligence (AGI)

Artificial neural networks (ANN) or connectionist systems are computing systems vaguely inspired by the biological neural networks that constitute animal brains. Such systems "learn" to perform tasks by considering examples, generally without being programmed with any task-specific rules. For example, in image recognition, they might learn to identify images that contain cats by analyzing images that have been manually labelled as "cat" or "no cat" and using the results to identify cats in other images. They do this without any prior knowledge about cats, e.g., that they have fur, tails, whiskers and cat-like faces. Instead, they automatically generate identifying characteristics from the learning material that they process. An ANN is based on a collection of connected units or nodes called artificial neurons which loosely model the neurons in a biological brain. Each connection, like the synapses in a biological brain, can transmit a signal from one artificial neuron to another. An artificial neuron that receives a signal can process it and then signal additional artificial neurons connected to it. In common ANN implementations, the signal at a connection between artificial neurons is a real number. The connections between artificial neurons are called 'edges'. Artificial neurons and edges typically have a weight that adjusts as learning proceeds. The weight increases or decreases the strength of the signal at a connection. Artificial neurons may have a threshold such that the signal is only sent if the aggregate signal crosses that threshold. Typically, artificial neurons are aggregated into layers. Different layers may perform different kinds of transformations on their inputs. Signals travel from the first layer (the input layer), to the last layer (the output layer), possibly after traversing the layers multiple times.

Artificial neuron

An artificial neuron is a mathematical function conceived as a model of biological neurons in a neural network. Artificial neurons are the elementary units of artificial neural networks. The artificial neuron receives one or more inputs (representing excitatory postsynaptic potentials and inhibitory postsynaptic potentials at neural dendrites) and sums them to produce an output (or activation, representing a neuron's action potential which is transmitted along its axon).

Association rule learning

Association rule learning is a method for discovering interesting relationships between variables in large databases.

Attention

Attention was developed to address the weaknesses of recurrent neural networks, where words in a sentence are slowly processed one at a time. Recurrent neural networks favor more recent words at the end of a sentence while earlier words fade away in volatile neural activations. Attention gives all words equal access to any part of a sentence in a faster parallel scheme and no longer suffers the wait time of serial processing. Earlier uses attached this mechanism to a serial recurrent neural network's language translation system, but later uses in large language models removed the recurrent neural network and relied heavily on the faster parallel attention scheme.

Automated planning and scheduling

Automated planning and scheduling, sometimes denoted as simply AI planning, is a branch of artificial intelligence that concerns the realization of strategies or action sequences, typically for execution by intelligent agents, autonomous robots and unmanned vehicles. Unlike classical control and classification problems, the solutions are complex and must be discovered and optimized in multidimensional space.

Automated reasoning

Automated reasoning is dedicated to understanding different aspects of reasoning. The study of automated reasoning helps produce computer programs that allow computers to reason completely, or nearly completely, automatically.

Backpropagation

Backpropagation, or backward propagation of errors, is an algorithm that is designed to test for errors working back from output nodes to input nodes. It is an important mathematical tool for improving the accuracy of predictions in data mining and machine learning. Backpropagation computes the gradient of a loss function with respect to the weights of the network for a single input–output example, and does so efficiently, computing the gradient one layer at a time, iterating backward from the last layer to avoid redundant calculations of intermediate terms in the chain rule.

Bayesian inference

This is a method of statistical inference in which Bayes' theorem is used to update the probability for a hypothesis as more evidence or information becomes available. Bayesian inference is an important technique in statistics, and especially in mathematical statistics. Bayesian updating is particularly important in the dynamic analysis of a sequence of data. Bayesian inference has found application in a wide range of activities, including science, engineering, philosophy, medicine, sport, and law. In the philosophy of decision theory, Bayesian inference is closely related to subjective probability, often called "Bayesian probability". An example is "If the current patient has a fever, adjust the probability they have influenza in such-and-such way".

Bayesian network

Bayesian network, belief network or directed acyclic graphical model is a probabilistic graphical model that represents a set of random variables and their conditional independencies via a directed acyclic graph (DAG). For example, a Bayesian network could represent the probabilistic relationships between diseases and symptoms. Given symptoms, the network can be used to compute the probabilities of the presence of various diseases. Efficient algorithms exist that perform inference and learning. A Bayesian network is a type of graphical model that uses probability to determine the occurrence of an event. It is also known as a belief network or a causal network. It consists of directed cyclic graphs (DCGs) and a table of conditional probabilities to find out the probability of an event happening. Bayesian networks are a very general tool that can be used for a large number of problems: reasoning (using the Bayesian inference algorithm), learning (using the expectation-maximization algorithm), planning (using decision networks) and perception (using dynamic Bayesian networks). Probabilistic algorithms can also be used for filtering, prediction, smoothing and finding explanations for streams of data, helping perception systems to analyze processes that occur over time. Compared with symbolic logic, formal Bayesian inference is computationally expensive. For inference to be tractable, most observations must be conditionally independent of one another.

Bayesian probability

This is an interpretation of the concept of probability, in which, instead of frequency or propensity of some phenomenon, probability is interpreted as reasonable expectation representing a state of knowledge or as quantification of a personal belief.

Beam search

This is a heuristic search algorithm that explores a graph by expanding the most promising node in a limited set. Beam search is an optimization of best-first search that reduces its memory requirements. Best-first search is a graph search which orders all partial solutions (states) according to some heuristic. However, in beam search, only a predetermined number of best partial solutions are kept as candidates. Beam search is thus a “greedy” algorithm.

A *heuristic* In mathematical optimization and computer science is a technique designed for problem solving more quickly when classic methods are too slow for finding an exact or approximate solution, or when classic methods fail to find any exact solution in a search space. This is achieved by trading optimality, completeness, accuracy, or precision for speed. In a way, it can be considered a shortcut.

Bees algorithm

This is a population-based search algorithm which mimics the food foraging behaviour of honey bee colonies. In its basic version the algorithm performs a kind of neighbourhood search combined with global search, and can be used for both combinatorial optimization and continuous optimization. The only condition for the application of the bees algorithm is that some measure of topological distance between the solutions is defined. The effectiveness and specific abilities of the bees algorithm have been proven in a number of studies. The biological basis for this is as follows: a colony of honey bees can extend itself over long distances (over 14 km) and in multiple directions simultaneously to harvest nectar or pollen from multiple food sources (flower patches). A small fraction of the colony constantly searches the environment looking for new flower patches. These scout bees move randomly in the area surrounding the hive, evaluating the profitability (net energy yield) of the food sources encountered. When they return to the hive, the scouts deposit the food harvested. Those individuals that found a highly profitable food source go to an area in the hive called the “dance floor”, and perform a ritual known as the waggle dance. Through the waggle dance a scout bee communicates the location of its discovery to idle onlookers, which join in the exploitation of the flower patch. Since the length of the dance is proportional to the scout’s rating of the food source, more foragers get recruited to harvest the best rated flower patches. After dancing, the scout returns to the food source it discovered to collect more food. As long as they are evaluated as profitable, rich food sources will be advertised by the scouts when they return to the hive. Recruited foragers may waggle dance as well, increasing the recruitment for highly rewarding flower patches. Thanks to this autocatalytic process, the bee colony is able to quickly switch the focus of the foraging effort to the most profitable flower patches.

Behavior-based robotics or behavioral robotics

This is an approach in robotics that focuses on robots that are able to exhibit complex-appearing behaviors despite little internal variable state to model its immediate environment, mostly gradually correcting its actions via sensory-motor links. Behavior-based robotics sets itself apart from traditional artificial intelligence by using biological systems as a model. Classic artificial intelligence typically uses a set of steps to solve problems: it follows a path based on internal representations of events compared to the behaviour-based approach. Rather than use preset calculations to tackle a situation, behavior-based robotics relies on adaptability. This advance has allowed behaviour-based robotics to become commonplace in research and data gathering.

Black box

In science, computing, and engineering a black box is a device, system or object which can be viewed in terms of its inputs and outputs (or transfer characteristics), without any knowledge of its internal workings. Its implementation is "opaque" (black). Almost anything might be referred to as a black box: a transistor, an algorithm, or the human brain.

Boids

This is an artificial life program which simulates the flocking behaviour of birds. The name "boid" corresponds to a shortened version of "bird-oid object". As with most artificial life simulations, boids is an example of emergent behavior; that is, the complexity of boids arises from the interaction of individual agents (the boids, in this case) adhering to a set of simple rules. It has been shown that the assumption that each bird in a flock adjusts its velocity and position to the other birds within a fixed radius, the time it takes to converge to a steady state is an iterated exponential of height logarithmic in the number of birds. This means that if the number of birds is large enough, the convergence time will be so great that it might as well be infinite. This result applies only to convergence to a steady state. For example, arrows fired into the air at the edge of a flock will cause the whole flock to react more rapidly than can be explained by interactions with neighbors.

Boolean algebra

This is the branch of algebra in which the values of the variables are the truth values true and false, usually denoted 1 and 0 respectively. Instead of elementary algebra where the values of the variables are numbers, and the prime operations are addition and multiplication, the main operations of Boolean algebra are the conjunction and denoted as ∧, the disjunction or denoted as ∨, and the negation not denoted as ¬. It is thus a formalism for describing logical relations in the same way that ordinary algebra describes numeric relations.

Boolean satisfiability problem

This is sometimes called propositional satisfiability problem and abbreviated as SATISFIABILITY or SAT). It is the problem of determining if there exists an interpretation that satisfies a given Boolean formula. In other words, it asks whether the variables of a given Boolean formula can be consistently replaced by the values TRUE or FALSE in such a way that the formula evaluates to TRUE. If this is the case, the formula is called satisfiable. On the other hand, if no such assignment exists, the function expressed by the formula is FALSE for all possible variable assignments and the formula is unsatisfiable.

Causal calculus

When experimental interventions are not feasible or illegal, the derivation of cause-effect relationship from observational studies must rest on some qualitative theoretical assumptions, for example, that symptoms do not cause diseases, usually expressed in the form of missing arrows in causal graphs such as Bayesian networks

Ceteris paribus or caeteris paribus

This is a Latin phrase meaning "other things equal". English translations of the phrase include "all other things being equal" or "other things held constant" or "all else unchanged". A prediction or a statement about a causal, empirical, or logical relation between two states of affairs is ceteris paribus if it is acknowledged that the prediction, although usually accurate in expected conditions, can fail or the relation can be abolished by intervening factors.

Chlorophyll

This is any of several related green pigments found in cyanobacteria and the chloroplasts of algae and plants. Chloroplasts are organelles (specialized compartments) in plant and algal cells. The main role of chloroplasts is to conduct photosynthesis, in which the photosynthetic pigment chlorophyll captures the energy from sunlight and converts it and stores it in the energy-storage molecules ATP and NADPH while freeing oxygen from water.

Circumscription logic

This is a non-monotonic logic used to formalize the common sense assumption that things are as expected unless otherwise specified.

Classification

Given a population whose members each belong to one of a number of different sets or classes, a classification rule or classifier is a procedure by which the elements of the population set are each predicted to belong to one of the classes. A perfect classification is one for which every element in the population is assigned to the class it really belongs to. Classifiers can be trained in various ways; there are many statistical and machine learning approaches. The decision tree is perhaps the most widely used machine learning algorithm. Other widely used classifiers are the neural network, k-nearest neighbour algorithm, kernel methods such as the support vector machine (SVM), Gaussian mixture model, and the very popular naive Bayes classifier. Classifier performance depends greatly on the characteristics of the data to be classified, such as the dataset size, the dimensionality, and the level of noise. Model-based classifiers perform well if the assumed model is an extremely good fit for the actual data. Otherwise, if no matching model is available, and if accuracy (rather than speed or scalability) is the sole concern, conventional wisdom is that discriminative classifiers (especially SVM) tend to be more accurate than model-based classifiers such as "naive Bayes" on most practical data sets.

Cluster analysis

Cluster analysis is the assignment of a set of observations into subsets (called clusters) so that observations within the same cluster are similar according to some predesignated criterion or criteria, while observations drawn from different clusters are dissimilar. Different clustering techniques make different assumptions on the structure of the data, often defined by some similarity metric and evaluated for example by internal compactness (similarity between members of the same cluster) and separation between different clusters. Other methods are based on estimated density and graph connectivity. Clustering is a method of unsupervised learning, and a common technique for statistical data analysis.

Cognition

This is "the mental action or process of acquiring knowledge and understanding through thought, experience, and the senses". It encompasses processes such as attention, the formation of knowledge, memory, judgment and evaluation, reasoning and "computation", problem solving and decision making, comprehension and production of language. Cognitive processes use existing knowledge and generate new knowledge.

Cognitive simulation AI

The economists Herbert Simon and Allen Newell studied human problem-solving skills and attempted to formalize them; their work laid the foundations of the field of artificial intelligence, as well as cognitive science, operations research and management science. Their research team used the results of psychological experiments to develop programs that simulated the techniques that people used to solve problems. This tradition, centered at Carnegie Mellon University, would eventually culminate in the development of the SOAR architecture in the mid-1980s.

Combinatorial explosion

In mathematics this is the rapid growth of the complexity of a problem due to how the combinatorics of the problem are affected by the input, constraints, and bounds of the problem.

Common sense

This is sound practical judgment concerning everyday matters, or a basic ability to perceive, understand, and judge that is shared by nearly all people. Common sense reasoning is one of the branches of artificial intelligence (AI) that is concerned with simulating the human ability to make presumptions about the type and essence of ordinary situations they encounter every day. These assumptions include judgments about the physical properties, purpose, intentions and behavior of people and objects, as well as possible outcomes of their actions and interactions.

Competitive learning

This is a form of unsupervised learning in artificial neural networks, in which nodes compete for the right to respond to a subset of the input data. A variant of Hebbian learning, competitive learning works by increasing the specialization of each node in the network. It is well suited to finding clusters within data.

Computational computing and soft computing

Computational statistics, or statistical computing is the interface between statistics and computer science. It provides solutions to problems which cannot be solved with complete logical certainty, and where an approximate solution is often sufficient. Other soft computing approaches to AI include fuzzy systems, evolutionary computation and many statistical tools. Computational intelligence and soft computing, including interest in neural networks and "connectionism", was revived by David Rumelhart and others in the middle of the 1980s. Artificial neural networks are an example of soft computing - they are solutions to problems which cannot be solved with complete logical certainty, and where an approximate solution is often sufficient. The application of soft computing to AI is studied collectively by the emerging discipline of computational intelligence.

Computational intelligence

This is the application of soft computing to AI.

Computational learning theory (or just learning theory)

This is a subfield of artificial intelligence devoted to studying the design and analysis of machine learning algorithms.

Computer program

This is a collection of instructions for performing a specific task that is designed to solve a specific class of problems. The instructions of a program are designed to be executed by a computer and it is required that a computer is able to execute programs in order for it to function.

Computer science

This is the study of the theory, experimentation, and engineering that form the basis for the design and use of computers. It is the scientific and practical approach to computation and its applications and the systematic study of the feasibility, structure, expression, and mechanization of the methodical procedures (or algorithms) that underlie the acquisition, representation, processing, storage, communication of, and access to, information

Computer vision

This is an interdisciplinary field that deals with how computers can be made for gaining high-level understanding from digital images or videos. From the perspective of engineering, it seeks to automate tasks that the human visual system can perform. Computer vision is the ability to analyze visual input. Such input is usually ambiguous; a giant, fifty-meter-tall pedestrian far away may produce exactly the same pixels as a nearby normal-sized pedestrian, requiring AI to judge the relative likelihood and reasonableness of different interpretations, for example by using its "object model" to assess that fifty-meter pedestrians do not exist.

Configuration space

Configuration space is a transformation from the physical space in which the robot is of finite-size into another space in which the robot is treated as a point.

Conjunctive normal form (CNF) is a formula in which a conjunction of one or more clauses occurs, where a clause is a disjunction of literals.

Connectionism is an approach in the fields of cognitive science that hopes to represent mental phenomena using artificial neural networks.

Content delivery network or content distribution network (CDN) is a geographically distributed network of proxy servers and their data centres. The goal is to distribute service spatially relative to end-users to provide high availability and high performance.

Control theory in control systems engineering deals with the control of continuously operating dynamic systems in engineered processes and machines. The objective is to develop a control model for controlling such systems using a control action in an optimum manner without delay or overshoot and ensuring control stability.

Convolutional neural network (CNN, or ConvNet) is a class of deep, feed-forward artificial neural networks, most commonly applied to analyzing visual imagery. CNNs use a variation of multilayer perceptrons designed to require minimal preprocessing. They are also known as shift invariant or space invariant artificial neural networks (SIANN), based on their shared-weights architecture and translation invariance characteristics. Convolutional networks were inspired by biological processes in that the connectivity pattern between neurons resembles the organization of the mammalian visual cortex. Individual cortical neurons respond to stimuli only in a restricted region of the visual field known as the receptive field. The receptive fields of different neurons partially overlap such that they cover the entire visual field. CNNs use relatively little pre-processing compared to other image classification algorithms. This means that the network learns the filters that in traditional algorithms were hand-engineered. This independence from prior knowledge and human effort in feature design is a major advantage. They have applications in image and video recognition, recommender systems and natural language processing. CNNs with 12 convolutional layers were used in conjunction with reinforcement learning by Deepmind's "AlphaGo Lee", the program that beat a top Go champion in 2016.

Central processing unit (CPU)

The CPU is the most important processor in a computer. Its electronic circuitry executes instructions of a computer program, such as arithmetic, logic, controlling, and input/output (I/O) operations. This role contrasts with that of external components, such as main memory and specialized coprocessors such as graphics processing units.

Computer programming languages

Computer programs can be categorized by the programming language paradigm used to produce them. Two of the main paradigms are imperative and declarative.

Imperative languages

Imperative programming languages specify a sequential algorithm using declarations, expressions, and statements:

A *declaration* couples a variable name to a datatype – for example, var x: integer;

An *expression* yields a value – for example, 2 + 2 yields 4

A *statement* might assign an expression to a variable or use the value of a variable to alter the program's control flow – for example: x := 2 + 2; if x = 4 then do something.

One criticism of imperative languages is the side effect of an assignment statement on a class of variables called non-local variables.

Declarative languages

Declarative programming languages describe what computation should be performed and not how to compute it. Declarative programs omit the control flow and are considered sets of instructions. Two broad categories of declarative languages are functional languages and logical languages. The principle behind functional languages (like Haskell) is to not allow side effects, which makes it easier to reason about programs like mathematical functions. The principle behind logical languages (like Prolog) is to define the problem to be solved – the goal – and leave the detailed solution to the Prolog system itself. The goal is defined by providing a list of subgoals. Then each subgoal is defined by further providing a list of its subgoals. If a path of subgoals fails to find a solution, then that subgoal is backtracked and another path is systematically attempted.

Cybernetics is a transdisciplinary approach for exploring regulatory systems—their structures, constraints, and possibilities. Norbert Wiener defined cybernetics in 1948 as "the scientific study of control and communication in the animal and the machine." In the 21st Century, the term is often used in a rather loose way to imply "control of any system using technology." In other words, it is the scientific study of how humans, animals and machines control and communicate with each other.

Cyc and the Japanese Fifth Computer Systems

Cyc is the world's longest-lived artificial intelligence project, attempting to assemble a comprehensive ontology and knowledge base that spans the basic concepts and "rules of thumb" about how the world works (think common sense knowledge but focusing more on things that rarely get written down or said, in contrast with facts one might find somewhere on the internet or retrieve via Google or Wikipedia), with the goal of enabling AI applications to perform human-like reasoning and be less "brittle" when confronted with novel situations that were not preconceived.

Historically, projects such as the Cyc knowledge base (1984 -) and the massive Japanese Fifth Generation Computer Systems initiative (1982 - 1992) attempted to cover the breadth of human cognition. These early projects failed to escape the limitations of non-quantitative symbolic logic models and, in retrospect, greatly underestimated the difficulty of cross-domain AI. Nowadays, the vast majority of current AI researchers work instead on tractable "narrow AI" applications (such as medical diagnosis or automobile navigation).

Cyc knowledge base

Cyc (pronounced syke) is a long-term artificial intelligence project that aims to assemble a comprehensive ontology and knowledge base that spans the basic concepts and rules about how the world works.

Data (plural of datum) are a set of values of qualitative or quantitative variables.

Data analysis, or data analytics, is the process of inspecting, cleansing, transforming, and modelling data with the goal of discovering useful information, informing conclusions, and supporting decision-making.

Data compression is the process of reducing the size of a data file. In signal processing, data compression, source coding, or bit-rate reduction this involves encoding information using fewer bits than the original representation. Compression can be either lossy or lossless. Lossless compression reduces bits by identifying and eliminating statistical redundancy. No information is lost in lossless compression.

Lossy compression reduces bits by removing unnecessary or less important information.

Data mining

This is the process of discovering patterns in large data sets involving methods at the intersection of machine learning, statistics, and database systems. Data mining is an interdisciplinary subfield of computer science with an overall goal of extracting information from a data set and transforming the information into a comprehensible structure for further use. Data mining is the analysis step of the "knowledge discovery in databases" process. Aside from the raw analysis step, it also involves database and data management aspects, data preprocessing, model and inference considerations, interestingness metrics, complexity considerations, post-processing of discovered structures, visualization, and online updating. Data mining evolved from the study of pattern recognition and computational learning theory.

Data structure

This refers to a data organization, management and storage format that enables efficient access and modification. More precisely, a data structure is a collection of data values, the relationships among them, and the functions or operations that can be applied to the data.

Davis–Putnam–Logemann–Loveland (DPLL) algorithm is a complete, backtracking-based search algorithm for deciding the satisfiability of propositional logic formulae in conjunctive normal form.

Decision theory (or the theory of choice)

This is the study of the reasoning underlying an agent's choices. Decision theory can be broken into three branches: normative decision theory, which gives advice on how to make the best decisions, given a set of uncertain beliefs and a set of values; descriptive decision theory, which analyzes how existing, possibly irrational agents actually make decisions; and prescriptive decision theory, which tries to guide or give procedures on how or what we should do in order to make best decisions in line with the normative theory.

Decision tree learning

Decision tree learning uses a decision tree as a predictive model, which maps observations about an item to conclusions about the item's target value. Decision tree learning uses a decision tree (as a predictive model) to go from observations about an item (represented in the branches) to conclusions about the item's target value (represented in the leaves). It is one of the predictive modelling approaches used in statistics, data mining and machine learning. Tree models where the target variable can take a discrete set of values are called classification trees; in these tree structures, leaves represent class labels and branches represent conjunctions of features that lead to those class labels.

Deep learning algorithms

These discover multiple levels of representation, or a hierarchy of features, with higher-level, more abstract features defined in terms of (or generating) lower-level features. It has been argued that an intelligent machine is one that learns a representation that disentangles the underlying factors of variation that explain the observed data. This approach uses artificial "neurons" that can learn by comparing themselves to the desired output and altering the strengths of the connections between their internal neurons to "reinforce" connections that seemed to be useful. The four main approaches can overlap with each other and with evolutionary systems; for example, neural nets can learn to make inferences, to generalize, and to make analogies. Some systems implicitly or explicitly use multiples of these approaches, alongside many other AI and non-AI algorithms.

Learning algorithms work on the basis that strategies, algorithms, and inferences that worked well in the past are likely to continue working well in the future. These inferences can be obvious, such as "since the sun rose every morning for the last 10,000 days, it will probably rise tomorrow morning as well". Learners also work on the basis of "Occam's razor" (explained above) that the simplest theory that explains the data is the likeliest to be correct. Therefore, to be successful, a learner must be designed such that it prefers simpler theories to complex theories, except in cases where the complex theory is proven substantially better.

Deep learning consists of multiple hidden layers in an artificial neural network. Deep learning is any artificial neural network that can learn a long chain of causal links. For example, a feedforward network with six hidden layers can learn a seven-link causal chain (six hidden layers + output layer) and has a "credit assignment path" (CAP) depth of seven. Many deep learning systems need to be able to learn chains ten or more causal links in length. Deep learning has transformed many important subfields of artificial intelligence, including computer vision, speech recognition, natural language processing and others. The first functional Deep Learning networks were trained one layer at a time. Ivakhnenko's 1971 paper describes the learning of a deep feedforward multilayer perceptron with eight layers, already much deeper than many later networks. In 2006, a publication by Geoffrey Hinton and Ruslan Salakhutdinov introduced another way of pre-training many-layered feedforward neural networks (FNNs) one layer at a time, treating each layer in turn as an unsupervised restricted Boltzmann machine, then using supervised backpropagation for fine-tuning. Similar to shallow artificial neural networks, deep neural networks can model complex non-linear relationships. Over the last few years, advances in both machine learning algorithms and computer hardware have led to more efficient methods for training deep neural networks that contain many layers of non-linear hidden units and a very large output layer. Deep learning often uses convolutional neural networks (CNNs), whose origins can be traced back to the Neocognitron introduced by Kunihiko Fukushima in 1980. In 1989, Yann LeCun and colleagues applied backpropagation to such an architecture. In the early 2000s CNNs processed an estimated 10% to 20% of all the cheques written in the US. Since 2011 fast implementations of CNNs on graphic processing units (GPUs) have won many visual pattern recognition competitions.

Deep recurrent neural networks (RNNs) applied to sequence learning can run arbitrary programs to process arbitrary sequences of inputs. The depth of an RNN is unlimited and depends on the length of its input sequence; thus, an RNN is an example of deep learning. RNNs can be trained by gradient descent but suffer from the vanishing gradient problem. In 1992 it was shown that unsupervised pre-training of a stack of recurrent neural networks can speed up subsequent supervised learning of deep sequential problems. Numerous researchers now use variants of a deep learning recurrent NN called the *long short-term memory* (LSTM) network published by Hochreiter & Schmidhuber in 1997.

Connectionist Temporal Classification (CTC)

At Google, Microsoft and Baidu this approach has revolutionised speech recognition. For example, in 2015 Google's speech recognition experienced a dramatic performance jump of 49% through CTC-trained LSTM, which is now available through Google Voice to billions of smartphone users. Google also used LSTM to improve machine translation. LSTM combined with CNNs also improved automatic image captioning and many other applications.

DeepMind Technologies Limited is a British artificial intelligence company founded in September 2010. The company is based in London, but has research centres in California and Canada. Acquired by Google in 2014, the company has created a neural network that learns how to play video games in a fashion similar to that of humans, as well as a Neural Turing machine, or a neural network that may be able to access an external memory like a conventional Turing machine, resulting in a computer that mimics the short-term memory of the human brain. The company made headlines in 2016 after its AlphaGo program beat a human professional Go player for the first time in October 2015 and again when AlphaGo beat Lee Sedol, the world champion, in a five-game match, which was the subject of a documentary film. A more generic program, AlphaZero, beat the most powerful programs playing go, chess and shogi (Japanese chess) after a few hours of play against itself using reinforcement learning.

Default logic

This is a non-monotonic logic used to formalize reasoning with default assumptions. Default logic can express facts like “by default, something is true”; by contrast, standard logic can only express that something is true or that something is false. This is a problem because reasoning often involves facts that are true in the majority of cases but not in every case.

Density estimation

This is the construction of an estimate, based on observed data, of an unobservable underlying probability density function. The unobservable density function is thought of as the density according to which a large population is distributed; the data are usually thought of as a random sample from that population.

Description logics (DL) are a family of formal knowledge representation languages. Many DLs are more expressive than propositional logic but less expressive than first-order logic. In contrast to the latter, the core reasoning problems for DLs are (usually) decidable, and efficient decision procedures have been designed and implemented for these problems.

Dimensionality reduction, or dimension reduction

This is the process of reducing the number of random variables under consideration by obtaining a set of principal variables. It can be divided into feature selection and feature extraction.

Domain and Application domain

A domain is the targeted subject area of a computer program. Formally it represents the target subject of a specific programming project, whether narrowly or broadly defined. For example, for a particular programming project that has as a goal the creation of a program for a particular hospital, that hospital would be the domain. the project can be expanded in scope to include all hospitals as its domain. In a computer programming design, a domain is defined by delineating a set of common requirements, terminology, and functionality. The word domain is also taken as a synonym of application domain.

Dynamic Bayesian Network (DBN) is a Bayesian network which relates variables to each other over adjacent time steps. This is often called a Two-Timeslice BN (2TBN) because it says that at any point in time T, the value of a variable can be calculated from the internal regressors and the immediate prior value (time T-1).

Economic theory relies upon a priori quantitative economic models, which employ a variety of concepts. The theory typically proceeds with an assumption of *ceteris paribus*, which means holding constant explanatory variables other than the one under consideration. When creating theories, the objective is to find ones which are at least as simple in information requirements, more precise in predictions, and more fruitful in generating additional research than prior theories.

Embodied agents

Also known as interface agents, intelligent agents interact with the environment through a physical body within that environment.

Embodied intelligence

This includes embodied, situated, behaviour-based, and nouvelle AI. Researchers from the related field of robotics rejected symbolic AI and focused on the basic engineering problems that would allow robots to move and survive. This work revived the non-symbolic viewpoint of the early cybernetics researchers of the 1950s and reintroduced the use of control theory in AI. This coincided with the development of the embodied mind thesis in the related field of cognitive science: the idea that aspects of the body (such as movement, perception and visualization) are required for higher intelligence.

Estimation of distribution algorithms (EDAs), sometimes called probabilistic model-building genetic algorithms (PMBGAs), are stochastic optimization methods that guide the search for the optimum by building and sampling explicit probabilistic models of promising candidate solutions. Optimization is viewed as a series of incremental updates of a probabilistic model, starting with the model encoding the uniform distribution over admissible solutions and ending with the model that generates only the global optima.

Eukaryotes are organisms whose cells have a nucleus enclosed within membranes, (unlike prokaryotes such as bacteria and other archaea). Eukaryotic cells also contain other membrane-bound organelles such as mitochondria and the Golgi apparatus, and in addition, some cells of plants and algae contain chloroplasts. Unlike unicellular archaea and bacteria, eukaryotes may also be multicellular and include organisms consisting of many cell types forming different kinds of tissue.

Event calculus

This is similar to other languages for reasoning about change: the event calculus represents the effects of actions on fluents. However, events can also be external to the system. In event calculus, one can specify the value of fluents at some given time points, the events that take place at given time points, and their effects.

Evolutionary algorithm (EA)

Evolutionary computation is a family of algorithms for global optimization inspired by biological evolution, and the subfield of artificial intelligence and soft computing studying these algorithms. In technical terms, they are a family of population-based trial and error problem solvers with a metaheuristic or stochastic optimization character. Evolutionary computation uses a form of optimization search. For example, they may begin with a population of organisms (the guesses) and then allow them to mutate and recombine, selecting only the fittest to survive each generation (refining the guesses). Classic evolutionary algorithms include genetic algorithms, gene expression programming, and genetic programming. Alternatively, distributed search processes can coordinate via swarm intelligence algorithms. Two popular swarm algorithms used in search are particle swarm optimization (inspired by bird flocking) and ant colony optimization(inspired by ant trails).

Expert systems

These are computer systems that emulate the decision-making ability of a human expert. Expert systems are designed to solve complex problems by reasoning through bodies of knowledge, represented mainly "as if - then rules" rather than through conventional procedural code. The first expert systems were created in the 1970s and then proliferated in the 1980s. Expert systems were among the first truly successful forms of artificial intelligence (AI) software. An expert system is divided into two subsystems: the inference engine and the knowledge base. The knowledge base represents facts and rules. The inference engine applies the rules to the known facts to deduce new facts. Inference engines can also include explanation and debugging abilities.

Explainable AI

Explainability (also referred to as "interpretability") is the concept that a machine learning model and its output can be explained in a way that "makes sense" to a human being at an acceptable level.

Exploratory data analysis (EDA)

This is an approach to analysing data sets to summarize their main characteristics, often with visual methods. A statistical model can be used or not, but primarily EDA is for seeing what the data can reveal beyond the formal modelling or hypothesis testing task.

Extended mind thesis (EMT) states that an agent's mind and associated cognitive processing are neither skull-bound nor even body-bound but extend into the agent's world. Within developmental robotics, developmental learning approaches are elaborated upon to allow robots to accumulate repertoires of novel skills through autonomous self-exploration, social interaction with human teachers, and the use of guidance mechanisms (such as active learning, maturation, and motor synergies).

Falling hardware prices and the development of graphics processing units (GPUs) for personal use in the last few years have contributed to the development of the concept of deep learning. This approach tries to model the way the human brain processes light and sound into vision and hearing. Some successful applications of deep learning are computer vision and speech recognition.

Feature selection approach

Feature selection is the process of selecting an optimal subset of relevant features for use in model construction. It is assumed the data contain some features that are either redundant or irrelevant and can thus be removed to reduce calculation cost without incurring much loss of information. Common optimality criteria include accuracy, similarity and information measures.

Feedforward neural network

This is an artificial neural network wherein connections between the nodes do not form a cycle. As such, it is different from recurrent neural networks. Feedforward neural networks were the first and simplest type of artificial neural network devised. In this network, the information moves in only one direction, forward, from the input nodes, through the hidden nodes (if any) and to the output nodes. There are no cycles or loops in the network. As such, it is different from recurrent neural networks.

Fifth Generation Computer Systems

This was an initiative by Japan's Ministry of International Trade and Industry, begun in 1982, to create a computer using massively parallel computing/processing. It aimed to create an "epoch-making computer" with supercomputer-like performance and to provide a platform for future developments in artificial intelligence.

In the history of computing hardware, computers using vacuum tubes were called the first generation; transistors and diodes, the second; integrated circuits, the third; and those using microprocessors, the fourth. Whereas previous computer generations had focused on increasing the number of logic elements in a single CPU, it was widely believed at the time, that the fifth generation would instead turn to massive numbers of CPUs for added performance.

First-order logic, also known as first-order predicate calculus and predicate logic, is a collection of formal systems used in mathematics, philosophy, linguistics, and computer science. First-order logic uses quantified variables over non-logical objects and allows the use of sentences that contain variables, so that rather than propositions such as “Socrates is a man’ one can have expressions in the form "there exists X such that X is Socrates and X is a man". This distinguishes it from propositional logic, which does not use quantifiers or relations. First-order logic adds quantifiers and predicates, and can express facts about objects, their properties, and their relations with each other.

Fitness function is a particular type of objective function that is used to summarise how close a given design solution is to achieving the set aims. Fitness functions are used in genetic programming and genetic algorithms to guide simulations towards optimal design solutions.

Fluent calculus is a formalism for expressing dynamical domains in first-order logic. It is a variant of situation calculus; the main difference is that situations are considered representations of states.

Fluents in artificial intelligence are conditions that can change over time.
In logical approaches to reasoning about actions, fluents can be represented in first-order logic by predicates having an argument that depends on time.

Formal language

Formalism is a theory that holds that statements of mathematics and logic can be considered to be statements about the consequences of certain string manipulation rules.

Frame problem in artificial intelligence describes an issue with using *first-order logic* (FOL) to express facts about a robot in the world. Representing the state of a robot with traditional FOL requires the use of many axioms that simply imply that things in the environment do not change arbitrarily. Fuzzy logic is a form of many-valued logic in which the truth values of variables may be any real number between 0 and 1. It is employed to handle the concept of partial truth, where the truth value may range between completely true and completely false. By contrast, in Boolean logic, the truth values of variables may only be the integer values 0 or 1.

Fuzzy logic is successfully used in control systems to allow experts to contribute vague rules such as "if you are close to the destination station and moving fast, increase the train's brake pressure"; these vague rules can then be numerically refined within the system. Fuzzy logic is a fuzzy control system based on fuzzy logic - a mathematical system that analyzes analog input values in terms of logical variables that take on continuous values between 0 and 1, in contrast to classical or digital logic, which operates on discrete values of either 1 or 0 (true or false, respectively).

Fuzzy logic fails to scale well in knowledge bases; many AI researchers question the validity of chaining fuzzy-logic inferences.

Fuzzy set theory assigns a "degree of truth" (between 0 and 1) to vague statements such as "Alice is old" (or rich, or tall, or hungry) that are too linguistically imprecise to be completely true or false. In classical set theory, the membership of elements in a set is assessed in binary terms according to a bivalent condition - an element either belongs or does not belong to the set. By contrast, fuzzy set theory permits the gradual assessment of the membership of elements in a set; this is described with the aid of a membership function valued in the real unit interval – 0 or 1.

Game theory is the study of mathematical models of strategic interaction between rational decision-makers. It has applications in all fields of social science, as well as in logic and computer science. Originally, it addressed zero-sum games, in which one person's gains result in losses for the other participants. Today, game theory applies to a wide range of behavioural relations, and is now an umbrella term for the science of logical decision making in humans, animals, and computers.

Gene expression programming (GEP) is an evolutionary algorithm that creates computer programs or models. These computer programs are complex tree structures that learn and adapt by changing their sizes, shapes, and composition, much like a living organism. And like living organisms, the computer programs of GEP are also encoded in simple linear chromosomes of fixed length. Thus, GEP is a genotype–phenotype system, benefiting from a simple genome to keep and transmit the genetic information and a complex phenotype to explore the environment and adapt to it.

Generalized coordinates: in classical mechanics the parameters that define the configuration of a system are called generalized coordinates, and the vector space defined by these coordinates is called the configuration space of the physical system.

Genetic algorithm (GA) is a search heuristic that mimics the process of natural selection, and uses methods such as mutation and crossover to generate new genotypes in the hope of finding good solutions to a given problem. Conversely, machine learning techniques have been used to improve the performance of genetic and evolutionary algorithms.

Genetic programming (GP) is a technique whereby computer programs are encoded as a set of genes that are then modified (evolved) using an evolutionary algorithm (often a genetic algorithm, (GA); it is an application of genetic algorithms where the space of solutions consists of computer programs. The results are computer programs that are able to perform well in a predefined task. The methods used to encode a computer program in an artificial chromosome and to evaluate its fitness with respect to the predefined task are central in the GP technique.

Genetic recombination (also known as *genetic reshuffling*) is the production of offspring with combinations of traits that differ from those found in either parent. In eukaryotes, genetic recombination during meiosis can lead to a novel set of genetic information that can be passed on from the parents to the offspring. Most recombination is naturally occurring.

Group method of data handling (GMDH) is used in such fields as data mining, knowledge discovery, prediction, complex systems modelling, optimization and pattern recognition.

Golgi apparatus is an organelle found in most eukaryotic cells. Part of the endomembrane system in the cytoplasm, the Golgi apparatus packages proteins into membrane-bound-vesicles inside the cell before the vesicles are sent to their destination. The Golgi apparatus resides at the intersection of the secretory, lysosomal, and endocytic pathways. It is of particular importance in processing proteins for secretion, containing a set of glycosylation enzymes that attach various sugar monomers to proteins as the proteins move through the apparatus.

Gradient descent and *gradient ascent*

This is a first order iterative optimization algorithm for finding the minimum of a function. To find a local minimum of a function using gradient descent, one takes steps proportional to the negative of the gradient (or approximate gradient) of the function at the current point. If instead one takes steps proportional to the positive of the gradient, one approaches a local maximum of that function; the procedure is then known as gradient ascent.

Greedy algorithm is an algorithmic paradigm that follows the problem-solving heuristic of making the locally optimal choice at each stage with the intent of finding a global optimum. In many problems, a greedy strategy does not usually produce an optimal solution, but nonetheless a greedy heuristic may yield locally optimal solutions that approximate a globally optimal solution in a reasonable amount of time.

Hebbian theory is a neuroscientific theory claiming that an increase in synaptic efficacy arises from a presynaptic cell's repeated and persistent stimulation of a postsynaptic cell. It is an attempt to explain synaptic plasticity such as the adaptation of brain neurons during the learning process.

Hidden Markov Model (HMM) is a statistical Markov model in which the system being modelled is assumed to be a Markov process with unobserved (i.e. hidden) states.

The hidden Markov model can be represented as the simplest dynamic Bayesian network.

Hierarchical temporal memory (HTM) is a biologically constrained theory (or model) of intelligence. HTM is rigorously based on neuroscience and the physiology and interaction of pyramidal neurons in the neocortex of the mammalian (in particular, human) brain. At the core of HTM are learning algorithms that can store, learn, infer and recall high-order sequences. Unlike most other machine learning methods, HTM learns (in an unsupervised fashion) time-based patterns in unlabelled data on a continuous basis. HTM is robust to noise, and it has high capacity, meaning that it can learn multiple patterns simultaneously. When applied to computers, HTM is well suited for prediction, anomaly detection, classification and ultimately sensorimotor applications. Hierarchical temporal memory is an approach that models some of the structural and algorithmic properties of the neocortex.

Hill climbing is a mathematical optimization technique which belongs to the family of local search. It is an iterative algorithm that starts with an arbitrary solution to a problem, then attempts to find a better solution by making an incremental change to the solution. If the change produces a better solution, another incremental change is made to the new solution, and so on until no further improvements can be found.

Artificial general intelligence

Currently the vast majority of current AI researchers work on tractable "narrow AI" applications (such as medical diagnosis or automobile navigation). Many researchers predict that such "narrow AI" work in different individual domains will eventually be incorporated into a machine with *artificial general intelligence* (AGI), combining narrow skills and at some point even exceeding human ability in most or all these areas. Many advances have general, cross-domain significance. One high-profile example is that DeepMind in the 2010s developed a "generalized artificial intelligence" that could learn many diverse Atari games on its own, and later developed a variant of the system which succeeded at sequential learning. Besides transfer learning, hypothetical AGI breakthroughs could include the development of reflective architectures that can engage in decision-theoretic meta-reasoning, and figuring out how to "slurp up" a comprehensive knowledge base from the entire unstructured Web. Some argue that some kind of (currently undiscovered) conceptually straightforward, but mathematically difficult, "Master Algorithm" could lead to AGI.

A few "emergent" approaches look to simulating human intelligence extremely closely, and believe that anthropomorphic features like an artificial brain or simulated child development may someday reach a critical point where general intelligence emerges. Many of the problems with this is that it may also require general intelligence, if machines are to solve the problems as well as people do. For example, even specific straightforward tasks, like machine translation, require that a machine read and write in both languages, follow the author's argument (reason), know what is being talked about (knowledge), and faithfully reproduce the author's original intent (social intelligence). A problem like machine translation is considered "AI-complete", because all of these problems need to be solved simultaneously in order to reach human-level machine performance.

In AGI research some researchers caution against over-reliance on statistical learning, and argue that continuing research into GOFAI will still be necessary to attain general intelligence.

Explainable AI (XAI) or *Transparent AI* is an artificial intelligence whose actions can be easily understood by humans. It contrasts with the concept of the "black box" in machine learning, where even their designers cannot explain how the AI arrived at a specific decision. XAI can be used to implement a social right to explanation. Transparency rarely comes for free; there are often trade-offs between how "smart" an AI is and how transparent it is, and these trade-offs are expected to grow larger as AI systems increase in internal complexity. The technical challenge of explaining AI decisions is sometimes known as the interpretability problem.

Labelling

In machine learning, data labelling is the process of identifying raw data (images, text files, videos, etc.) and adding one or more meaningful and informative labels to provide context so that a machine learning model can learn from it.

Noise

In machine learning, noise refers to unwanted behaviours within the data that provide a low signal-to-noise ratio. Noise refers to random or unpredictable fluctuations in data that disrupt the ability to identify target patterns or relationships. The result is decreased accuracy or reliability of a model's predictions or output. Essentially, data = signal + noise. While a minority of the noise in data is irreducible, most can be prevented by understanding its causes and correcting them.

Formal language

This is a set of strings of symbols together with a set of rules that are specific to it.

Inductive logic programming

Inductive logic programming (ILP) is an approach to rule learning using logic programming as a uniform representation for input examples, background knowledge, and hypotheses. Given an encoding of the known background knowledge and a set of examples represented as a logical database of facts, an ILP system will derive a hypothesized logic program that entails all positive and no negative examples. Inductive programming is a related field that considers any kind of programming languages for representing hypotheses such as functional programs.

Inference engines

These are a component of the system that applies logical rules to the knowledge base to deduce new information. The first inference engines were components of expert systems. The typical expert system consisted of a knowledge base and an inference engine. The knowledge base stores facts about the world. The inference engine applies logical rules to the knowledge base and deduced new knowledge. This process would iterate as each new fact in the knowledge base could trigger additional rules in the inference engine. Inference engines work primarily in one of two modes: forward chaining and backward chaining.

Forward chaining and *backward chaining*

This starts with the known facts and asserts new facts. Backward chaining starts with goals and works backward to determine what facts must be asserted so that the goals can be achieved.

Information theory

This studies the quantification, storage, and communication of information. It was originally proposed by Claude E. Shannon in 1948 to find fundamental limits on signal processing and communication operations such as data compression in a landmark paper entitled "A Mathematical Theory of Communication". Applications of fundamental topics of information theory include lossless data compression (e.g. ZIP files), lossy data compression (e.g. MP3s and JPEGs), and channel coding (e.g. for digital subscriber line (DSL)). Information theory studies the quantification, storage, and communication of information.

Integer

An integer is a whole number (not a fractional number) that can be positive, negative, or zero.

Intelligent agent

An intelligent agent is an autonomous entity which observes through sensors and acts upon an environment using actuators (i.e. it is an agent) and directs its activity towards achieving goals (i.e. it is "rational", as defined in economics). Intelligent agents may also learn or use knowledge to achieve their goals. They may be very simple or very complex. A reflex machine, such as a thermostat, is considered an example of an intelligent agent. The simplest intelligent agents are programs that solve specific problems. More complicated agents include human beings and organizations of human beings (such as firms). The paradigm allows researchers to directly compare or even combine different approaches to isolated problems, by asking which agent is best at maximizing a given "goal function". An agent that solves a specific problem can use any approach that works – some agents are symbolic and logical, some are sub-symbolic artificial neural networks and others may use new approaches. The paradigm also gives researchers a common language to communicate with other fields - such as decision theory and economics - that also use concepts of abstract agents. Building a complete agent requires researchers to address realistic problems of integration; for example, because sensory systems give uncertain information about the environment, planning systems must be able to function in the presence of uncertainty. The intelligent agent paradigm became widely accepted during the 1990s. Intelligent agent must be able to set goals and achieve them. They need a way to visualize the future - a representation of the state of the world and be able to make predictions about how their actions will change it - and be able to make choices that maximize the utility (or "value") of available choices. In classical planning problems, the agent can assume that it is the only system acting in the world, allowing the agent to be certain of the consequences of its actions. However, if the agent is not the only actor, then the agent must be able to reason under uncertainty. This calls for an agent that can not only assess its environment and make predictions, but also evaluate its predictions and adapt based on its assessment. Multi-agent planning uses the cooperation and competition of many agents to achieve a given goal. Emergent behavior such as this is used by evolutionary algorithms and swarm intelligence.

k-NN classification

An object is classified by a majority vote of its neighbours, with the object being assigned to the class most common among its k-nearest neighbours (k is a positive integer, typically small). If k = 1, then the object is simply assigned to the class of that single nearest neighbour. In k-NN regression, the output is the property value for the object. This value is the average of the values of its k-nearest neighbours. k-nearest neighbours algorithm is a non-parametric method used in pattern recognition for classification and regression. In both cases the input consists of the k closest training examples in the feature space. The output depends on whether k-NN is used for classification or regression: k-NN is a type of instance-based learning or lazy learning, where the function is only approximated locally and all computation is deferred until classification. The k-NN algorithm is among the simplest of all machine learning algorithms.

Knowledge bases

These represent a technology used to store complex structured and unstructured information used by a computer system. The initial use of the term was in connection with expert systems which were the first knowledge-based systems.

Knowledge representation and reasoning (KR, KR², KR&R)

This is a field of artificial intelligence dedicated to representing information about the world in a form that a computer system can utilize to solve complex tasks such as diagnosing a medical condition or having a dialogue in a natural language.

Knowledge representation incorporates findings from psychology about how humans solve problems and represent knowledge in order to design formalisms that will make complex systems easier to design and build. Knowledge representation and reasoning also incorporates findings from logic to automate various kinds of reasoning, such as the application of rules or the relations of sets and subsets. Examples of knowledge representation formalisms include semantic nets, systems architecture, frames, rules, and ontologies. Examples of automated reasoning engines include inference engines, theorem provers, and classifiers. Knowledge representation and knowledge engineering are central to classical AI research. Some expert systems attempt to gather together explicit knowledge possessed by experts in a narrow domain. In addition, some projects have attempted to gather the "commonsense knowledge" known to the average person into a database containing extensive knowledge about the world. Among the things a comprehensive commonsense knowledge base would contain are objects, properties, categories and relations between objects; situations, events, states and time; causes and effects; knowledge about knowledge (what we know about what other people know); and many other, less well researched domains. A representation of "what exists" is an *ontology*: the set of objects, relations, concepts, and properties formally described so that software agents can interpret them. The semantics of these are captured as description logic concepts, roles, and individuals, and typically implemented as classes, properties, and individuals in the Web Ontology Language. The most general ontologies are called upper ontologies, which attempt to provide a foundation for all other knowledge by acting as mediators between domain ontologies that cover specific knowledge about a particular knowledge domain (field of interest or area of concern). Such formal knowledge representations can be used in content-based indexing and retrieval, scene interpretation, clinical decision support, knowledge discovery (mining "interesting" and actionable inferences from large databases), and other areas.

Knowledge

Much of what people know is not represented as "facts" or "statements" that they could express verbally. For example, a chess master will avoid a particular chess position because it "feels too exposed" or an art critic can take one look at a statue and realize that it is a fake. These are non-conscious and sub-symbolic intuitions or tendencies in the human brain. Knowledge like this informs, supports and provides a context for symbolic, conscious knowledge. As with the related problem of sub-symbolic reasoning, it is hoped that situated AI, computational intelligence, or statistical AI will provide ways to represent this kind of knowledge.

Knowledge-based AI

When computers with large memories became available around 1970, researchers began to build knowledge into AI applications. This "knowledge revolution" led to the development and deployment of expert systems, the first truly successful form of AI software. The knowledge revolution was also driven by the realization that enormous amounts of knowledge would be required by many simple AI applications.

Large language model (LLM)

Large language model is a type of language model notable for its ability to achieve general-purpose language understanding and generation. LLMs acquire these abilities by using massive amounts of data to learn billions of parameters during training and consuming large computational resources during their training and operation. LLMs are artificial neural networks (mainly transformers) and are (pre-) trained using self-supervised learning and semi-supervised learning.

Learning classifier systems

Learning classifier systems (LCS) are a family of rule-based machine learning algorithms that combine a discovery component (e.g. typically a genetic algorithm) with a learning component (performing either supervised learning, reinforcement learning, or unsupervised learning). They seek to identify a set of context-dependent rules that collectively store and apply knowledge in a piecewise manner in order to make predictions.

Learning to learn, or meta learning

This is a subfield of machine learning in which automatic learning algorithms are applied to metadata about machine learning experiments. The main goal is to use such metadata to understand how automatic learning can become flexible in solving learning problems in order to improve the performance of existing learning algorithms or to learn (induce) the learning algorithm itself.

Metadata

Metadata is "data that provides information about other data", but not the content of the data itself, such as the text of a message or the image itself. There are many distinct types of metadata.

Learning to rank or machine-learned ranking (MLR)

This is the application of machine learning, typically supervised, semi-supervised or reinforcement learning, in the construction of ranking models for information retrieval systems

Lidar (also called LIDAR, LiDAR, and LADAR)

This is a surveying method that measures distance to a target by illuminating the target with pulsed laser light and measuring the reflected pulses with a sensor. Differences in laser return times and wavelengths can then be used to make digital 3-D representations of the target. The name lidar, now used as an acronym of light detection and ranging (sometimes light imaging, detection, and ranging), was originally a portmanteau of light and radar. Lidar is sometimes called laser scanning and 3-D scanning, with terrestrial, airborne and mobile applications.

Logic

This is used for knowledge representation and problem solving, but it can be applied to other problems as well. For example, the satplan algorithm uses logic for planning and inductive logic programming is a method for learning. (Satplan (also known as Planning as Satisfiability) is a method for automated planning. It converts the planning problem instance into an instance of the Boolean satisfiability problem, which is then solved using a method for establishing satisfiability such as the DPLL algorithm or WalkSAT). Logic consists of the systematic study of the form of valid inference. A valid inference is one where there is a specific relation of logical support between the assumptions of the inference and its conclusion. In ordinary discourse, inferences may be signified by words like therefore, hence, and ergo. Logic originally meant "the word" or "what is spoken", but is coming to mean "thought" or "reason" and is a subject concerned with the most general laws of truth, and is now generally held to consist of the systematic study of the form of valid inference. A valid inference is one where there is a specific relation of logical support between the assumptions of the inference and its conclusion.

Logic-based AI

John McCarthy felt that machines did not need to simulate human thought, but should instead try to find the essence of abstract reasoning and problem-solving, regardless of whether people used the same algorithms. His laboratory at Stanford University focused on using formal logic to solve a wide variety of problems, including knowledge representation, planning and learning. Logic was also the focus of work at the University of Edinburgh and elsewhere in Europe which led to the development of the programming language Prolog and the science of logic programming.

Long short-term memory (LSTM)

These are units of a recurrent neural network (RNN). An RNN composed of LSTM units is often called an LSTM network. A common LSTM unit is composed of a cell, an input gate, an output gate and a forget gate. The cell remembers values over arbitrary time intervals and the three gates regulate the flow of information into and out of the cell. LSTM networks are well-suited to classifying, processing and making predictions based on time series data, since there can be lags of unknown duration between important events in a time series. LSTMs were developed to deal with the exploding and vanishing gradient problems that can be encountered when training traditional RNNs

Loss of function.

Loss function or cost function in mathematical optimization, statistics, econometrics, decision theory, machine learning and computational neuroscience, is a function that maps an event or values of one or more variables onto a real number intuitively representing some "cost" associated with the event. An optimization problem seeks to minimize a loss function. An objective function is either a loss function or its negative (in specific domains, variously called a reward function, a profit function, a utility function or a fitness function), in which case it is to be maximized.

Lossless compression

This is a class of data compression algorithms that allows the original data to be perfectly reconstructed from the compressed data.

Lossy compression

This permits reconstruction only of an approximation of the original data, though usually with improved compression rates (and therefore reduced file sizes).

Machine learning

A categorization of machine learning tasks arises when one considers the desired output of a machine-learned system. Machine learning tasks are typically classified into two broad categories, depending on whether there is a learning "signal" or "feedback" available to a learning system. Machine learning is a subset of artificial intelligence in the field of computer science that often uses statistical techniques to give computers the ability to "learn" (i.e., progressively improve performance on a specific task) with data, without being explicitly programmed. Machine learning-based attention is a mechanism mimicking cognitive attention. It calculates "soft" weights for each word, more precisely for its embedding, in the context window. It can do it either in parallel (such as in transformers) or sequentially (such as recurrent neural networks). "Soft" weights can change during each runtime, in contrast to "hard" weights, which are (pre-)trained and fine-tuned and remain frozen afterwards.

Machine perception

This is the ability to use input from sensors (such as cameras (visible spectrum or infrared), microphones, wireless signals, and active lidar, sonar, radar, and tactile sensors) to deduce aspects of the world. Applications include speech recognition, facial recognition, and object recognition. Machine perception is the capability of a computer system to interpret data in a manner that is similar to the way humans use their senses to relate to the world around them. The basic method that the computers take in, and respond to, their environment is through the attached hardware. Until recently input was limited to a keyboard, or a mouse, but advances in technology, both in hardware and software, have allowed computers to take in sensory input in a way similar to humans.

Many of the things people know take the form of "working assumptions". For example, if a bird comes up in conversation, people typically picture a creature that is fist-sized, sings, and flies. None of these things are true about all birds. This problem was identified in 1969 as the qualification problem: for any commonsense rule that AI researchers care to represent, there tend to be a huge number of exceptions. Almost nothing is simply true or false in the way that abstract logic requires. AI research has explored a number of solutions to this problem. Many problems in AI (in reasoning, planning, learning, perception, and robotics) require the agent to operate with incomplete or uncertain information. AI researchers have devised a number of powerful tools to solve these problems using methods from probability theory and economics.

Manifold learning algorithms (Markov process)

Markov process, named after the Russian mathematician Andrey Markov, is a stochastic process that satisfies the Markov property (sometimes characterized as "memorylessness"). Roughly speaking, a process satisfies the Markov property if it can make predictions for the future of the process based solely on its present state just as well as it could knowing by knowing the process's full history.

Massively parallel

This is a term which refers to the use of a large number of processors (or separate computers) to perform a set of coordinated computations in parallel (simultaneously).

Mathematical optimization or mathematical programming

This is the selection of a best element (with regard to a specific criterion) from some set of available alternatives.

Means-ends analysis (MEA) is a problem-solving technique used commonly in artificial intelligence for limiting search in AI programs.

Meiosis

Meiosis is a specialized type of cell division that reduces the chromosome number by half, creating four haploid cells, each genetically distinct from the parent cell that gave rise to them. This process occurs in all sexually reproducing single-celled and multicellular eukaryotes, including animals, plants, and fungi. Meiosis is a special type of cell division of germ cells in sexually-reproducing organisms that produces the gametes - sperm or egg cells.

Metaheuristic

This is a higher-level procedure or a heuristic designed to find, generate, or select a heuristic (partial search algorithm) that may provide a sufficiently good solution to an optimization problem, especially with incomplete or imperfect information or limited computation capacity. Metaheuristics sample a set of solutions which is too large to be completely sampled. Metaheuristics may make few assumptions about the optimization problem being solved, and so they may be usable for a variety of problems.

Methodological individualism

This is the requirement that causal accounts of social phenomena explain how they result from the motivations and actions of individual agents, at least in principle.

Mitochondria

These are double-membrane-bound organelles found in most eukaryotic organisms. Mitochondria generate most of the cell's supply of adenosine triphosphate (ATP), used as a source of chemical energy. Mitochondria are commonly between 0.75 and 3 μm in diameter but vary considerably in size and structure. Unless specifically stained, they are not visible. In addition to supplying cellular energy, mitochondria are involved in other tasks, such as cell signalling, cellular differentiation, and cell death, as well as maintaining control of the cell cycle and cell growth.

Modal logic

This is a type of formal logic which extends classical propositional and predicate logic to include operators expressing modality. A modal - a word that expresses a modality - qualifies a statement. For example, the statement "John is happy" might be qualified by saying that John is usually happy, in which case the term "usually" is functioning as a modal.

Monolithic architecture

Related to software, monolithic architecture is one in which functionally distinguishable aspects (for example data input and output, data processing, error handling, and the user interface) are all interwoven, rather than containing architecturally separate components.

Motion planning (also known as the navigation problem)

This is a term used in robotics for the process of breaking down a desired movement task into discrete motions that satisfy movement constraints and possibly optimize some aspect of the movement. Motion planning is the process of breaking down a movement task into "primitives" such as individual joint movements. Such movement often involves compliant motion, a process where movement requires maintaining physical contact with an object. Moravec's paradox generalizes that low-level sensorimotor skills that humans take for granted are, counterintuitively, difficult to program into a robot; the paradox is named after Hans Moravec, who stated in 1988 that "it is comparatively easy to make computers exhibit adult level performance on intelligence tests or playing checkers, and difficult or impossible to give them the skills of a one-year-old when it comes to perception and mobility". This is attributed to the fact that, unlike checkers, physical dexterity has been a direct target of natural selection for millions of years.

Multi-agent system (MAS or "self-organized system") is a computerized system composed of multiple interacting intelligent agents. Multi-agent systems can solve problems that are difficult or impossible for an individual agent or a monolithic system to solve.

Multimodal sentiment analysis

This is a new dimension of the traditional text-based sentiment analysis, which goes beyond the analysis of texts, and includes other modalities such as audio and visual data. It can be bimodal, which includes different combinations of two modalities, or trimodal, which incorporates three modalities. With the extensive amount of social media data available online in different forms such as videos and images, the conventional text-based sentiment analysis has evolved into more complex models of multimodal analysis of news videos, and emotion recognition (sometimes known as emotion detection) such as depression monitoring, among others.

Nany-valued logic (also multi- or multiple-valued logic) is a propositional calculus in which there are more than two truth values.

Natural language processing (NLP) gives machines the ability to read and understand human language. A sufficiently powerful natural language processing system would enable natural language user interfaces and the acquisition of knowledge directly from human-written sources, such as newswire texts. Some straightforward applications of natural language processing include information retrieval, text mining, question answering and machine translation. Many current approaches use word co-occurrence frequencies to construct syntactic representations of text. "Keyword spotting" strategies for search are popular and scalable but dumb: a search query for "dog" might only match documents with the literal word "dog" and miss a document with the word "poodle". "Lexical affinity" strategies use the occurrence of words such as "accident" to assess the sentiment of a document. Modern statistical NLP approaches can combine all these strategies as well as others, and often achieve acceptable accuracy at the page or paragraph level but continue to lack the semantic understanding required to classify isolated sentences well. Besides the usual difficulties with encoding semantic commonsense knowledge, existing semantic NLP sometimes scales too poorly to be viable in business applications. Beyond semantic NLP, the ultimate goal of "narrative" NLP is to embody a full understanding of commonsense reasoning.

Natural language understanding (NLU) or natural language interpretation (NLI)

This is a subtopic of natural language processing in artificial intelligence that deals with machine reading comprehension.

Natural-language user interfaces (NLUI)

These are a type of computer human interface where linguistic phenomena such as verbs, phrases and clauses act as user interface controls for creating, selecting and modifying data in software applications.

Neural network (NN)

This is an interconnected group of nodes, akin to the vast network of neurons in the human brain. Neural networks, or neural nets, were inspired by the architecture of neurons in the human brain. A simple "neuron" N accepts input from multiple other neurons, each of which, when activated (or "fired"), cast a weighted "vote" for or against whether neuron N should itself activate. Learning requires an algorithm to adjust these weights based on the training data. One simple algorithm (dubbed "fire together, wire together") is to increase the weight between two connected neurons when the activation of one triggers the successful activation of another. The net forms "concepts" that are distributed among a subnetwork of shared neurons that tend to fire together: a concept meaning "leg" might be coupled with a subnetwork meaning "foot" that includes the sound for "foot". Neurons have a continuous spectrum of activation; in addition, neurons can process inputs in a nonlinear way rather than weighing straightforward votes. Modern neural nets can learn both continuous functions and, surprisingly, digital logical operations. Neural networks' early successes included predicting the stock market and (in 1995) a mostly self-driving car. In the 2010s, advances in neural networks using deep learning thrust AI into widespread public consciousness and contributed to an enormous upshift in corporate AI spending; for example, AI-related company mergers and acquisitions in 2017 was over 25 times as large as in 2015.

Node

A node is an artificial neuron which makes up part of an artificial neural network.

Noise in AI

Humans are prone to making mistakes when collecting data, and data collection instruments may be unreliable, resulting in dataset errors. The errors are referred to as noise. Data noise in machine learning can cause problems since the algorithm interprets the noise as a pattern and can start generalizing from it.

Non-monotonic logic is a formal logic whose consequence relation is not monotonic. In other words, non-monotonic logics are devised to capture and represent defeasible inferences, i.e., a kind of inference in which reasoners draw tentative conclusions, enabling reasoners to retract their conclusion(s) based on further evidence.

Nouvelle AI differs from classical AI by aiming to produce robots with intelligence levels similar to insects. Researchers believe that intelligence can emerge organically from simple behaviours as these intelligences interacted with the "real world," instead of using the constructed worlds which symbolic AIs typically needed to have programmed into them.

Nucleus

This is a membrane-enclosed organelle found in eukaryotic cells.

Occam's razor

This is the problem-solving principle that the simplest solution tends to be the right one. When presented with competing hypotheses to solve a problem, one should select the solution with the fewest assumptions. The idea is attributed to William of Ockham (c. 1287–1347), who was an English Franciscan friar, scholastic philosopher, and theologian. In science, Occam's razor is used as an abductive heuristic in the development of theoretical models, rather than as a rigorous arbiter between candidate models.

Opinion mining

Opinion mining (sometimes known as sentiment analysis or emotion AI) refers to the use of natural language processing, text analysis, computational linguistics, and biometrics to systematically identify, extract, quantify, and study affective states and subjective information. Sentiment analysis is widely applied to voice of the customer materials such as reviews and survey responses, online and social media, and healthcare materials for applications that range from marketing to customer service to clinical medicine.

Optical character recognition (OCR)

Optical character recognition is the mechanical or electronic conversion of images of typed, handwritten or printed text into machine-encoded text, whether from a scanned document, a photo of a document, a scene-photo (for example the text on signs and billboards in a landscape photo) or from subtitle text superimposed on an image

Optimization

In mathematics, computer science and operations research, optimization is the selection of a best element (with regard to a specific criterion) from some set of available alternatives. For many problems, it is possible to begin the search with some form of a guess and then refine the guess incrementally until no more refinements can be made. These algorithms can be visualized as blind hill climbing: the search is initiated at a random point on the landscape, and then, by jumps or steps, it keeps moving the guess uphill, until the top is reached. Other optimization algorithms are simulated annealing, beam search and random optimization.

P versus NP

The general class of questions for which some algorithm can provide an answer in polynomial time is called "class P" or just "P". For some questions, there is no known way to find an answer quickly, but if one is provided with information showing what the answer is, it is possible to verify the answer quickly. The class of questions for which an answer can be verified in polynomial time is called NP, which stands for "nondeterministic polynomial time. The P versus NP problem is a major unsolved problem in computer science. It asks whether every problem whose solution can be quickly verified (technically, verified in polynomial time) can also be solved quickly (again, in polynomial time).

Partial derivative of a function of several variables

This is the derivative with respect to one of those variables, with the others held constant (as opposed to the total derivative, in which all variables are allowed to vary).

Pattern recognition is a branch of machine learning that focuses on the recognition of patterns and regularities in data, although it is in some cases considered to be nearly synonymous with machine learning

Perceptron

This is a learning network with a single layer, similar to the old concept of linear regression. The main categories of networks are acyclic or feedforward neural networks (where the signal passes in only one direction) and recurrent neural networks (which allow feedback and short-term memories of previous input events). Among the most popular feedforward networks are perceptrons, multi-layer perceptrons and radial basis networks. Neural networks can be applied to the problem of intelligent control (for robotics) or learning, using such techniques as Hebbian learning ("fire together, wire together"), GMDH or competitive learning. Today, neural networks are often trained by the backpropagation algorithm.

Pheromone (see ant colony organization)

Pheromones are chemical signals, that is, carriers of information between individuals within a species. Pheromones induce a physiological or behavioural response in the receiving individual, and often play a crucial role in mate finding and other interactions among animals.

Pixel

In digital imaging a pixel is the smallest addressable element in a raster image, or the smallest addressable element in a dot matrix display device. In most digital display devices, pixels are the smallest element that can be manipulated through software. In computer graphics and digital photography, a raster image represents a two-dimensional picture as a rectangular matrix or grid of square pixels, viewable via a computer display, paper, or other display medium. A raster is technically characterized by the width and height of the image in pixels and by the number of bits per pixel. Each pixel is a sample of an original or synthetic image; more samples typically provide more accurate representations of the original. The intensity of each pixel is variable. In color imaging systems, a color is typically represented by three or four component intensities such as red, green, and blue, or cyan, magenta, yellow, and black.

Predictive analytics

This encompasses a variety of statistical techniques from data mining, predictive modelling, and machine learning, that analyze current and historical facts to make predictions about future or otherwise unknown events

Probabilistic logic (also probability logic and probabilistic reasoning) is the combination of capacity of probability theory to handle uncertainty and the capacity of deductive logic to exploit structure of formal argument. The result is a richer and more expressive formalism with a broad range of possible application areas. Probabilistic logics attempt to find a natural extension of traditional logic truth tables: the results they define are derived through probabilistic expressions.

Probability

This measure is a real-valued function defined on a set of events in a probability space that satisfies measure properties such as countable additivity. The difference between a probability measure and the more general notion of measure (which includes concepts like area or volume) is that a probability measure must assign value 1 to the entire probability space.

Probability space

This is a mathematical construct that models a real-world process (or “experiment”) consisting of states that occur randomly. A probability space is constructed with a specific kind of situation or experiment in mind. It proposes that each time a situation of that kind arises, the set of possible outcomes is the same and the probabilities are also the same.

Probability theory is the branch of mathematics concerned with probability. Although there are several different probability interpretations, probability theory treats the concept in a rigorous mathematical manner by expressing it through a set of axioms. Typically these axioms formalise probability in terms of a probability space, which assigns a measure taking values between 0 and 1, termed the probability measure, to a set of outcomes called the sample space. Any specified subset of these outcomes is called an event. The first axiom of probability theory is a non-negative real number.

Probability is the measure of the likelihood that an event will occur.

Processor or processing units

These are electronic circuits which performs operations on some external data source, usually memory or some other data stream.

Prokaryotes

These are unicellular organism that lacks a membrane-bound nucleus, mitochondria, or any other membrane-bound organelle. Bacteria and algae are examples.

Propositional calculus

This is a branch of logic and is also called propositional logic, statement logic, sentential calculus, or sentential logic. It deals with propositions (which can be true or false) and argument flow. Compound propositions are formed by connecting propositions by logical connectives. The propositions without logical connectives are called atomic propositions. Unlike first-order logic, propositional logic does not deal with non-logical objects, predicates about them, or quantifiers. However, all the machinery of propositional logic is included in first-order logic and higher-order logics. In this sense, propositional logic is the foundation of first-order logic and higher-order logic.

Propositional logic

This is also known as statement logic, sentential calculus, or sentential logic. It deals with propositions (which can be true or false). Propositional calculus is a branch of logic. It deals with propositions (which can be true or false) and argument flow. Several different forms of logic are used in AI research. Propositional logic involves truth functions such as "or" and "not". Several extensions of logic have been designed to handle specific domains of knowledge, such as description logics, situation calculus, event calculus and fluent calculus (for representing events and time), causal calculus, belief calculus and modal logics.

Qualification problem

In philosophy and AI (especially in knowledge-based systems) this is concerned with the impossibility of listing all the preconditions required for a real-world action to have its intended effect. It might be posed as how to deal with the things that prevent the achievement of an intended result. It is strongly connected to, and opposite the ramification side of, the frame problem.

Radial basis function (RBF)

This is a real-valued function whose value depends only on the distance from the origin. A radial basis function network is an artificial neural network that uses radial basis functions as activation functions. The output of the network is a linear combination of radial basis functions of the inputs and neuron parameters. Radial basis function networks have many uses, including function approximation, time series prediction, classification, and system control.

Random forest or random decision forests

This is an ensemble learning method for classification, regression and other tasks that operates by constructing a multitude of decision trees at training time. For classification tasks, the output of the random forest is the class selected by most trees. For regression tasks, the mean or average prediction of the individual trees is returned.

Random optimization (RO)

This is a family of numerical optimization methods that do not require the gradient of the problem to be optimized and RO can hence be used on functions that are not continuous or differentiable. Such optimization methods are also known as direct-search, derivative-free, or black-box methods.

Random variables, (also known as random quantities, aleatory variables, or stochastic variables)

These are variables whose possible values are outcomes of a random phenomenon. As a function, a random variable is required to be measurable, which rules out certain pathological cases where the quantity which the random variable returns is infinitely sensitive to small changes in the outcome. Random variables have a lack of pattern or predictability in events.

Rational choice theory

Also known as choice theory or rational action theory, this is a framework for understanding, and often formally modelling, social and economic behaviour. The basic premise of rational choice theory is that aggregate social behaviour results from the behaviour of individual actors, each of whom is making their individual decisions. The theory also focuses on the determinants of the individual choices (methodological individualism).

Reasoning

This was an early approach to searching using developed algorithms that imitated step-by-step the reasoning that humans use when they solve puzzles or make logical deductions. Simple exhaustive searches are rarely sufficient for most real-world problems: the search space (the number of places to search) quickly grows to astronomical numbers. The result is a search that is too slow or that never completes. The solution, for many problems, is to use heuristics or "rules of thumb" that prioritize choices in favour of those that are more likely to reach a goal and to do so in a shorter number of steps. In some search methodologies heuristics can also serve to entirely eliminate some choices that are unlikely to lead to a goal (called "pruning the search tree"). Heuristics supply the program with a "best guess" for the path on which the solution lies. Heuristics limit the search for solutions into a smaller sample size.

Recurrent neural network (RNN)

This is a class of artificial neural network where connections between nodes form a directed graph along a sequence. This allows it to exhibit temporal dynamic behaviour for a time sequence. Unlike feedforward neural networks, RNNs can use their internal state (memory) to process sequences of inputs. This makes them applicable to tasks such as unsegmented, connected handwriting recognition or speech recognition.

*Reinforcement learnin*g (RL)

Reinforcement learning is concerned with how an agent ought to take actions in an environment so as to maximize some notion of long-term reward. Reinforcement learning algorithms attempt to find a policy that maps states of the world to the actions the agent ought to take in those states. Reinforcement learning differs from the supervised learning problem in that correct input/output pairs are never presented, nor sub-optimal actions explicitly corrected. Training data (in the form of rewards and punishments) is given only as feedback to the program's actions in a dynamic environment, such as driving a vehicle or playing a game against an opponent.

Representation learning

Researchers at the Massachusetts Institute of Technology (MIT) found that solving difficult problems in vision and natural language processing required ad-hoc solutions – they argued that there was no simple and general principle (like logic) that would capture all the aspects of intelligent behavior. Roger Schank described their "anti-logic" approaches as "scruffy" (as opposed to the "neat" paradigms used at universities such as Carnegie Mellon and Stanford Universities). Commonsense knowledge bases are an example of "scruffy" AI, since they must be built by hand, one complicated concept at a time. Representation learning algorithms often attempt to preserve the information in their input but transform it in a way that makes it useful, often as a pre-processing step before performing classification or predictions, allowing reconstruction of the inputs coming from the unknown data generating distribution, while not being necessarily faithful for configurations that are implausible under that distribution.

Restricted Boltzmann machine (RBM) is a generative stochastic artificial neural network that can learn a probability distribution over its set of inputs.

Robotics

This is an interdisciplinary branch of engineering and science that includes mechanical engineering, electronics engineering, computer science, and others. Robotics deals with the design, construction, operation, and use of robots, as well as computer systems for their control, sensory feedback, and information processing. AI is heavily used in robotics. Advanced robotic arms and other industrial robots, widely used in modern factories, can learn from experience how to move efficiently despite the presence of friction and gear slippage. A modern mobile robot, when given a small, static, and visible environment, can easily determine its location and map its environment; however, dynamic environments, such as in endoscopy (examining the interior of a patient's breathing body) pose a greater challenge. Robots can be guided by an external control device or the control may be embedded within. Robots may be constructed to take on human form but most robots are machines designed to perform a task with no regard as to how they look.

Rule of inference

Also known as inference rule or transformation rule), rule of inference is a logical form consisting of a function which takes premises, analyzes their syntax, and returns a conclusion (or conclusions).

Rule-based machine learning

Rule-based systems are used as a way to store and manipulate knowledge to interpret information in a useful way. They are often used in artificial intelligence applications and research.

Sample space

In probability theory of an experiment or random trial this is the set of all possible outcomes or results of that experiment.

Satplan

(Better known as Planning as Satisfiability), this is a method for automated planning. It converts the planning problem instance into an instance of the Boolean satisfiability problem, which is then solved using a method for establishing satisfiability such as the DPLL algorithm or WalkSAT.

Search and optimization

Many problems in AI can be solved in theory by intelligently searching through many possible solutions: Reasoning can be reduced to performing a search. For example, logical proof can be viewed as searching for a path that leads from premises to conclusions, where each step is the application of an inference rule. Planning algorithms search through trees of goals and subgoals, attempting to find a path to a target goal, a process called means-ends analysis. Robotics algorithms for moving limbs and grasping objects use local searches in configuration space. Many learning algorithms use search algorithms based on optimization.

Semi-supervised learning

The computer is given only an incomplete training signal: a training set with some (often many) of the target outputs missing.

Sequence learning

In cognitive psychology, this is inherent to human ability because it is an integrated part of conscious and nonconscious learning as well as activities. Sequences of information or sequences of actions are used in various everyday tasks: from sequencing sounds in speech, to sequencing movements in typing or playing instruments, to sequencing actions in driving an automobile. Sequence learning can be used to study skill acquisition and in studies of various groups. According to Ritter and Nerb, “The order in which material is presented can strongly influence what is learned, how fast performance increases, and sometimes even whether the material is learned at all.” Sequence learning, more known and understood as a form of explicit learning, is now also being studied as a form of implicit learning as well as other forms of learning. Sequence learning can also be referred to as sequential behaviour, behaviour sequencing, and serial order in behavior.

Set theory

This is a branch of mathematical logic that studies sets, which informally are collections of objects. Although any type of object can be collected into a set, set theory is applied most often to objects that are relevant to mathematics. The language of set theory can be used in the definitions of nearly all mathematical objects.

Similarity and metric learning

Similarity learning is closely related to distance metric learning. Metric learning is the task of learning a distance function over objects. A metric or distance function has to obey four axioms: non-negativity, identity of indiscernibles, symmetry and subadditivity (or the triangle inequality).

Simulated annealing (SA)

This is a probabilistic technique for approximating the global optimum of a given function. Specifically, it is a metaheuristic to approximate global optimization in a large search space. It is often used when the search space is discrete (e.g., all tours that visit a given set of cities). For problems where finding an approximate global optimum is more important than finding a precise local optimum in a fixed amount of time, simulated annealing may be preferable to alternatives such as gradient descent.

Situated agents

These are agents which are embedded in an environment. The term situated is commonly used to refer to robots, but some researchers argue that software agents can also be situated.

Situation calculus

This represents changing scenarios as a set of first-order logic formulae. It is a logic formalism designed for representing and reasoning about dynamical domains.

SOAR is a cognitive architecture, originally created by John Laird, Allen Newell, and Paul Rosenbloom at Carnegie Mellon University. The goal of the SOAR project is to develop the fixed computational building blocks necessary for general intelligent agents – agents that can perform a wide range of tasks and encode, use, and learn all types of knowledge to realize the full range of cognitive capabilities found in humans, such as decision making, problem solving, planning, and natural language understanding. It is both a theory of what cognition is and a computational implementation of that theory.

Social intelligence (also known as Affective computing)

This is an interdisciplinary umbrella that comprises systems which recognize, interpret, process, or simulate human affects. Moderate successes related to affective computing include textual sentiment analysis and, more recently, multimodal affect analysis, in which AI classifies the affects displayed by a videotaped subject. In the long run, social skills and an understanding of human emotion and game theory would be valuable to a social agent. Being able to predict the actions of others by understanding their motives and emotional states would allow an agent to make better decisions. Some computer systems mimic human emotion and expressions to appear more sensitive to the emotional dynamics of human interaction, or to otherwise facilitate human - computer interaction. Similarly, some virtual assistants are programmed to speak conversationally or even to banter humorously; this tends to give naive users an unrealistic conception of how intelligent existing computer agents actually are. Social intelligence comprises social skills and an understanding of human emotion and game theory. Some computer systems mimic human emotion and expressions to appear more sensitive to the emotional dynamics of human interaction, or to otherwise facilitate human–computer interaction.

Soft Computing (SC)

This has as its principal constituents Fuzzy Logic, Evolutionary Computation, Machine Learning and Probabilistic Reasoning, with the latter subsuming belief networks and parts of learning theory. Soft computing (sometimes referred to as computational intelligence, is the use of inexact solutions to computationally hard tasks, for which there is no known algorithm that can compute an exact solution in polynomial time. Soft computing differs from conventional (hard) computing in that, unlike hard computing, it is tolerant of imprecision, uncertainty, partial truth, and approximation. In effect, the role model for soft computing is the human mind.

AI planning

Sometimes denoted as AI Planning, automated planning and scheduling is a branch of artificial intelligence that concerns the realization of strategies or action sequences, typically for execution by intelligent agents, autonomous robots and unmanned vehicles. Unlike classical control and classification problems, the solutions are complex and must be discovered and optimized in a multidimensional space.

Sparse dictionary learning

Statistical learning in AI is the adoption of sophisticated mathematical tools, such as hidden Markov models, information theory, and normative Bayesian decision theory to compare or to unify competing architectures. The shared mathematical language permits a high level of collaboration with more established fields (like mathematics, economics or operations research).

Stochastic neural network

This is a type of artificial neural networks built by introducing random variations into the network, either by giving the network's neurons stochastic transfer functions, or by giving them stochastic weights. This makes them useful tools for optimization problems, since the random fluctuations help it escape from local minima. An example of a neural network using stochastic transfer functions is a Boltzmann machine. Each neuron is binary valued, and the chance of it firing depends on the other neurons in the network. Stochastic neural networks have found applications in risk management, oncology, bioinformatics, and other similar fields.

Stochastic optimization (SO) methods

These are optimization methods that generate and use random variables. For stochastic problems, the random variables appear in the formulation of the optimization problem itself, which involve random objective functions or random constraints. Stochastic optimization methods also include methods with random iterates. Some stochastic optimization methods use random iterates to solve stochastic problems, combining both meanings of stochastic optimization. Stochastic optimization methods generalize deterministic methods for deterministic problems. Stochastic optimization methods are optimization methods that generate and use random variables. For stochastic problems, the random variables appear in the formulation of the optimization problem itself, which involve random objective functions or random constraints. Stochastic optimization methods also include methods with random iterates.

Stochastic

This is an adjective that describes something that was randomly determined.

Sub-symbolic AI

By the 1980s progress in symbolic AI seemed to stall and many believed that symbolic systems would never be able to imitate all the processes of human cognition, especially perception, robotics, learning and pattern recognition. A number of researchers began to look into "sub-symbolic" approaches to specific AI problems. Sub-symbolic methods manage to approach intelligence without specific representations of knowledge.

Supervised learning

The computer is presented with example inputs and their desired outputs, given by a "teacher", and the goal is to learn a general rule that maps inputs to outputs; the input signal can be only partially available, or restricted to special feedback.

Supervised learning

The computer is presented with example inputs and their desired outputs, given by a "teacher", and the goal is to learn a general rule that maps inputs to outputs; the input signal can be only partially available, or restricted to special feedback:

Support vector machines

Support vector machines (SVMs) are a set of related supervised learning methods used for classification and regression. Given a set of training examples, each marked as belonging to one of two categories, an SVM training algorithm builds a model that predicts whether a new example falls into one category or the other. Support vector machines, also known as support vector networks in machine learning, are supervised learning models with associated learning algorithms that analyse data used for classification and regression analysis. Given a set of training examples, each marked as belonging to one or the other of two categories, an SVM training algorithm builds a model that assigns new examples to one category or the other, making it a non-probabilistic binary linear classifier.

Swarm intelligence (SI)

This is the collective behaviour of decentralized, natural or artificial self-organized systems. SI systems consist typically of a population of simple agents or boids interacting locally with one another and with their environment. The inspiration often comes from nature, especially biological systems. The agents follow very simple rules, and although there is no centralized control structure dictating how individual agents should behave, local, and to a certain degree random, interactions between such agents lead to the emergence of "intelligent" global behavior, unknown to the individual agents. Examples in natural systems of SI include ant colonies, bird flocking, animal herding, bacterial growth, fish schooling and microbial intelligence.

Symbolic AI

When access to digital computers became possible in the middle 1950s, AI research began to explore the possibility that human intelligence could be reduced to symbol manipulation. The research was centered in three institutions: Carnegie Mellon University, Stanford and the Massachusetts Institute of Technology (MIT), and each one developed its own style of research. John Haugeland named these symbolic approaches to AI "good old fashioned AI" or "GOFAI". During the 1960s symbolic approaches had achieved great success at simulating high-level thinking in small demonstration programs. Approaches based on cybernetics or artificial neural networks were abandoned or pushed into the background. Symbolic artificial intelligence is the term for the collection of all methods in artificial intelligence research that are based on high-level "symbolic" (human-readable) representations of problems, logic and search. Symbolic AI was the dominant paradigm of AI research from the mid-1950s until the late 1980s.

Syntax

This is anything having to do with formal languages or formal systems without regard to any interpretation or meaning given to them. Syntax is concerned with the rules used for constructing, or transforming the symbols and words of a language, as contrasted with the semantics of a language which are concerned with its meaning.

Sparse coding algorithms

These represent an attempt to work under the constraint that the learned representation is low-dimensional. They attempt to do so under the constraint that the learned representation is sparse (ie has many zeros). Multilinear subspace learning algorithms aim to learn low-dimensional representations directly from tensor representations for multidimensional data, without reshaping them into high-dimensional vectors.

Transfer learning

Transfer learning is a research problem in machine learning that focuses on storing knowledge gained while solving one problem and applying it to a different but related problem. For example, knowledge gained while learning to recognize cars could apply when trying to recognize trucks.

Transformer

Transformer is a deep learning architecture based on the multi-head attention mechanism. It is notable for not containing any recurrent units, and thus requires less training time than previous recurrent neural architectures.

Truth value

This is sometimes called a logical value, in logic and mathematics, and is a value indicating the relationship of a proposition to truth.

U-net

U-Net architecture stems from the so-called "fully convolutional network" The main idea is to supplement a usual contracting network by successive layers, where pooling operations are replaced by upsampling operators. In contrast, with CNN the image is converted into a vector which is largely used in classification problems. In U-Net an image is converted into a vector and then the same mapping is used to convert it again to an image. This reduces the distortion by preserving the original structure of the image.

Unstructured data (or unstructured information)

This is information that either does not have a pre-defined data model or is not organized in a pre-defined manner. Unstructured information is typically text-heavy, but may contain data such as dates, numbers, and facts as well. This results in irregularities and ambiguities that make it difficult to understand using traditional programs as compared to data stored in fielded form in databases or annotated (semantically tagged) in documents.

Unsupervised learning

This is a machine learning task of inferring a function that describes the structure of "unlabelled" data (i.e. data that have not been classified or categorized). Since the examples given to the learning algorithm are unlabelled, there is no straightforward way to evaluate the accuracy of the structure that is produced by the algorithm - one feature that distinguishes unsupervised learning from supervised learning and reinforcement learning. No labels are given to the learning algorithm, leaving it on its own to find structure in its input. Unsupervised learning can be a goal in itself (discovering hidden patterns in data) or a means towards an end (feature learning)

Vanishing gradient problem

This is a difficulty found in training artificial neural networks with gradient-based learning methods and backpropagation. In such methods, each of the neural network's weights receives an update proportional to the partial derivative of the error function with respect to the current weight in each iteration of training. The problem is that in some cases, the gradient will be vanishingly small, effectively preventing the weight from changing its value. In the worst case, this may completely stop the neural network from further training.

Waggle dance

This is a term used in beekeeping and ethology for a particular figure-eight dance of the honey bee. By performing this dance, successful foragers can share, with other members of the colony, information about the direction and distance to patches of flowers yielding nectar and pollen, to water sources, or to new nest-site locations.

WalkSAT (and *GSAT*) are local search algorithms to solve Boolean satisfiability problems. Both algorithms work on formulae in Boolean logic that are in, or have been converted into, conjunctive normal form. They start by assigning a random value to each variable in the formula. If the assignment satisfies all clauses, the algorithm terminates, returning the assignment. Otherwise, a variable is flipped and the above is then repeated until all the clauses are satisfied.

Zero-sum game

In game theory and economic theory a zero-sum game is a mathematical representation of a situation in which each participant's gain or loss of utility is exactly balanced by the losses or gains of the utility of the other participants. If the total gains of the participants are added up and the total losses are subtracted, they will sum to zero.

Chapter 2. An introduction to artificial intelligence and machine learning

Introduction

Artificial intelligence (AI) is the use of data to solve complex problems.

It involves the use of machines (ie computers) that can learn by themselves, rather than being taught (programmed) by humans to perform tasks normally requiring human intelligence, such as visual perception, speech recognition, decision-making, and translation between languages. In simple terms AI is the capability of a machine to imitate intelligent human behaviour. AI is comprised of a number of algorithms and computer code. AI involves logic and data input, all resulting in data output.

What is an algorithm?

A programming algorithm can be thought of as a recipe that describes the exact steps needed for the computer to solve a problem or reach a goal. An algorithm can be compared to a food recipe with a list of the ingredients needed and a set of steps on how to make the intended meal. In computer terms, the word for a recipe is a procedure, and the ingredients are called inputs. A programming algorithm describes what the computer should do, and the computer will do it exactly that way every time. The process of folding a shirt or a pair of trousers is an algorithm, as are the activities people do when they wake up: these would be the inputs for the latter:

Wake up

Take shower

Do exercises

Have breakfast

Dress for work

Wait for transport to work

The output would be “Typical activities early on a weekday morning”.

Another simple example of an algorithm would be to find the largest number in an unsorted list of numbers. If there was a list of five different numbers, this can be easily done without the help of a computer, but if there are five million different numbers a computer will be required, and a computer needs an algorithm. This is what the algorithm could look like: the input consists of a list of numbers, and this list is called L. The number L1 would be the first number in the list, L2 the second number, and so on. Thus, the input to the algorithm is a list of numbers, and the output would be the largest number in the list.

Algorithms can perform calculations, data processing and automated reasoning tasks.

Another way to describe an algorithm is a sequence of unambiguous instructions. A procedure for solving a mathematical problem (such as finding the highest common factor) is a finite number of steps in a step-by-step procedure. An algorithm can be expressed within a finite amount of space and time and in a well-defined formal language for calculating a function. Starting from an initial state and initial input, the instructions describe a computation that, when executed, proceeds through a finite number of well-defined successive states, eventually producing an output. The transition from one state to the next is not necessarily deterministic; some algorithms, known as randomized algorithms, incorporate random input.

It is important, however, to note that a programming algorithm is not computer code. It can be written in everyday language. It has a start, a middle, and an end. It includes only what is needed to carry out the task. It does not include anything that is unclear or ambiguous. Although algorithms can be written in regular language, it takes a long time to do so. Therefore, algorithms are now usually written in programming languages such as Cobal, Fortran or Python.

Computer programming

Computer programming or coding is the composition of sequences of instructions, called programs, that computers follow to perform tasks. It involves designing and implementing algorithms, step-by-step specifications of procedures, by writing code in one or more programming languages. Programmers typically use high-level programming languages that are more easily intelligible to humans than machine code, which is directly executed by the central processing unit of the computer. Proficient programming usually requires expertise in several different subjects, including knowledge of the application domain, details of programming languages and generic code libraries, specialized algorithms, and formal logic.

What is computer code?

Source code, or simply code, is any collection of text written using a human-readable programming language, usually as plain text. The source code of a program is specially designed to facilitate the work of computer programmers, who specify the actions to be performed by a computer mostly by writing source code. Source code is the version of software as it is originally written (i.e., typed into a computer) by a human in plain text (i.e., human readable alphanumeric characters).

How do machines learn?

In one of two ways:

1. by having their incorrect outputs revised by human input

This is straightforward: for example, if 10,000 images of a melanoma are uploaded into the computer's memory labelled as "melanoma" and then 10,000 images of a benign freckle labelled as "benign freckle" are uploaded, a photograph of a dark skin lesion can then be uploaded and the computer can be asked to diagnose it as either "melanoma" or 'benign freckle". If it gets the diagnosis incorrectly, this can be corrected and the computer's learning ability is thereby increased and improved.

2. by insertion of a length of computer code

This is more difficult but useful: insertion of a length of computer code picks up errors in output and automatically improves the computer's output ability.

Computers are learning how to code themselves

Snyk is a company focused on an all-in-one platform for securing computer code. Snyk's DeepCoder is a machine learning system that can write its own code. It does this using a technique called program synthesis. Essentially, it creates new programs by combining existing lines of code taken from other software, which is what human coders do. With a particular output in mind, DeepCoder is able to determine which lines or pieces of code are likely to be particularly useful. The approach is to train a neural network to predict properties of the program that generated the outputs from the inputs. DeepCoder can trawl through the basic, input-output style challenges usually set by programming competitions. It is able to search through lines of code more thoroughly and widely than a human coder could, quickly piecing together code in a manner humans might not think of. Because DeepCoder is essentially a deep learning algorithm, every time it is given a new problem, it gets better at combining lines from source codes. Ultimately, this algorithm can make programming accessible to non-coders, allowing anyone to easily build simple programs. DeepCoder's current version only allows it to handle programming challenges with around five lines of code. Future versions of DeepCode may facilitate building routine programs that take information from websites without the need for human coders.

Modifying/Improving programs

It is now possible for a computer program to write its own programs.

Types of artificial intelligence

AI can be categorized in any number of ways; here are two examples. The first classifies AI systems as either weak AI or strong AI. Weak AI, also known as narrow AI, is an AI system that is designed and trained for a particular task. Virtual personal assistants, such as Apple's Siri, are a form of weak AI. Strong AI, also known as artificial general intelligence, is an AI system with generalized human cognitive abilities so that when presented with an unfamiliar task, it has enough intelligence to find a solution.

Arend Hintze categorized AI into four types, from the kind of AI systems that exist today to sentient systems, which do not yet exist. His categories are as follows:

Type 1: Reactive machines. An example is Deep Blue, the IBM chess program that beat Garry Kasparov in the 1990s. Deep Blue can identify pieces on the chess board and make predictions, but it has no memory and cannot use past experiences to inform future ones. It analyzes possible moves - its own and those of its opponent - and chooses the most strategic move. Deep Blue and Google's AlphaGo were designed for narrow purposes and cannot easily be applied to other situations.

Type 2: Limited memory. These AI systems can use past experiences to inform future decisions. Some of the decision-making functions in autonomous vehicles have been designed this way. Observations can be used to inform actions such as a car that has changed lanes. These observations are not stored permanently.

Type 3: Theory of mind. This is a psychology term. It refers to the understanding that others have their own beliefs, desires and intentions that impact the decisions they make. This kind of AI does not yet exist.

Type 4: Self-awareness. In this category, AI systems have a sense of self and consciousness. Machines with self-awareness understand their current state and can use the information to infer what others are feeling. This type of AI does not yet exist.

Examples of AI technology

Automation is the process of making a system or process function automatically. Robotic process automation (RPA), for example, can be programmed to perform high-volume, repeatable tasks normally performed by humans. RPA is different from IT automation in that it can adapt to changing circumstances.

There are three types of machine learning algorithms

Supervised learning, in which data sets are labelled so that patterns can be detected and used to label new data sets; unsupervised learning, in which data sets are not labelled and are sorted according to similarities or differences; and reinforcement learning, in which data sets are not labelled but, after performing an action or several actions, the AI system is given feedback.

Machine vision

Machine vision is the science of making computers see. Machine vision captures and analyzes visual information using a camera, analog-to-digital conversion and digital signal processing. It is often compared to human eyesight, but machine vision is not bound by biology and can be programmed to see through walls, for example. It is used in a range of applications from signature identification to medical image analysis. There are four key tasks required of the computer. They are

1. image classification – assigning labels to the images, for example, liver metastases

2. object detection - locating and outlining specific entities on the image

3. semantic segmentation - assigning object category to each pixel in the image

4. instance segmentation - segmenting and labelling individual objects at the pixel level

Object recognition (also called object classification)

One or several pre-specified or learned objects or object classes can be recognized, usually together with their 2D positions in the image or 3D poses in the scene.

Identification

An individual instance of an object is recognized. Examples include identification of a specific person's face or fingerprint, identification of handwritten digits, or identification of a specific vehicle.

Detection

The image data are scanned for specific objects along with their locations. Examples include the detection of an obstacle in the car's field of view and possible abnormal cells or tissues in medical images or the detection of a vehicle in an automatic road toll system. Detection based on relatively simple and fast computations is sometimes used for finding smaller regions of interesting image data which can be further analyzed by more computationally demanding techniques to produce a correct interpretation.

Natural language processing (NLP)

This is the processing of human - and not computer - language by a computer program. One of the older and best-known examples of NLP is spam detection, which looks at the subject line and the text of an email and decides if it is spam. Current approaches to NLP are based on machine learning. NLP tasks include text translation, sentiment analysis and speech recognition.

Pattern recognition

This is a branch of machine learning that focuses on identifying patterns in data.

Robotics is a field of engineering focused on the design and manufacturing of robots. Robots are often used to perform tasks that are difficult for humans to perform or perform consistently. They are used in assembly lines for car production or by NASA to move large objects in space. More recently, researchers are using machine learning to build robots that can interact in social settings.

Improving patient outcomes and reducing costs

Companies are applying machine learning to make better and faster diagnoses than humans. One of the best-known healthcare technologies is IBM Watson. IBM Watson is designed for a wide range of uses, including data analysis, healthcare, finance, and customer service. It understands natural language and is capable of responding to questions asked of it. The system mines patient data and other available data sources to form a hypothesis, which it then presents with a confidence scoring schema. In contrast, ChatGPT is primarily designed for natural language processing tasks, such as chatbots, language translation, and text generation. In 2022 IBM divested and spun-off their Watson Health division into Merative. As of 2023, it remains a standalone company headquartered in Ann Arbor, Michigan.

Chatbots

Other AI applications include chatbots, a computer program used online to answer questions and assist customers, to help schedule follow-up appointments or aiding patients through the billing process, and virtual health assistants that provide basic medical feedback.

Current status of AI

In 2012 a series of experiments showed that neural networks fuelled with large sets of data and powerful computer chips gave machines new powers of perception. Deep learning, the rocket fuel of the current AI boom, is a revival of one of the oldest ideas in AI. The technique involves passing data through webs of mathematics loosely inspired by how brain cells work (known as artificial neural networks). As the network processes training data, connections between the parts of the network adjust, building up an ability to interpret future data.

Multimodal generative AI

The dream of precision health is to develop a continuous learning health system where new health information is instantly incorporated to optimize care delivery and accelerate biomedical discovery. Multimodal generative AI has the potential to drastically accelerate progress toward precision health by supercharging the structuring of health data and scaling population-level insight generation. Health data is inherently multimodal and longitudinal, comprising physical measurements and natural-language narratives. Only a fraction of such data is available in structured forms, as manual curation is costly and hard to scale. Multimodal generative AI can alleviate the curation bottleneck by leveraging self-supervision from cross-modal correspondence and help extract predictive signals not available in standalone modalities (Poon, 2024).

Modern generative AI takes self-supervision to the web scale, thus acquiring emergent capabilities not seen in smaller scale of pretraining. In a truly generalist fashion, large language models (LLMs) such as GPT-4 have demonstrated unprecedented prowess in conversation, reasoning, and instruction-following for new tasks without specialized training.

In health applications GPT-4 has already demonstrated its potentially transformative power from drafting in-basket responses to automating clinical documentation, and from scaling clinical trial matching to analyzing population-level real-world data (Fernandes et al., 2023). However, to fulfill the potential of generative AI in precision health, there are still big challenges, especially as the scope of multimodal data such as medical imaging and multi-omics is broadened.

Scaling Benchmark Creation and Evaluation

Perhaps counterintuitively, the most fundamental challenge facing health generative AI lies less in model building, but in creating realistic benchmarks that reflect real-world use cases, as well as scaling evaluation for complex generation tasks. Without reliable goalposts, it is hard to measure progress, especially for modern foundation models with open-ended capabilities, such as GPT-4V.

It is exciting to see a plethora of medical AI explorations in diagnostics. However, the potential impact of health generative AI is much broader, encompassing many low-risk yet high-value scenarios across the entire health system, from clerical and documentation tasks in health delivery, to clinical trials and post-market surveillance in drug development, to early biomedical discovery and value-based care.

To sustain and accelerate progress in health generative AI, it is thus necessary to invest in comprehensive benchmark creation and evaluation that represent diverse populations and real-world scenarios. Manual effort is not scalable, especially for accurate evaluation. Interestingly, generative AI itself may be harnessed to address this challenge. Powerful LLMs such as GPT-4 have already demonstrated remarkable capabilities in self-verifying its own output. It may seem paradoxical at first sight, but verification is often easier than generation, akin to P vs NP in computer science. Developing self-improving LLM-based agent systems to supercharge domain experts in benchmark creation and evaluation represents a key direction forward for health generative AI.

Bridging the health competency gap in large multimodal models (LMMs)

Generalist LLMs such as GPT-4 have demonstrated astonishing capabilities in various health applications, but they still have significant growth areas. In multimodal generative AI, the potential gap in health competency may be even larger, as there is scarce availability of multimodal, longitudinal health data in the public web for pretraining.

Contrastive learning

A standard approach to multimodal learning is contrastive learning. Contrastive learning has a long history in NLP and computer vision, initially focusing on unimodal scenarios (e.g., by creating semantic-equivalent variants of an image and training the encoder to map them closer to each other). It can be extended to the multimodal regime by pushing corresponding instances across modalities (e.g., image-text pairs) closer and non-corresponding ones farther apart, akin to machine translation.

To sustain and accelerate progress in health generative AI, it is thus important to invest in comprehensive benchmark creation and evaluation that represent diverse populations and real-world scenarios.

For precision health, a major bottleneck lies in the scarcity of biomedical data in common resources for multimodal pretraining. One way to address this deficiency is by extracting cross-modal data from publicly available resources. By extracting biomedical figures and their corresponding captions and citations from PubMed-Central articles, the BiomedCLIP project has assembled one of the largest datasets for biomedical vision-language pretraining, with 15 million image-text pairs across diverse categories and 46 million fine-grained pairs after splitting composite figures.

Standard contrastive learning treats all modalities equally. In practice, text captures a large swath of digitized knowledge, whereas data for other modalities is much scarcer by comparison. Multimodal input is tokenized and embedded in the natural-language instruction for output generation by a large language model. Subsequent biomedical large multimodal models (such as MedPaLM-M) all follow the same general recipe to align image and text, but LLaVA-Med stands out by using GPT-4 to generate multimodal instruction-following data. Similar approaches can also be applied to other modalities such as single-cell data and protein sequences.

Ultimately, routinely collected real-world clinical data represents the biggest growth opportunity for multimodal generative AI. For example, a cancer patient may have hundreds of clinical notes with their corresponding imaging, multi-omics, and other medical tests, across the disease trajectory from diagnosis to treatment to outcome. Such naturally occurring multimodal, longitudinal data can be leveraged to bridge the health competency gap in LLMs, following the general recipe of LLaVA-Med.

Ongoing research in digital pathology exploration has demonstrated promise. Researchers have collaborated to train real-world pathology foundation models using over one billion images from hundreds of thousands of slides along with clinical reports, with initial promising results in pathomics and progression modeling. Meanwhile, the BiomedJourney project extended the LLaVA-Med approach to image generation, by using GPT-4 to generate instruction-following data from multimodal patient journeys. This enables BiomedJourney to help answer what-if questions for in silico medical imaging.

By encapsulating multimodal and longitudinal dependencies from population-level real-world data, LMMs can potentially unlock a slew of high-value applications, from cross-modal retrieval and generation, to multimodal conversational copilots (enabling stakeholders to “talk to” multimodal data), to the ultimate dream of precision health: learning from multimodal real-world observational data to predict longitudinal treatment outcome and adverse events.

The AI market in healthcare is estimated to grow from a $5 billion industry in 2020 to $45 billion in 2026.

Chapter 3. How AI will improve the interpretation of radiological images

In 2023 there are AI applications for all major medical diagnostic imaging modalities. There are two artificial intelligence methods used for a representative classification task, such as the diagnosis of a suspicious object on an x-ray as either benign or malignant. The first method relies on engineered features extracted from regions of interest from the image on the basis of expert knowledge. Examples of these features in cancer characterization include tumour volume, shape, texture, intensity and location. The most robust features are selected and fed into machine learning classifiers.

The second method uses deep learning and does not require region annotation — rather, localization is usually sufficient. It comprises several layers where feature extraction, selection and ultimate classification are performed simultaneously during training. As layers learn increasingly higher-level features, earlier layers might learn abstract shapes such as lines and shadows, while other deeper layers might learn entire organs or objects. Both methods fall under radiomics, the data-centric, radiology-based research field (Hosny et al, 2018).

In the realm of image acquisition, AI augments scanning procedures, optimises image fidelity, and fosters sophisticated image reconstruction across MRI, CT, and PET modalities. Foremost among these advancements, deep learning accelerates MRI scanning, harmonising efficiency and quality, with commensurate progress witnessed in CT and PET image reconstruction (Najjar, R. 2023).

Chest x-rays

AI significantly streamlines the acquisition of radiologist analyses on chest X-rays, as evidenced by a study in which an AI system reduced interpretation delivery times from 11.2 days to 2.7 days, reinforcing the potency of automated triaging systems in streamlining healthcare workflows and amplifying patient care standards (Annarumma et al., 2019).

In a study published in 2019, The European Society of Radiology reviewed the basis for the application of AI in radiology, discussed the immediate ethical and professional impact of AI in radiology, and considered its possible future evolution (European Society of Radiology, 2019). The authors drew these conclusions:

in radiomics AI can foster the analysis of the features and help in the correlation with other omics data. Imaging biobanks will become a necessary infrastructure to organise and share the image data on which AI models can be trained. AI can be used as an optimising tool to assist the technologist and radiologist in choosing a personalised patient's protocol, tracking the patient's dose parameters and providing an estimate of the radiation risks. AI can also aid the reporting workflow and help the linking between words, images, and quantitative data. Additionally, AI coupled with a clinical decision support (CDS) system can improve the clinical decision process and thus optimise clinical and radiological workflow.

The key factor of AI performance is training with big and high-quality data to avoid overfitting and underfitting. If AI is used in clinical practice, the main medico-legal issue that arises is "who is responsible for the diagnosis."

AI can be understood as a set of tools and programs that make software "smarter" to the extent that an outside observer thinks the output is generated by a human. It operates similarly to the way a normal human brain functions during regular tasks like common-sense reasoning, forming an opinion, or social behaviour.

The term machine learning (and its subcategories) involves a situation in which an agent (anything that can be viewed as perceiving its environment through sensors and acting upon that environment through actuators) is learning if it improves its performance on future tasks after making observations about the world. Machine learning has been extensively applied to big data analysis. Machine learning algorithms evolve with increasing exposure to data; they are not based exclusively on rules, but improve with experience, learning to give specific answers by evaluating large amounts of data.

The learning can be unsupervised, reinforced, supervised, or semi-supervised. In unsupervised learning, the agent learns patterns in the input even though no explicit feedback is supplied. In reinforcement learning, the agent learns from a series of reinforcements. Supervised learning provides the agent with a teacher's output that the agent then learns. In semi-supervised learning, fewer teacher's outputs are given to the agent. In this context, the concept of "ground truth," which means checking the results of machine learning for accuracy against the real world, is fundamental for validating AI performance. In a radiology context this might mean confirming diagnoses suggested by AI by comparison to pathological or surgical diagnoses. Ground truth is the data that is assumed to be true. Machine learning has been likened to training a dog: reinforcing good behaviour, ignoring bad, and giving her/him enough practice to work out what to do for herself/himself.

Deep learning is a subset of machine learning and is the basis of most AI tools for image interpretation. Deep learning means that the computer has multiple layers of algorithms interconnected and stratified into hierarchies of importance. These layers accumulate data from inputs and provide an output that can change step by step once the AI system learns new features from the data. Such multi-layered algorithms form large artificial neural networks.

Artificial neural networks are composed of nodes or units (thousands to millions) connected by links. A link propagates activation from one unit to another, and each link activation is weighted by a numeric value which determines the strength of the connection. The activation function can be based on a threshold of activation (the strength), and the unit that receives the activation is called a perceptron. Perceptrons are connected by links and create a network; the network can be feed-forward (where connections are only in one direction) or it can be a recurrent network, which feeds its outputs back into its own inputs (a loop). Feed-forward networks are usually arranged in layers. The goal is that the answer for each examination should match the examination's labels. Mathematically, the algorithm is designed to maximise the number of right answers as the inputs are processed through its layers.

Artificial neural networks must be "trained" using training data sets from which the network "learns." In radiology, these usually consist (at least initially) of hand-labelled image data sets used by the algorithm to improve its fit to match the ground truth. Once a network has been trained using a training data set, it would then be tested using a different set of data (validation data sets), designed to evaluate the fit of the model to new data. In this step, it is common to observe "overfitting" of the model. The consequence of overfitting is that the network will not be generalisable to never-seen-before data and will be a source of more interpretation errors than those which occurred in the training data set.

The best solution for reducing overfitting is to obtain more training data. Multiple rounds of training and testing on different datasets may be performed, gradually improving network performance, and permitting assessment of the accuracy and generalisability of the algorithm, before the algorithm is released for general use. Another solution is so-called “data augmentation” which means modifying the training data by adding some variability so that the model will not see the exact same inputs from the training data set during the training iterations. If the network is being trained to recognise a cystic lesion on ultrasound, on the training data set the lesion could be perfectly cystic, but in a further iteration of training, some internal hyperechoic spots caused by artifacts could be added in order to train or fine-tune the network to recognise a “non-perfect cyst” in the validation data sets.

As a general rule, the “deeper” the network (more layers) and the more rounds of training, the better the performance of the network.

Use cases

The term “use case” describes a specific clinical application of AI in radiology. Use cases can be considered as precise scenarios within the radiology service chain where automation can add significant value and establish standards. Computer-aided detection (CAD) represents the earliest clinical applications of basic AI in radiology. CAD system has been progressively implemented in radiological practice over the last two decades in the detection of lung, colon, breast, and prostate cancer.

The main difference between CAD and AI is that CAD only makes diagnoses for which it has been specifically trained and bases its performance on a training dataset and a rigid scheme of recognition that can only be improved if more datasets are added to the CAD algorithm. In contrast, AI is characterised by the process of autonomous learning, without explicit programming of each step, based on a network of algorithms and connections.

In the last decade there has been an explosion in studies employing artificial intelligence for image interpretation that embrace disease detection and classification, organ and lesion segmentation (determining the boundaries of an organ or lesion), and assessment of response to treatment. Some of many recent applications of AI include the Radiology Society of North America (RSNA) paediatric bone age machine learning challenge on plain radiographs, breast cancer detection in mammography and MRI, chest radiograph interpretation, liver lesion characterisation on ultrasound and CT, brain tumour and prostate cancer detection.

A step beyond disease detection is disease classification into low or high risk, with good or poor prognosis. Much of the work in this field has been in brain imaging, in both benign and malignant disease. There has been considerable effort to develop AI classifiers in pediatrics, where brain mapping and functional connectivity can be linked to neurodevelopmental outcome. In a study evaluating resting state functional MRI data from 50 preterm-born infants, binary support vector machines distinguished them from term infants with 84% accuracy ($p < 0.0001$), based primarily on inter- and intra-hemispheric connections throughout the brain (Smyser et al., 2016). In multiple sclerosis, AI has been used to evaluate the performance of combinations of MRI sequences to optimise brain lesion detection (Aslam et al, 2022). Classification of glioma grade based on MR images has been attempted with some success (Cho et al., 2018).

Automated segmentation is crucial in AI for reducing the burden on radiology workflow, obviating the need to perform segmentation manually. It also provides important information on the functional performance of tissues and organs, disease extent, and burden.

Avendi et al. (2016) developed a deep learning and deformable model for left ventricular (LV) segmentation from cardiac MRI datasets, to obtain an automated calculation of clinical indices such as ventricular volume and ejection fraction.

AI significantly streamlines the acquisition of radiologists' analyses of chest X-rays, , reinforcing the potency of automated triaging systems in streamlining healthcare workflows and amplifying patient care standards (Annarumma et al., 2019).

Other applications of AI in radiology

Outside the traditional radiology activities of lesion detection and characterisation, and assessment of response to treatment, AI is likely to impact other areas of radiologists' and other healthcare professionals' work.

Radiomics

In medicine, radiomics is a method that extracts a large number of features from medical images using data-characterisation algorithms. These features, termed radiomic features, have the potential to uncover tumor patterns and characteristics that cannot be appreciated by the human eye.

A radiomics analysis can extract over 400 features from a region of interest in a CT, MRI, or PET study, and correlate these features with each other and other data, far beyond the capability of the human eye or brain to appreciate. Such features may be used to predict prognosis and response to treatment. AI can support analysis of radiomics features and help in the correlation between radiomics and other data (such as proteomics, genomics, biopsy results) by building patients' signatures.

Imaging biobanks

The constantly enlarging memory capacity of computers permits storage of large amounts of data. In radiology, the need to store native images and big data derived from quantitative imaging represents the main cause of overloading picture archiving and communication system (PACS). Quantitative imaging can produce imaging biomarkers that can be stored and organised in large imaging biobanks, available to be processed, analysed, and used to predict the risk of disease and treatment response in large population studies. Such banks could potentially use data from many institutions and locations. Large biobanks also have the potential to become the repository of digital patients (avatars or digital twins of humans) that can be used by AI to perform simulations of disease development and progression. Imaging biobanks will be a necessary infrastructure to organise and share the image data on which AI models can be trained.

Dose optimisation

The European Society of Radiology (ESR) EuroSafe Imaging initiative is designed to support and strengthen medical radiation protection across Europe following a holistic, inclusive approach (www.eurosafeimaging.org). EuroSafe Imaging promotes the adoption of clinical diagnostic reference levels in CT that should be customised based on appropriateness criteria and on patient characteristics, such as body mass index (BMI) and circulation time. The choice of protocol, however, is subject to variability since it is frequently operator-dependent, and consequently the quality of the examination are subject to variability at both intra- and inter-institutional levels. In this setting, AI can be an optimising tool for assisting the technologist and radiologist in choosing a personalised patient's protocol, in tracking the patient's dose parameters, and in providing an estimate of the radiation risks associated with cumulative dose and the patient's susceptibility (age and other clinical parameters).

Structured reporting

AI can aid the reporting workflow and help link words, images, and quantitative data, finally suggesting the most probable diagnosis. The structured reporting initiative of RSNA, in which ESR is a partner, is proposing the adoption of common data elements (CDEs) that define the attributes and allowable values of a unit of information so that information can be collected and stored uniformly across institutions and studies. CDEs are defined in a data dictionary and make biomedical data interoperable for a variety of applications, including clinical radiology reports, computer-assisted reporting systems, structured image annotations, case report forms for clinical research, and radiology case collections. Thus, CDEs can be the vocabulary of AI to build a patient's specific structured report.

AI tools can also impact the daily workflow by filtering examination priority based on appropriateness criteria. ESR has implemented the "ESR iGuide," a clinical decision support system (CDS) that assists referring physicians to choose the most appropriate imaging procedure based on the level of evidence for appropriateness, and the level of emergency. AI coupled with CDS can improve the decision process and thereby optimise clinical and radiological workflow.

Barriers to AI in radiology and challenges

Data sets and training

The availability of large amounts (big data) of medical images in the imaging domain (from PACS systems) offers great potential for AI training, but such data need a curation process in which the data are stratified by patient cohorts, segmented to extract the region of interest for AI interpretation, filtered to assess the quality of acquisition and reconstructions.

Data set annotation, however, is very time- and labour-intensive, and the validation of ground truth diagnosis must be very robust. Rare findings are a potential weakness. If a condition or a finding is very rare, it is difficult to obtain enough examples to train an algorithm to identify it with confidence. Also, variation in findings can lead to inadvertent overfitting, where random noise is interpreted by the algorithm as an abnormality. Conversely, if the training data set used to train an algorithm contains inherent biases (for example, ethnic-, age- or gender-based), the algorithm may underfit findings from data derived from a different patient population.

Regulatory issues

Isaac Asimov's fictional three laws of robotics should be applied to AI in radiology, where the "robot" is the "AI medical imaging software":

1. A robot may not injure a human being or, through inaction, allow a human being to come to harm.

2. A robot must obey the orders given it by human beings except where such orders would conflict with the First Law.

3. A robot must protect its own existence as long as such protection does not conflict with the First or Second Laws.

The first law implies that AI tools should achieve the best possible diagnosis to improve patient's healthcare; however, AI failure or inaction could result in harm to the patient.

The second law suggests that AI must be properly trained and that the learning process of any AI software must be supervised by a radiologist, to ensure appropriate and clinically applicable outputs.

The third law may be an issue when considering the inevitable eventual obsolescence of any AI software. Imaging is evolving so rapidly that the training of a software, with specific imaging data, can be insufficient once a new development of imaging, or new modalities, are introduced into clinical practice.

Only by applying stringent standards of accountability, effectiveness, and validation of clinical usefulness that would be applied to a new drug or device can patient safety be assured when AI is applied to patient diagnosis.

Medico-legal responsibility

CAD, as applied to CT colonography, lung cancer, and breast cancer detection, can be used as a first reader (not generally recommended), second reader (mostly recommended) or as a concurrent reader (few recommendations), but not as an independent reader of studies.

The medico-legal issue that arises is the question of "who is responsible for the diagnosis," especially if it is wrong. Whether data scientists or manufacturers involved in development, marketing, and installation of AI systems will carry the ultimate legal responsibility for adverse outcomes arising from AI algorithm use is a difficult legal question. If doctors are no longer the primary agents of interpretation of radiological studies, will they still be held accountable? If radiologists monitor AI system outputs and still have a role in validating AI interpretations, do they still carry the ultimate responsibility, even though they do not understand, and cannot interrogate the precise means by which a diagnosis was determined? This "black box" element of AI poses many challenges, not least to the basic human need to understand how and why important decisions were made.

Need for access to large volumes of data

Access to large volumes of data is necessary to develop and train AI algorithms; this can be one of the major factors limiting algorithm development. Software developers use a variety of methods to obtain training datasets; some liaise directly with patients, others with institutions or academic databases. Fundamentally, each patient whose data is used by a third party should provide consent for that use, and that consent may need to be obtained afresh if the data is re-used in a different context (for example, to train an updated software version). Moreover, ownership of imaging datasets varies from one jurisdiction to another. In many countries, the ultimate ownership of such personal data resides with the patient, although the data may be stored, with consent, in a hospital or imaging centre repository.

Anonymisation of data should be guaranteed; this involves more than de-identification and should ensure that there is no capability to re-identify the patient through Digital Imaging and Communications in Medicine (DICOM) tags or facial recognition software. DICOM is a technical standard for the digital storage and transmission of medical images and related information. It includes a file format definition, which specifies the structure of a DICOM file. The primary purpose of the standard is to facilitate communication between the software and hardware entities involved in medical imaging, especially those that are created by different manufacturers. Entities that utilize DICOM files include components of picture archiving and communication systems (PACS), such as imaging machines (modalities), radiological information systems (RIS), scanners, printers, computing servers, and networking hardware.

Data mining and radiomics

One of the exciting prospects for AI incorporation into radiology practice is the potential to extract data from many studies, unconstrained by location, and use those data to identify imaging markers that may predict outcome or response to treatment. Neural network analysis of large datasets can isolate important relationships that could never be perceived by visual interpretation of studies alone, and which may prove important in future personalised healthcare.

Other ethical issues

Some of the points considered above encompass ethical elements. Fundamentally, it must be remembered that AI tools are mathematical constructs, designed to optimise a mathematical function. Intrinsically, they are amoral. The challenge for humans is to anticipate how AI systems can go wrong or could be abused and to build in protections against this happening.

AI, radiology training and future directions

Radiologists' skills are based on many years of training during which the trainee is taught to interpret large numbers of examinations based on a combined process of reading coupled with knowledge of clinical information. Interpretation skills strongly depend on the number of exams interpreted and the accuracy of the visual image analysis. AI can perform image reading by exploiting deep learning tools and is able not only to extract visual information but also quantitative information, such as radiomic signatures or other imaging biomarkers, which would not be identified by the human brain. When software becomes part of the process of interpretation, trainees may not make enough direct interpretations during their training years and therefore may not acquire adequate interpretation skills. Alternatively, trainees will be helped by AI to perform better interpretations. Regardless, a strong dependence of future radiologists on aid from AI software is a significant risk.

A vast amount of AI research is ongoing; image interpretation is an attractive target for researchers, given that the tasks involved (at least in part) involve analysis of large amounts of data to produce an output. Radiologists should embrace this research and integrate it as much as possible into their daily work.

Another task that must be taken on is leadership in educating policymakers and payers about radiology, AI, their integration, and the associated pitfalls. In any rapidly developing industry, there is initial excitement, often followed by disappointment when early promises are unfulfilled.

Will radiologists be replaced by AI?

The simple answer is no. However, radiologists' working lives will undoubtedly change in the era of artificial intelligence. Many of the single routine tasks in the radiology workflow will be performed faster and better by AI algorithms, but the role of the radiologist is a complex one, focused on solving complex clinical problems. The real challenge is not to oppose the incorporation of AI into the professional lives (a futile effort) but to embrace the inevitable change of radiological practice, incorporating AI in the radiological workflow.

An excellent review of this field is given in Najjar R. Redefining Radiology: A Review of Artificial Intelligence Integration in Medical Imaging. Diagnostics. 2023; 13(17):2760. https://doi.org/10.3390/diagnostics13172760

Chapter 4 How AI will improve outcomes in dermatology

Nondermoscopic images

A CNN trained on 129,450 images achieved performance comparable to dermatologists on two binary classification tasks: carcinomas versus seborrheic keratoses and melanomas versus nevi, for both dermoscopic and nondermoscopic images (Esteva et al., 2017). Subsequently, dermatologist-level classification of malignant versus benign lesions using nondermoscopic datasets of predominantly East Asian participants was achieved. The investigators reported an area under the receiver operating characteristic curve of 0.94 for malignancy detection among 134 disorders, on par with dermatology residents; they also reported an area under the curve of 0.89–0.94 for predicting appropriate medications among four primary treatment options.

Dermoscopic images

CNNs have classified dermoscopic images of melanoma versus nevi with performances similar to or exceeding dermatologists (Brinker et al., 2019a, Brinker et al., 2019b). CNNs have also achieved expert-level diagnosis of nonpigmented skin cancer (Tschandl et al., 2019c) and outperformed dermatologists across five disease classes (Maron et al., 2019). Switching imaging modalities, a CNN trained only on dermoscopic images nonetheless achieved dermatologist-level melanoma classification performance on nondermoscopic images.

Alternative imaging modalities

AI coupled with hardware-based methods such as spectroscopy, multispectral imaging, or other specialized imaging modalities may augment dermatologists' capabilities. For example, early melanomas may not present morphologic differences detectable by conventional photography, but computer-assisted techniques such as dermatofluoroscopy may provide additional information for early diagnosis.

Emerging applications

Teledermatology

Telemedicine may be one of the first fields to embrace AI, driven by demand for services, the necessity of collecting fit-for-purpose high-quality images, and the availability of existing technology, although face-to-face diagnostic accuracy exceeds that of teledermatology.

AI may be integrated into smartphone apps to photograph skin lesions, collect relevant clinical information, and generate a referral if appropriate. Many smartphones already support on-device deep learning (DL) with Google's TensorFlow Lite (TensorFlow, 2020) or Apple's CoreML (Apple Inc, 2020), preserving privacy by keeping health information on the device.

Augmenting face-to-face assessments

Han et al. (2019) found that AI may enhance care by providing diagnostic support in real-time during a clinical visit. Using clinical images, the top-1 and top-3 accuracies (indicating the fraction of cases where the top-n diagnoses contained the correct diagnosis) of dermatologists in diagnosing 134 skin disorders were increased by 7.0% and 10.1%, respectively, with AI). For dermoscopic images, the combination of AI and humans achieved an accuracy of 83.0% (compared with 81.6% and 42.9% achieved by AI and humans alone, respectively).

AI can also expand physician differential diagnoses by retrieving images from a reference library with the most similar features to a concerning lesion. Further study is needed to assess the efficacy of such systems.

Current progress in applying deep learning to histopathologic data

Diagnostically important histomorphologic features can be subtle, subject to significant interobserver variability in assessment (such as melanocytic dysplasia and melanoma), or cumbersome for enumeration (such as mitotic figures). These considerations provide the impetus for leveraging DL for histopathology.

Early work in applying DL to the diagnosis of cutaneous diseases again demonstrated feasibility of CNN-based DL for the diagnosis of keratinocyte carcinomas (versus seborrheic keratoses) and melanomas (versus benign nevi) from clinical gross images, with performance on par with dermatologists. Exploratory studies using histopathologic images in dermatopathology have applied ML to melanocytic nevi, melanoma, basal cell carcinoma onychomycosis and psoriasis.

Skin cancers

Melanoma

A large study of melanoma detailed in two papers by Brinker et al. (2019a and 2019b) involved training a 'ResNet' model on the publicly available International Skin Imaging Collaboration (ISIC) database, which contains in excess of 20,000 labelled dermoscopic images and is required to meet some basic quality standards. This network was trained on over 12,000 images. The dermatologists were assessed using 200 test images. Additionally, the dermatologists' demographic data, such as experience and training level, were requested.

The method used to quantify the relative performance also consisted of drawing a mean receiver operating characteristic curve (ROC) curve by calculating the average predicted class probability for each test image. The dermatologists' performance for the same set of images was then plotted on the ROC curve. Barring a few individual exceptions, the dermatologists' performance fell below the CNN ROC curves in both the clinical and dermoscopic image classifications. The authors also used a second approach, whereby they set the sensitivity of the CNN at the level of the attending dermatologists, and compared the mean specificity achieved at equivalent sensitivity. In the dermoscopic test, at a sensitivity of 74·1%, the dermatologists' specificity was 60% whereas the CNN achieved a superior 86·5%.

An important consideration is the fact that training data lack sufficient quantities of certain types of lesions, particularly the rarer presentations of malignancy, such as amelanotic melanoma.

Figure 1. Melanoma of the skin

This image is by Unknown author - National Cancer Institute (AV Number: AV-8500-3850; Date Created: 1985; Date Entered: 1/1/2001), https://visualsonline.cancer.gov/details.cfm?imageid=9186, Public Domain, https://commons.wikimedia.org/w/index.php?curid=859342. https://en.wikipedia.org/wiki/Melanoma#/media/File:Melanoma.jpg. This work is in the public domain in the United States because it is a work prepared by an officer or employee of the United States Government as part of that person's official duties under the terms of Title 17, Chapter 1, Section 105 of the US Code. No changes were made to this image.

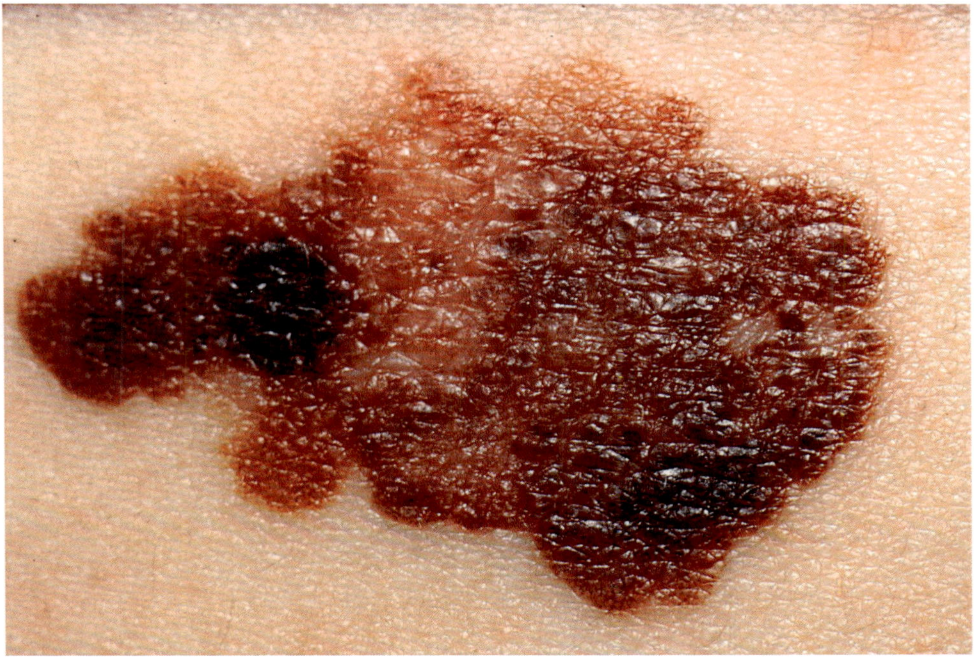

Figure 2. A comparison of malignant melanoma and benign pigmented freckles.

On the left side from top to bottom: melanomas showing (A) Asymmetry, (B) a border that is uneven, ragged, or notched, (C) colouring of different shades of brown, black, or tan and (D) diameter that had changed in size. The normal moles on the right side do not have abnormal characteristics (no asymmetry, even border, even color, no change in diameter).

Figure 2. A comparison of malignant and benign pigmented skin lesions.

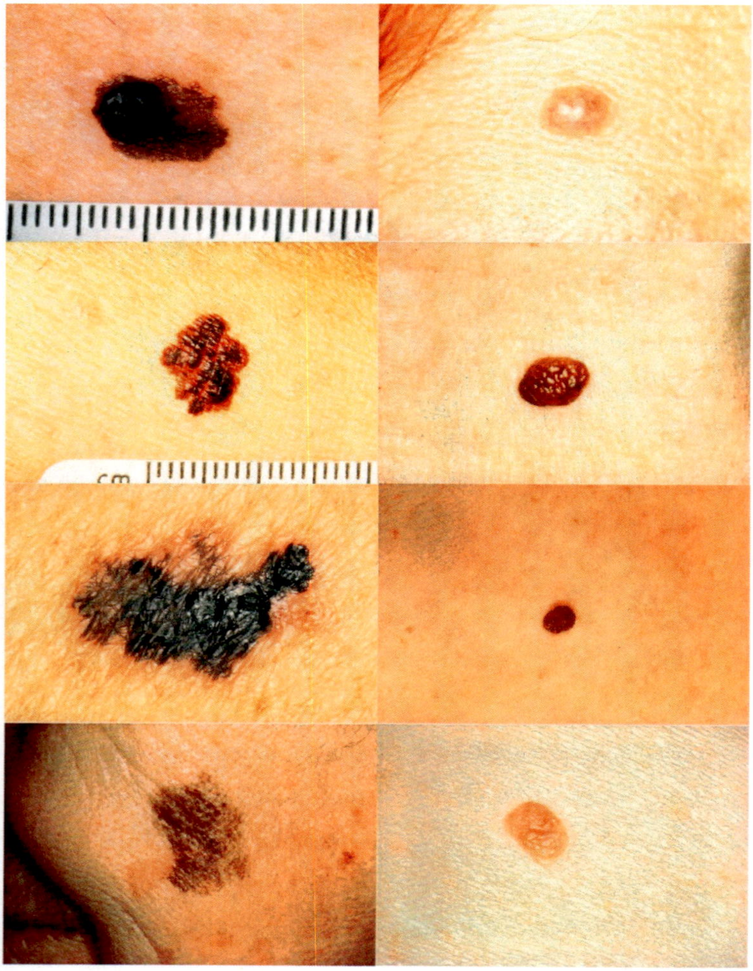

Numerous applications of DL to histopathologic images have been demonstrated. For example, a DL assistant can be used to aid a human pathologist in avoiding false negative diagnoses. In this context, DL has been shown to be feasible for detecting lymph node metastases and positive surgical margins for breast cancer. DL can be applied to enumerative tasks, such as mitotic counts and the Ki-67 proliferative index, as well as to other cumbersome tasks such as detection of acid-fast stained bacilli or quantification of hepatic steatosis.

Current progress in deep learning for dermatopathology

Presently, progress in DL for dermatopathology has been confined to proof-of-concept demonstrations of feasibility of using DL for diagnostic classification on digitized histopathology images. Early work investigated the technical feasibility of applying CNN to detection of basal cell carcinoma (BCC) from small image patches, demonstrating an AUC of up to 0.981 on this curated data set. Another investigation applied CNN to the detection of BCC from smartphone-captured microscopic ocular images (MOI) as well as whole-slide images (WSI), and demonstrated slightly superior maximal performance on MOIs as compared to WSIs (AUCs of 0.987 and 0.955, respectively). Another investigation applying the U-Net architecture, which is specifically designed for biomedical image analysis, to WSIs for detection of BCC reported sensitivity, specificity, and accuracy of >96%, although AUCs were not specifically reported. A study applying a weakly-supervised CNN-RNN algorithm to WSIs of skin biopsies with slide-level diagnostic labels, yielded an AUC of 0.988 for the detection of BCCs.

Figure 3. Basal cell carcinoma on a patient's back

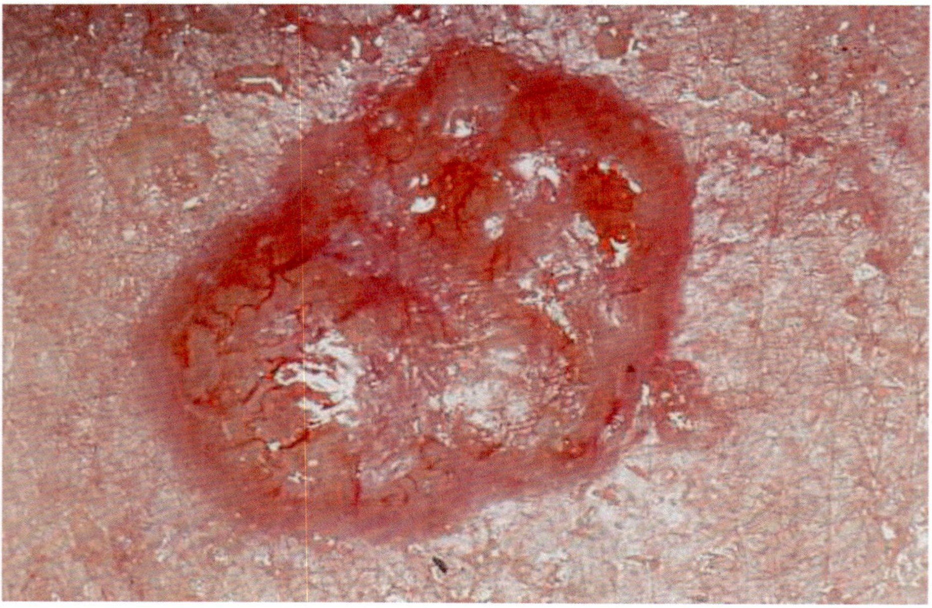

This image is by No machine-readable author provided. John Hendrix assumed (based on copyright claims). Own work assumed (based on copyright claims)., Public Domain, https://commons.wikimedia.org/w/index.php?curid=1216868; https://en.wikipedia.org/wiki/Basal-cell_carcinoma#/media/File:Basal_cell_carcinoma.jpg. the copyright holder of this work, release this work into the public domain. No changes were made to this image.

These studies of DL applied to histopathologic diagnosis of cutaneous neoplasia have been limited in scope, as each applies a unique DL workflow to perform a binary diagnostic classification task. Investigations of applying unified DL workflows to rendering multiple diagnoses have also emerged. An study utilizing a proprietary digital pathology and AI platform for developing separate CNN-based dichotomous diagnostic classifiers for detecting nodular BCCs, dermal melanocytic nevi, and seborrheic keratoses from WSIs, reported AUCs of 0.99, 0.97, and 0.99 respectively for these diagnoses.

While most investigations of applying DL to dermatopathology have focused on cutaneous solid neoplasia, especially BCCs and melanocytic lesions, preliminary work on applying DL to other diagnostic entities in dermatopathology has also emerged over the past few years. A CNN-based algorithm for diagnosing *onychomycosis* from WSI of periodic acid Schiff (PAS)-stained sections of nail clippings yielded diagnostic performance comparable to dermatopathologists, with an algorithmic AUC of 0.98.38

For *psoriasis*, a study comparing various traditional ML and DL-based approaches for segmenting WSIs of psoriatic skin biopsies demonstrated the superiority of a fully convolutional neural network (FCN)-based approach. Preliminary work on diagnostic distinction of *mycosis fungoides* (MF) from eczema by a modified U-Net-based algorithm applied to WSIs has also emerged, though with a modest accuracy of 68%.

Figure 4. Mycosis fungoides on sole of foot

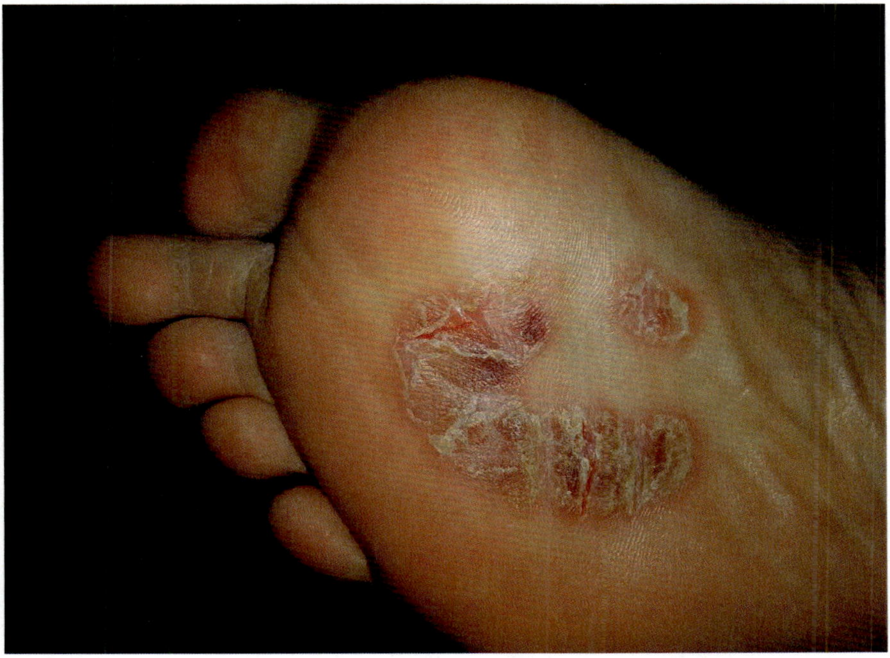

This image is by Public Domain, https://en.wikipedia.org/w/index.php?curid=59565181; https://en.wikipedia.org/wiki/Mycosis_fungoides#/media/File:Mycosis_fungoides_foor.JPG. The copyright holder of this work, hereby release it into the public domain. No changes were made to this image.

The amount of manual effort required to annotate large numbers of digital WSIs in sample data sets, poses another challenge for the development of DL algorithms by supervised learning methods. Recent developments in DL have offered potential solutions. In one approach, a separate DL algorithm can be trained to perform annotation, in an iterative human-in-the-loop framework. A pathologist would initially perform a limited set of manual annotations, from which the DL annotation algorithm learns to propose annotations to the pathologist for approval or correction. Iteratively, the DL annotation algorithm improves such that eventually little or no manual correction to the automated annotation is needed. This approach has been demonstrated for labeling Ki-67 staining, eosinophils, tumor cells, and tumor infiltrating lymphocytes. A second approach employs weakly supervised learning, which generally requires only a slide-level diagnosis as annotation for each WSI. Such diagnostic labels can be automatically imported from the electronic medical record and laboratory information system. DL algorithms rendering slide-level diagnoses using such approaches have been demonstrated to be feasible for BCCs as well as prostate cancers, lymph node metastases of breast cancers, and cancers of unknown primaries.

Challenges to the development of robust deep learning diagnostic algorithms

The development of high-performing DL algorithms that retain clinically acceptable diagnostic performance among diverse practice settings, requires the assembly of large, high-quality, and diversely sourced data for training, validation, and test data sets (henceforth referred to as sample data sets). Data should be acquired from multiple laboratories, employing different digital scanners as well as variable conditions for tissue fixation, processing, and staining. The availability of digital WSIs remains pegged to the adoption of digital pathology in pathology laboratories, affecting the quantity of available data.

Sample data must also be carefully reviewed to eliminate potential confounding factors, such as pen markings. In an example from clinical dermatology, a CNN-based DL assistant for analyzing dermoscopic images of melanocytic lesions was found to produce false-positive diagnoses on images with surgical skin markings, which were likely not properly eliminated as confounding features from sample data sets used in algorithmic development.

To effectively implement DL in clinical diagnostic practice, a high-quality DL algorithm needs to be incorporated into an easy-to-use interface that can be integrated seamlessly into a digital pathology workflow. Effective human-computer interaction (HCI) in the context of DL assistants would be important in ensuring widespread adoption and trust by pathologists using DL solutions. As DL algorithms themselves may make diagnostic errors, effective implementation of DL assistants entails minimizing pathologists' over-reliance on DL algorithmic outputs that are incorrect.

Prior to implementing a DL assistant, its diagnostic performance should be evaluated on locally sourced WSIs in a routine digital pathology workflow. The resilience of DL algorithmic performance to artifacts commonly encountered among clinical histopathology slides needs to be rigorously and locally assessed. While there are presently no guideline recommendations for validating AI algorithms for clinical use in pathology laboratories, it could be sensible to follow schema analogous to those for validating immunohistochemical or other clinical laboratory testing in current use. Future efforts by professional societies in producing formal practice guidelines for guiding the validation and implementation of DL solutions in pathology would be highly conducive to the widespread trust and adoption of DL in the field.

An ongoing concern that has been raised for deploying DL algorithms in real-world use is the black box problem of limited interpretability of DL algorithms. Recent developments of attention techniques in DL allow for the generation of heat maps (saliency maps) that differentially highlight areas of an image according to how much they have contributed to DL algorithmic analysis, but such surrogate measures do not directly reveal which features in the image are used by the DL algorithm to render an output.

The routine diagnosis of *basal cell carcinoma* is a straightforward and swift proposition, to which DL can add little value. However, detecting unusual *collision tumors*, or distinguishing between basal cell carcinoma and rare mimics, such as *basaloid squamous cell* or *Merkel cell carcinomas*, could be of great value to pathologists and patients alike. (A collision tumor is a neoplastic lesion comprised of two or more distinct cell populations that maintain distinct borders. Collision tumors, which are rare but well documented, can be composed of two benign tumors, a benign and malignant tumor, and two malignant tumors).

Merkel cell carcinoma (MCC) are rare aggressive neuroendocrine tumour of the skin. They can be considered a small round cell tumour. Most MCCs are caused by a virus - Merkel cell polyomavirus.

Figure 5. Merkel's carcinoma. Tumor cell nuclei are stained brown (arrow) by an antibody to the Merkel cell polyomavirus large T antigen.

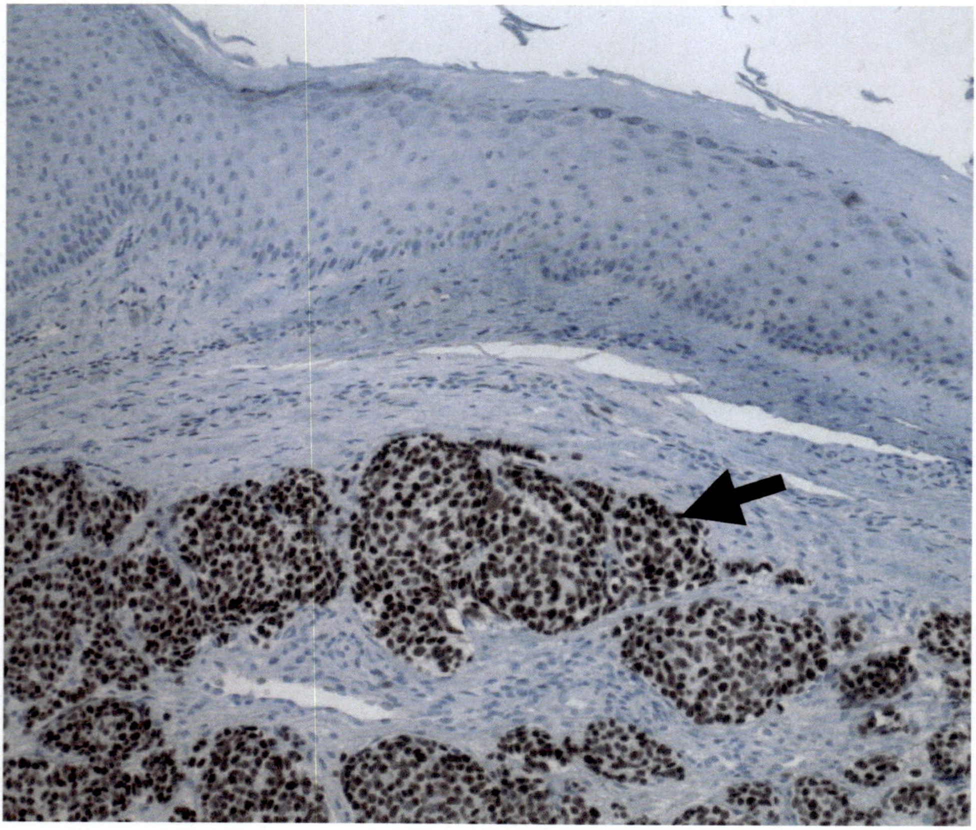

One study showed that entities that do not generally present with a crust (such as vascular lesions, dermatofibromas, and nevi) were frequently miscategorized in the presence of crusts. The same study showed that the presence of hair affected the misclassification of actinic keratosis (36 vs. 56% without hair). Finally, another study showed that the anatomic site of a lesion plays a critical role in the performance of CNN. Studies have shown the potential of CNN-based classification for special anatomic sites, such as face, palms, and soles that have different normal dermoscopic signs, but more extensive and diverse datasets as well as further research are needed to extend the application of AI in some anatomic sites and rare skin cancer subtypes. On the other side, banal-looking, benign lesions such as angiomas, dermatofibromas, or nevi are most often underrepresented or absent from studies' training sets, leading to underperformance of the algorithms.

Moreover, a study showed that rarer distributions of specific skin lesions such as non-pigmented nevi and non-pigmented melanomas decreased the accuracy of the algorithms' classifications compared to common distributions. These results highlight that algorithms should be tested on both usual and unusual types of lesions and imaging attributes. Together with histopathology immunohistochemical studies are useful in diagnosing *amelanotic melanoma,* for example the S100 protein.

Figure 6. Structure of the S100B protein

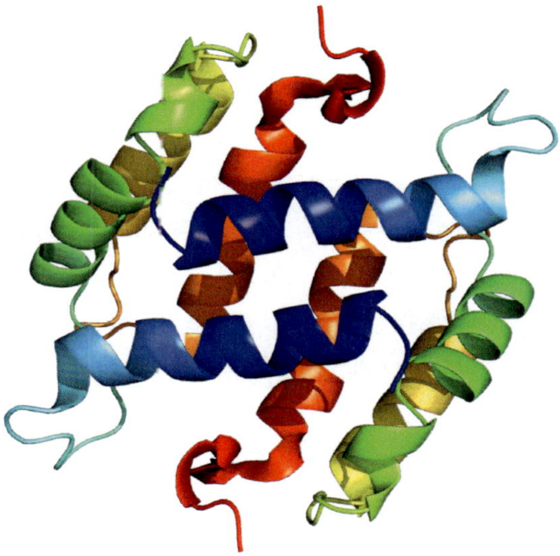

Neurofibroma

Neurofibromatosis (NF) is a rare group of three conditions in which tumors grow in the nervous system, and are called NF1, NF2 and schwannomatosis. NF1 is the most common neurofibroma. Most patients with NF1 have a normal life expectancy, but 10% of them develop malignant peripheral nerve sheath tumors (MPNST), which is a major cause of morbidity. Thus, the timely differentiation of benign and malignant lesions has direct significance for improving the survival rate of patients. Wei et al., (2020) successfully established a Keras-based machine-learning model that can discriminate between NF1-related benign and malignant craniofacial lesions with a very high accuracy (96.99 and 100%) in validation cohorts 1 and 2 and a 51.27% accuracy in various other body regions. Plexiform neurofibroma (PN) is the prototypical and most common NF1 tumor. Ho et al. (2020) created a DNN algorithm to conduct a semi-automated volume segmentation of PNs based on multiple b-value diffusion-weighted MRI. They evaluated the accuracy of semi-automated tumor volume maps constructed by a DNN compared to manual segmentation and revealed that the volumes generated by the DNN from multiple diffusion data on PNs had a good correlation with manual volumes, and that there is a significant difference between PN and normal tissue. Bashat and his colleagues (2018) also demonstrated that a quantitative image representation method based on machine learning may assist in the classification between benign PNs and MPNST in NF1. In a similar initiative, Duarte et al. (2014) used grey matter density maps obtained from magnetic resonance (MR) brain structure scans to create a multivariate pattern analysis algorithm to differentiate between NF1 patients and healthy controls. A total of 83% of participants were correctly classified, with 82% sensitivity and 84% specificity.

Figure 7. Dermal neurofibroma in a person whose lesions first appeared when he was a teenager.

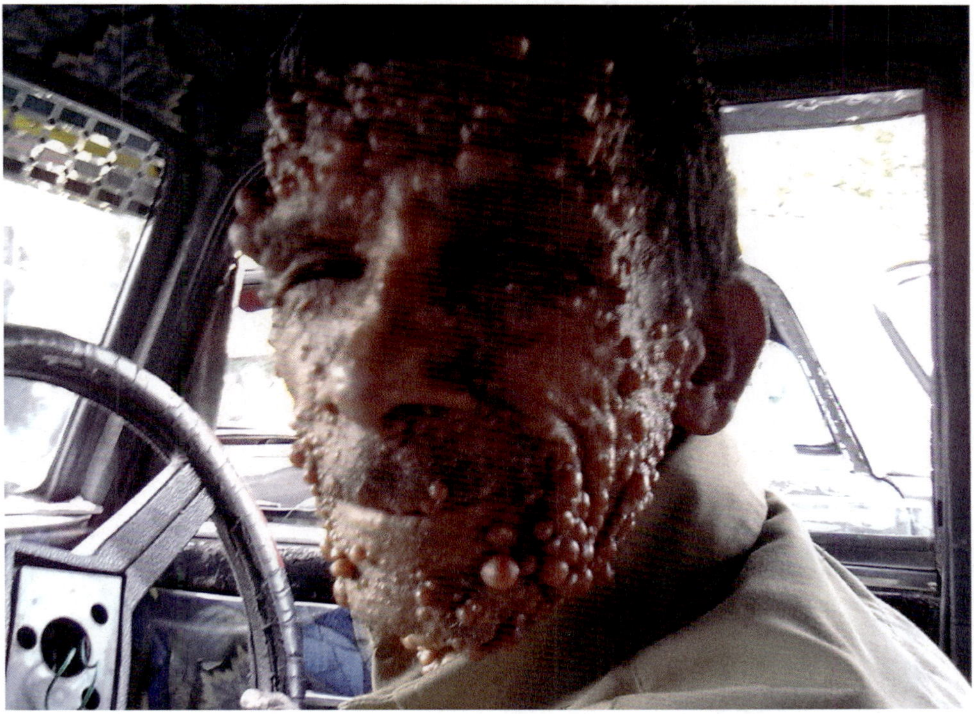

Infectious dermatoses

CNNs have also classified onychomycosis (Han et al., 2018b) at a level similar to dermatologists.

Figure 8. Onychomycosis involving the nail of the big toe.

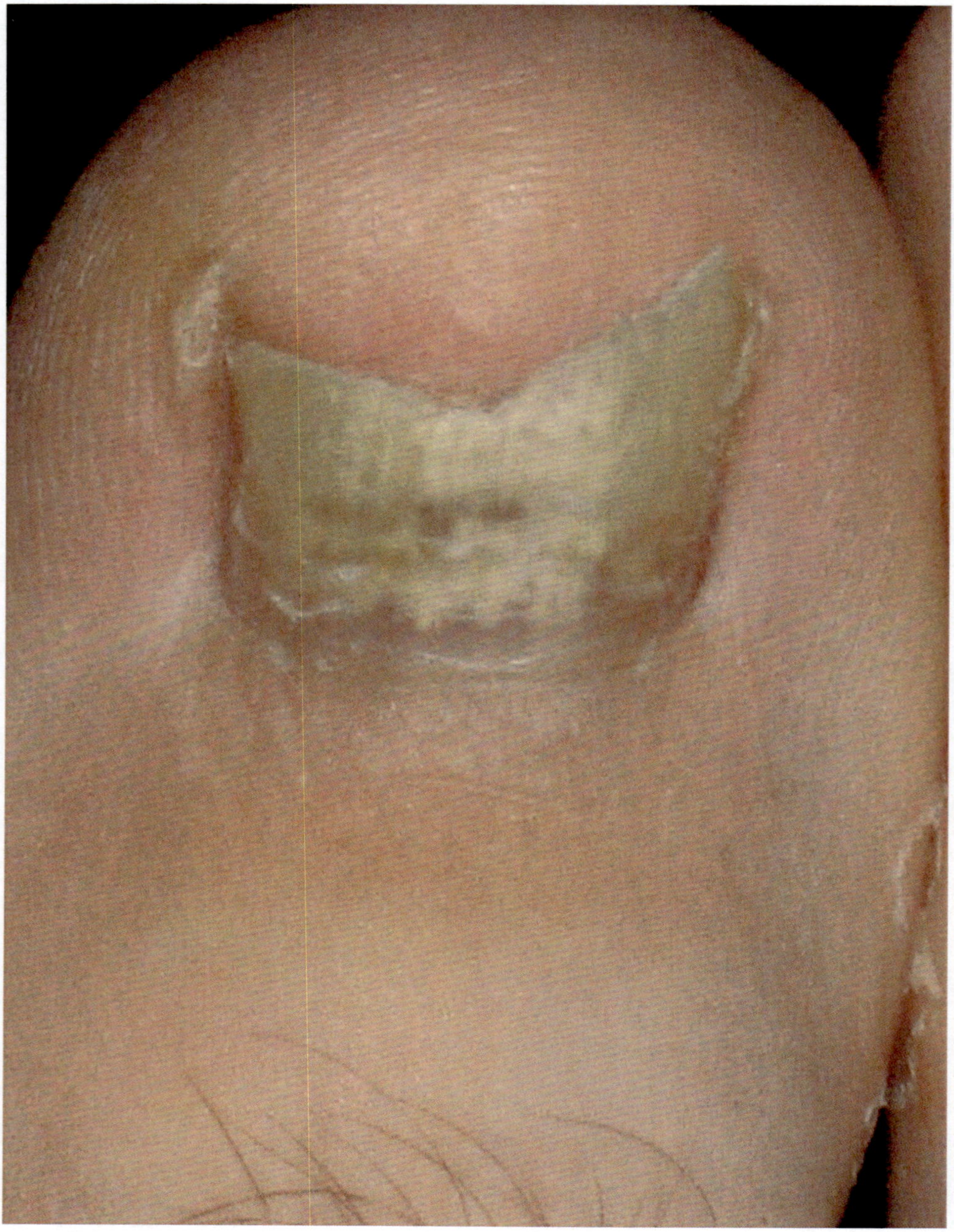

Inflammatory dermatoses

Psoriasis

Figure 9. Severe generalized pustular psoriasis

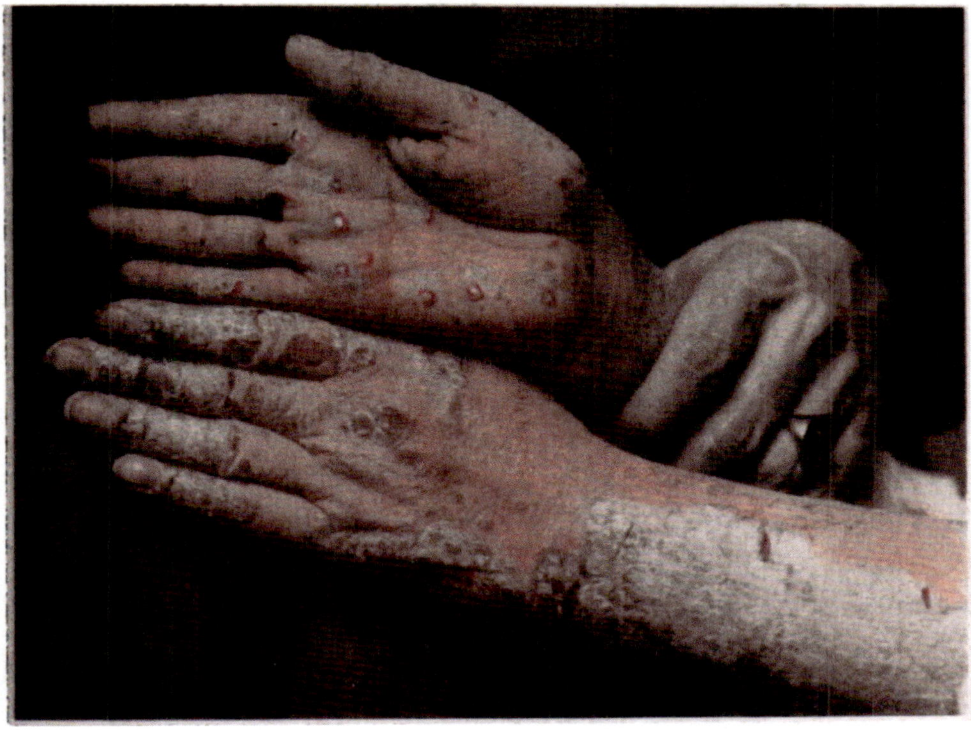

This image is by George Henry Fox - Fox, George Henry (1886) Photographic illustrations of skin diseases (2nd ed.), E.B. Treat Retrieved on 25 September 2010., Public Domain, https://commons.wikimedia.org/w/index.php?curid=11593519; https://en.wikipedia.org/wiki/Psoriasis#/media/File:Psoriasis_manum.jpg. This media file is in the public domain in the United States. This applies to U.S. works where the copyright has expired, often because its first publication occurred prior to January 1, 1928, and if not then due to lack of notice or renewal. No changes were made to this image.

The use of AI in psoriasis can help in clinical assessment and in the choice of personalized treatment protocols and outcome predictions. One of the most interesting and early use of AI in psoriasis was by Guo et al. (2014) who used an AI program to predict psoriasis. This system utilized microarray-based gene expression profiles from two datasets: GSE14905 and GSE13355. This study integrated the knowledge of three feature selection algorithms that revealed 21 features belonging to 18 genes as candidate markers. The final psoriasis classification model was established using the novel Incremental Feature Selection algorithm that utilizes only 3 features from 2 unique genes, IGFL1 and C10orf99. This model has demonstrated highly stable prediction accuracy (averaged at 99.81%) over three independent validation strategies.

In another study Shrivastava (2015) et al. built nine kinds of psoriasis risk assessment system (pRAS) utilizing different combinations of the key blocks. These nine pRAS systems use three classifiers [Support Vector Machine (SVM), Decision Tree (DT), and Neural Network (NN)] and three feature selection techniques [principal component analysis (PCA), Fisher discriminant ratio (FDR), and mutual information (MI)]. The two major experiments conducted using these nine systems were: (i) selection of best system combination based on classification accuracy and (ii) understanding the reliability of the system. This led to the computation of key systems performance parameters, such as feature retaining power, aggregated feature effect, and reliability index besides conventional attributes like accuracy, sensitivity, and specificity. The database used in this study consisted of 670 psoriasis images; the combination of SVM and FDR was revealed as the optimal pRAS system and yielded a classification accuracy of 99.84% using a cross-validation protocol. Further, SVM-FDR system provided a reliability of 99.99% using cross-validation protocol. They validated the pRAS system with automatically segmented lesions against manually segmented lesions showing comparable performance.

Eczema/atopic dermatitis

Many authors use the terms dermatitis and eczema synonymously, and various dictionaries that treat the terms as differentiable nonetheless do not provide explicit criteria for differentiating them, as the aspects of inflammation, pruritus, and either exogenous or endogenous provoking agent all can apply to either term.The challenge in the computer-aided image diagnosis of eczematous diseases is to correctly differentiate not only between disease and health, but also between different forms of eczema.

Figure 10. Severe eczema

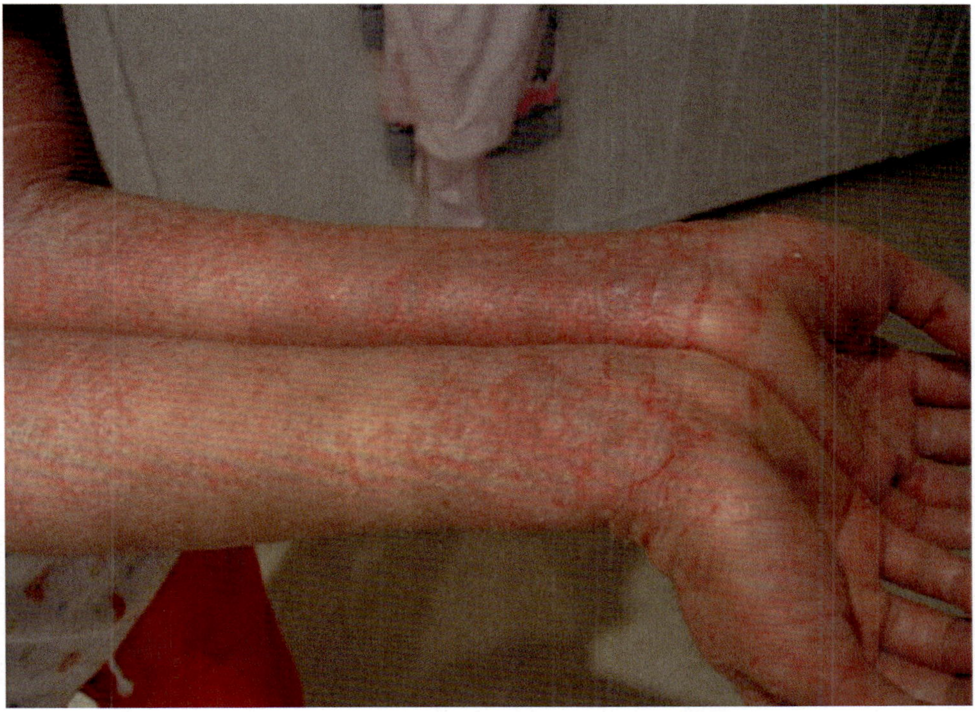

This image is by Jambula at English Wikipedia - Transferred from en.wikipedia to Commons., Public Domain, https://commons.wikimedia.org/w/index.php?curid=2042360; https://en.wikipedia.org/wiki/Dermatitis#/media/File:Eczema-arms.jpg. This work has been released into the public domain by its author, Jambula at English Wikipedia No changes were made to this image.

The eczema stage and affected area are the most essential factors in effectively assessing the dynamics of the disease. It is not trivial to accurately identify the eczema area and other inflammatory dermatoses on the basis of photographic documentation. The macroscopic forms of eczema are diverse, with different stages and varying degrees of distribution and severity. The prerequisite for training algorithms for the AI-supported image analysis of all of these various assessment parameters is therefore a correspondingly large initial quantity of image files that have been optimized and adjusted in terms of the recording technology. Forms of eczema with a disseminated eruption would also be linked to the availability of automated digital, serial whole-body photography for an efficient and time-saving AI-supported calculation of an area score. Han et al. (2020) trained a deep neural-network-based algorithm. The algorithm was able to differentiate between eczema and other skin diseases and to classify very rare skin lesions, which had direct clinical significance, as well as serving as augmented intelligence to empower medical professionals in diagnostic dermatology. They also showed that treatment recommendations (e.g., topical steroids versus antiseptics) could also be learned by differentiating between inflammatory and infectious causes. It remains to be seen and questioned, however, whether an AI-aided severity assessment and a clinically practicable area score can be derived from this as a prerequisite for a valid follow-up in the case of eczema. Schnüerle et al. designed a support-vector-machine-based image processing method for hand eczema segmentation with industry swiss4ward for operational use at the University Hospital Zurich. This system uses the F1-score as the primary measurement and is superior to a few advanced methods that were likewise tested on their gold standard dataset. It is likely that a combination of such an AI-aided image analysis and molecular diagnostics can optimize the future differential diagnostic classification of eczematous diseases.

Atopic dermatitis

Atopic dermatitis (AD) is the most common chronic inflammatory disease, with a prevalence of 10% to 20% in developed countries. It usually starts in childhood and recurs multiple times in adulthood, greatly affecting patients' quality of life.

In 2017 Gustafson et al. aimed to identify patients with atopic dermatitis for inclusion in genome-wide association studies. They described a machine learning-based phenotype algorithm. Using the electronic health record (EHR), they combined coded information with information extracted from encounter notes as features in a lasso logistic regression. (Lasso regression is also called Penalized regression method. This method is usually used in machine learning for the selection of the subset of variables. It provides greater prediction accuracy as compared to other regression models). Their algorithm achieved high positive predictive value and sensitivity, improving on previous algorithms with low sensitivity. These results demonstrate the utility of natural language processing and machine learning for electronic health record (HER)-based phenotyping.

In 2017 Gustofson's team identified patients with AD via a machine-learning-based phenotype algorithm. The algorithm combined code information with the collection of electronic health records to achieve a high positive predictive value and sensitivity.

These results demonstrated the utility of natural language processing and machine learning in EHR-based phenotyping. An ANN algorithm was developed to assess the influence of air contaminants and weather variation on AD patients; their results proved that the severity of AD symptoms was positively correlated with outdoor temperatures, as well as other factors. In the latest study, a fully automatic approach based on CNN was proposed to analyse multiphoton tomography (MPT) data. The proposed algorithm correctly diagnosed AD in 97.0 ± 0.2% of all images presenting living cells, with a sensitivity of 0.966 ± 0.003 and a specificity of 0.977 ± 0.003, indicating that MPT imaging can be combined with AI to successfully diagnose AD.

Acne

The assessment by AI has been very effective. Melina et al. (2018) showed an excellent correlation between the automatic and manual evaluation of the investigator's global assessment with r = 0.958. In the case of acne vulgaris in particular, such a procedure could prevent far-reaching consequences.

Figure 10. Teenager with acne causing permanent skin damage in the form of scar

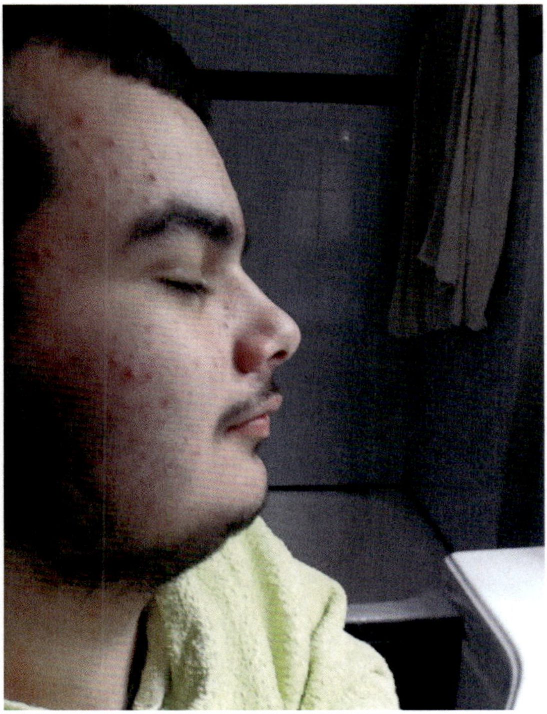

This image is by Nikos Likomitros - Own work, CC0, https://commons.wikimedia.org/w/index.php?curid=127724206; https://en.wikipedia.org/wiki/Acne#/media/File:Teenager_with_acne.jpg. The copyright holder of this file has made it available under the Creative Commons CC0 1.0 Universal Public Domain Dedication. No changes were made to this image.

Vitiligo

The depigmented macules of vitiligo are usually in marked contrast to unaffected skin (Figures 11 and 12). Vitiligo is more easily recognized by AI systems than features of eczema or psoriasis lesions with poorly defined borders. Computer-based algorithms used for the detection of vitiligo with an F1 score of 0.8462 demonstrated impressive performance. Li et al. (2020) designed a vitiligo AI diagnosis system employing cycle-consistent adversarial networks (cycle GANs) to generate images with Wood's lamp and improved the image resolution via an attention-aware dense net with residual deconvolution (ADRD). The system achieved a 9.32% improvement in classification performance accuracy compared to direct classification of the original images using Resnet50. Low and colleagues (2020) built a CNN that performs vitiligo skin lesion segmentation quickly and robustly. The network was trained on 308 images with various lesion sizes, intricacies and anatomical locations. The modified network outperformed the state-of-the-art U-Net with a much higher Jaccard index score (73.6% versus 36.7%) and shorter segmentation time than the previously proposed semi-autonomous watershed approach.

These novel systems have proved promising for clinical applications by greatly saving the testing time and improving the diagnostic accuracy.

Figure 11. Vitiligo of the hand in a person with dark skin

This image is by James Heilman, MD - Own work, CC BY-SA 3.0, https://commons.wikimedia.org/w/index.php?curid=10313925; https://en.wikipedia.org/wiki/Vitiligo#/media/File:Vitiligo2.JPG. This file is licensed under the Creative Commons Attribution-Share Alike 3.0 Unported license. No changes were made to this image.

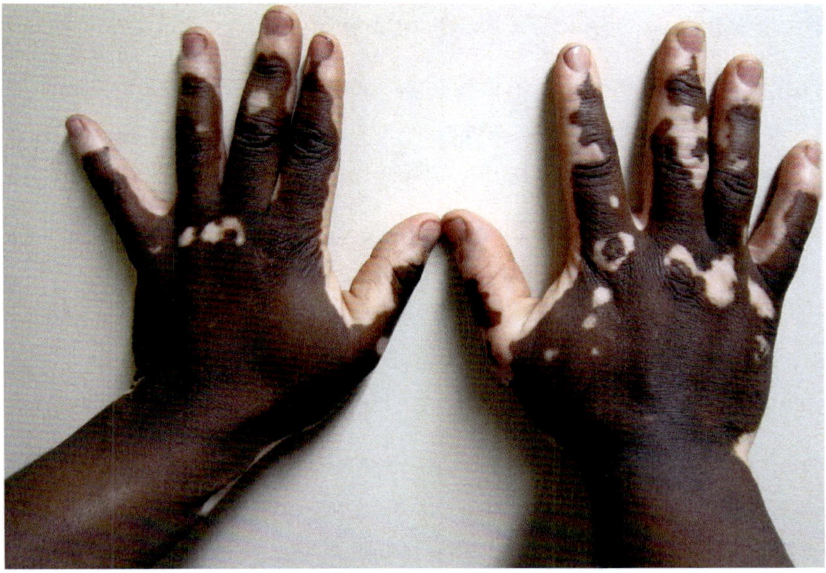

Figure 12. Vitiligo in a person with light skin

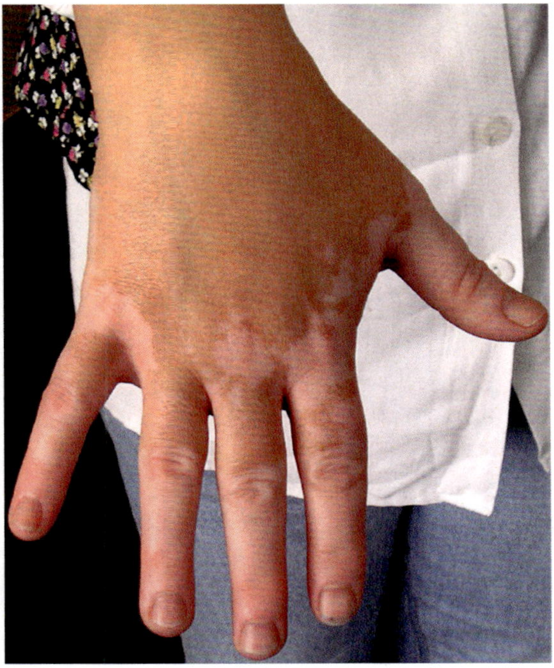

Chapter 5 How AI will improve outcomes in opthalmology

In ophthalmology a variety of multimodal imaging examinations are fundamental in the screening, diagnosis and monitoring of diseases and provide data input for AI development (Kras et al. 2020; Hogarty et al., 2018; Li et al, 2022).

Some applications, such as the IDx Technologies (Coralville, USA) which was approved by the Food and Drug Administration 3 years ago, are already used in clinical practice as a screening tool. Algorithms can even predict gender, age and cardiovascular risk through retinal images. AI may reduce subjectivity and interobserver disagreement in clinical practice.

Especially in low-income countries (LIC) and low-to-medium-income countries (LMIC), causes of preventable blindness such as diabetic retinopathy (DR) and age-related macular degeneration (AMD) could be prevented with screening programmes, home monitoring systems or telemedicine. AI-based screening could systematise screening and improve eye care in remote areas.

Machine learning (ML) requires high-quality, well-labelled, representative and large datasets, but at present, ophthalmological ML-ready datasets are only available in a few countries. Approximately, one hundred seventy-two countries do not have representation in training and validation cohorts.

Although data from all world countries are a distant goal, equivalent representation of all continents, ethnicities and the maximum number of countries is desired to reduce ML bias. Demographic information and other social determinants of health are typically not contained in these datasets, making it challenging to interrogate algorithms for bias. High-quality data are also fundamental for environmental-specific algorithm validation, which is necessary before AI implementation.

Available automated DR algorithm performance varies considerably in performance in the real world due to limited training data, including heterogeneity in disease presentations and suboptimal image quality. In LICs and LMICs, there is a growing gap between the ophthalmologist workforce and the population size. Two-thirds of ophthalmologists live in only 17 countries and in those countries, most practice in urban centres.

In addition to diversifying datasets to build AI technology in healthcare, it is necessary to invest in building capacity for health informatics and data science across countries. International collaboration between research groups should be incentivised to narrow disparities in AI research in order to reduce world blindness.

Artificial intelligence (AI) has emerged as a major frontier in computer science research. Although AI has broad application across many medical fields, it will have particular utility in ophthalmology and will dramatically change the diagnostic and treatment pathways for many eye conditions such as corneal ectasias, glaucoma, age-related macular degeneration and diabetic retinopathy.

Diabetic retinopathy

Diabetes affects more than 415 million people worldwide, meaning 1 in every 11 adults is affected. DR is a vasculopathy that affects one-third of diabetic patients and can lead to irreversible blindness. AI has been used to predict DR risk and DR progression in diabetic patients.

Figure 13. A fundus image showing several signs of diabetic retinopathy: hard exudates (scattered yellowish dots), microaneurysms (bulges off some blood vessels), and small hemorrhages (blurry red dots).

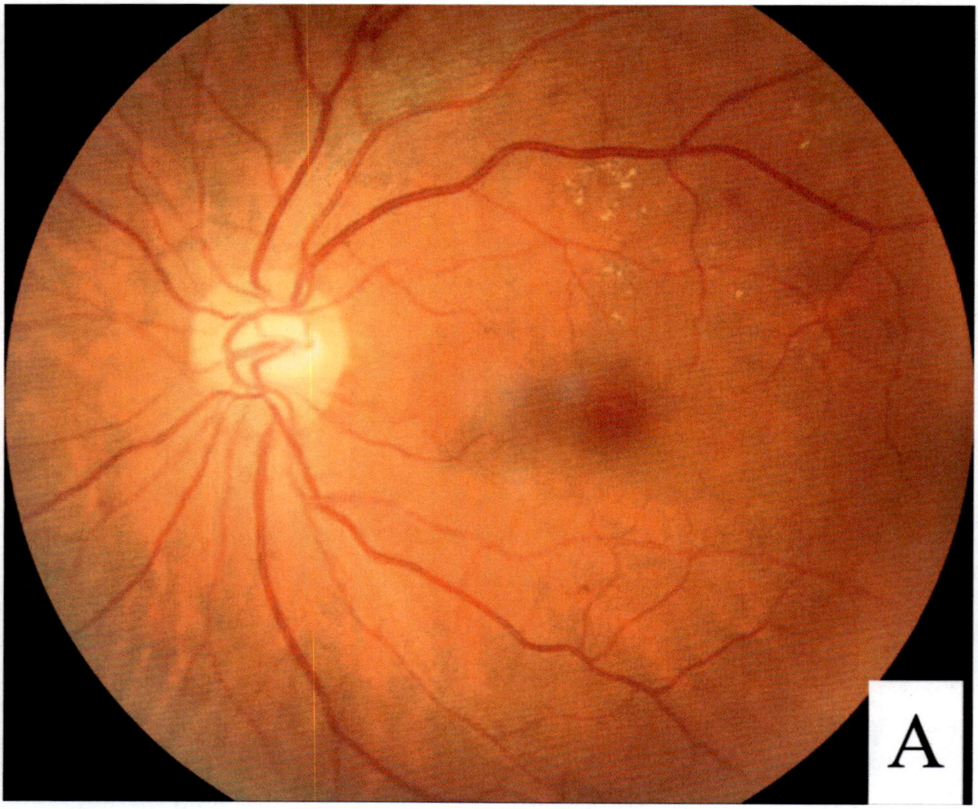

Community-based screening, timely referral, and appropriate treatment constitute the robust three-pronged strategy to prevent blindness from DR.Inadequate screening resources, however, remains a challenge. The application of AI can help screen large populations with minimal manpower and maximal efficiency, and accurately identify the pre-defined referrable disease for expedited treatment and thus can have far-reaching consequences. Investigators have reported a sensitivity of 96.8% and specificity of 87.0% with an area under the receiver operating characteristic curve (AUC) of 0.980 in the detection of referable DR. Another study reported excellent results using a Google AI-based DL system with an AUC was 0.990 and 0.991 for two different datasets. A third study validated the application of AI in DR screening using real-world data from 10 datasets in 6 countries with an AUC of 0.936, sensitivity of 90.5% and specificity of 91.6% in detecting referable DR and an AUC of 0.958, sensitivity of 100%, and specificity of 91.1% in detecting vision-threatening DR. In a prospective study, Abràmoff et al. achieved 87.2% sensitivity and 90.7% specificity. Their IDx-DR (Digital Diagnostics, Corville, Iowa, USA) was the first US Food and Drug Administration (FDA)-approved autonomous AI device in medicine, designed to detect diabetic retinopathy and diabetic macular edema. Topcon TRC-NW400 (Topcon, Tokyo, Japan) digital fundus camera incorporating IDx-DR (EyeArt, Eyenuk, Woodland Hills, Ca, USA) is also an FDA-approved autonomous AI system to detect more-than-mild and vision-threatening DR and works with with two non-mydriatic fundus cameras - Canon CR-2 AF and the Canon CR-2 Plus AF (Canon, Irvine, CA, USA). EyeArt achieved a high 96% sensitivity and a modest 88% specificity in detecting more-than-mild DR as compared to expert observers. It demonstrated 92% sensitivity and 94% specificity in detecting vision-threatening DR.

The specific abnormalities such as macular edema, exudates, cotton-wool spots, microaneurysms, and neovascularization on the optic disk can be detected by continuous machine learning (CML). Based on these hallmarks, the early diagnosis of DR in an automated fashion has been explored. Additionally, a system focused on timely detection has been developed to ensure immediate attention and intervention for proliferative DR (PDR).

Gulshan and colleagues (2016) were the first to report the application of DL for DR identification. They used large fundus image data sets to train a deep CNN (DCNN) in a supervised manner. They showed that the method based on DL techniques had very high sensitivity and specificity, and the AUC came up to 0.99 for detecting referable DR. In the past two years a number of DL models with impressive performance have been developed for the automated detection of DR. Additionally, some studies applied DL to automatically stage DR through fundus images, following up Gulshan's study that only detected referable DR but did not provide comparable data on sight-threatening DR or other stages of DR.

The majority of studies focused mainly on the analysis of fundus photographs. There were some other imaging modalities used to build models for DR. One developed a DL-based computer-aided system to detect DR through 52 OCT images, achieving an AUC of 0.98. A computer-aided diagnostic system based on CML algorithms using optical coherence tomography angiography (OCTA) images to automatically diagnose nonproliferative DR (NPDR) also achieved high accuracy and AUC.

The visualization of which pixels play an important role in the image-level predictions has been applied into DR diagnostic models. They intuitively represented the learning procedure of the DL network and highlighted important abnormal regions, thus providing better understanding by physicians of the DR predictions.

Age-related macular degeneration (AMD) and other macular diseases

AMD is the leading cause of irreversible blindness among older people in the developed world. The goal of using ML algorithms is to automatically identify AMD-related lesions to improve AMD diagnosis and treatment. Detection of drusen, fluid, reticular pseudodrusen and geographic atrophy from fundus images and SD-OCT using ML has been studied. The accuracy was usually over 80% and the agreement between the models and retina specialists could reach 90%.

Drusen regression, an anatomic endpoint of intermediate AMD and the onset of advanced AMD, can be predicted through the specifically designed, fully automated, ML-based classifier. Bogunovic et al. (2017a) developed a data-driven model to predict the progression risk in intermediate AMD. Automated image analysis steps were applied to identify and characterize individual drusen at baseline, and their development was monitored at every follow-up visit. Using such characterization and analysis, they developed an ML method based on survival analysis to estimate a risk score and predict the regression of individual drusen. These automated detections of the retinal lesions combined with interpretation of disease activity are feasible and have the potential to become a powerful tool in clinical practice.

Using ML to predict anti-vascular endothelial growth factor (anti-VEGF) injection requirements in eye diseases such as neovascular AMD and PDR can alleviate patients' economic burden and facilitate resource management. Bogunovic et al. (2017b) fed corresponding OCT images of patients with low or high anti-VEGF injection requirements into RF to obtain a predictive model. An AUC of 70% to 80% was achieved for treatment requirement prediction. Another study trained a DCNN neural network by OCT images to facilitate decision-making regarding anti-VEGF injection, and the outcomes were better than that of using CML. These studies are an important step toward image-guided prediction of treatment intervals in the management of neovascular AMD or PDR.

Multiple CML techniques have been applied for automated diagnosis and grading of AMD, but the most impressive work was based on DL techniques over the past several years. One study established a model to automatically detect exudative AMD from SD-OCT. In research studies based on fundus images, images with AMD were assigned into 4 classes of classification (no evidence of AMD, early-stage AMD, intermediate-stage AMD, and advanced AMD), or 2-class classification (no or early-stage AMD and intermediate or advanced stage AMD). The diagnostic accuracy was better in the 2-class classification. The DCNN appears to perform a screening function in these experiments, and the performance is comparable with physicians. DL algorithms have also been used to automatically detect abnormalities such as exudates, macular edema, drusen, and choroidal neovascularization.

With AMD becoming a significant public health problem, the application for AI for screening of referrable AMD is of immediate interest. One study, using the DR screening image set, demonstrated 0.932 AUC, 93.20% sensitivity and 88.70% specificity in detecting referable AMD. A diagnostic accuracy ranging from 88.4% and 91.6%, with an AUC between 0.94 and 0.96 was reported using image segmentation with the Age-Related Eye Disease Studies (AREDS) database.

Figure 14. A fundus photo showing intermediate age-related macular degeneration. Credit: National Eye Institute, National Institutes of Health Ref#: EDA2.

This image is by Unknown author - National Eye Institute of the NIH, http://www.nei.nih.gov/photo/eyedis/images/EDA22_72.jpg, Public Domain, https://commons.wikimedia.org/w/index.php?curid=19867518; https://en.wikipedia.org/wiki/Macular_degeneration#/media/File:Intermediate_age_related_macular_degeneration.jpg. This image is a work of the National Institutes of Health, part of the United States Department of Health and Human Services, taken or made as part of an employee's official duties. As a work of the U.S. federal government, the image is in the public domain. No changes were made to this image.

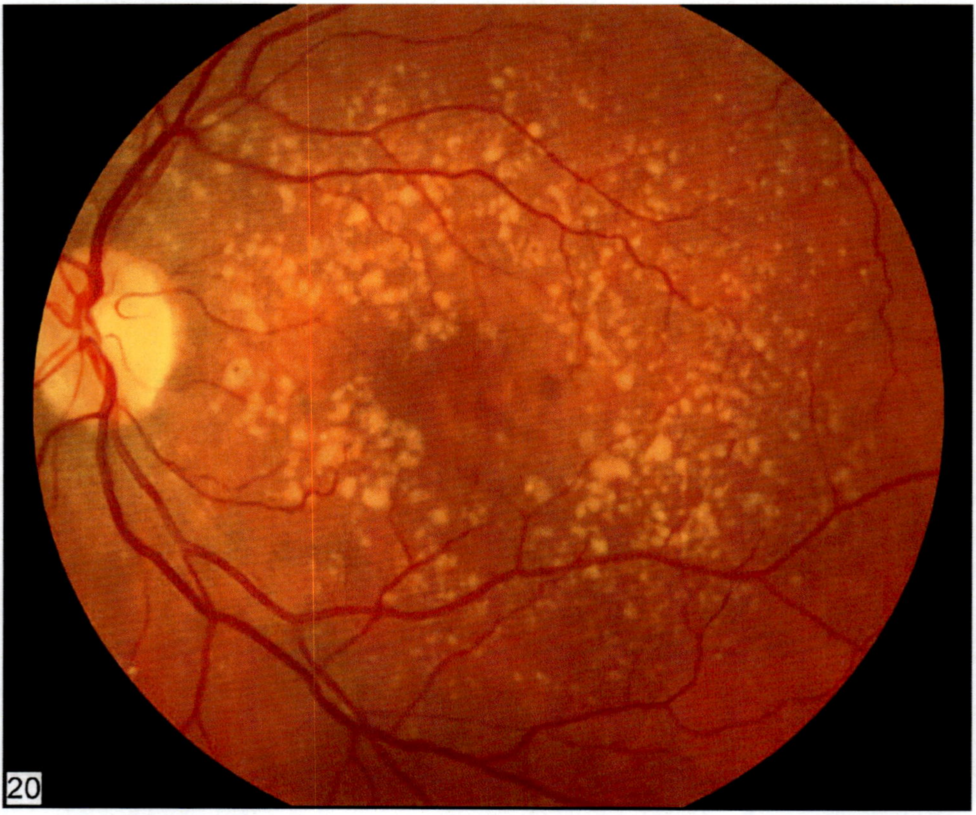

The large-scale availability of optical coherence tomography (OCT) images, relative consistency of OCT scans, and intricate structural details that OCT images provide make OCT an ideal tool for DL in macular diseases. Beginning with the automated classification of AMD using the two-dimensional OCT images, then progressing to segmentation of retinal anatomical boundaries and finally combining the power of segmentation and classification to identify standard retinal lesions, DL is now used to triage patients with macular pathologies (such as choroidal neovascularization, macular edema, *drusen*, geographic atrophy, epiretinal membrane, vitreomacular traction, macular hole, central serous chorioretinopathy), for triage and referral (urgent, semi-urgent, routine, observation) in the setting of an unsupervised virtual clinic with accuracy comparable to that of experts. (Drusen are yellow deposits under the retina. Drusen are made up of lipids and proteins. Drusen can be different sizes - small, medium, and large. Small drusen are common in those aged 50 and older without age-related macular degeneration but having many small drusen and larger drusen are often signs of AMD).

Retinopathy of prematurity

The management of retinopathy of prematurity is based on timely screening. While expert- and telemedicine-based screening are established strategies, a fully automated DL system was able to accurately identify Plus disease with an AUC of 0.98. The i-ROP DL system matched the consensus diagnosis more often than six of the eight international experts. It could also assign an objective severity score for monitoring of disease progression, regression, and response to treatment over time.

(Plus disease is a virulent form of the retinopathy of prematurity. It can be present as a major complicating factor at any stage of macular degeneration. It is characterised by

- Significant level of vascular dilation and tortuosity observed at the posterior retinal arterioles. This reflects the increase of blood flow through the retina.
- Vitreous haze and anterior chamber haze
- Iris vascular engorgement
- Persistent tunica vasculosa lentis or immature blood vessels growing over the lens which also restrict the dilatation of the pupils)

In being able to detect pre-plus or worse disease, the DL algorithm had 100% sensitivity and 94% specificity when compared that of the experts. Homegrown 3 nethra camera (Forus Health Incorporated, Bengaluru, Karnataka, India) has also demonstrated high performance in accurately identifying the ROP stage in retinal images.

Glaucoma

Glaucoma is the third largest sight-threatening eye disease around the world. Glaucoma patients suffer from high intraocular pressure, damage of the optic nerve head (ONH), retina nerve fiber layer (RNFL) defect, and gradual vision loss. Automatically detecting features related to glaucoma has great significance because of its timely diagnosis.

The optic cup-to-disc ratio (CDR) can be used to detect glaucoma. Based on automatic localization of the ONH and extraction of optic disc and optic cup from fundus images, CDR can be calculated to assist glaucoma diagnosis at an early stage by AI.

Spectrum domain OCT (SD-OCT) is another imaging modality for evaluation of CDR. After approximately locating the coarse disc margin by a spatial correlation smoothness constraint, a SVM model is trained to find the most likely patch on OCT images to determine a reference plane that can calculate the CDR. The proposed algorithm can achieve high segmentation accuracy and a low CDR evaluation error.

RNFL defects can serve as the earliest sign of glaucoma. Several researchers have explored the diagnostic accuracy of different methods using RNFL thickness parameters to diagnose glaucoma. However, severely myopic patients can also suffer from RNFL thickness reduction. Recently, reports on how to distinguish the normal retina from glaucoma in people with severe myopia via OCT parameters and optic disc morphology have been published.

Visual field (VF) defect is one of the main alterations of visual function during glaucoma progression. Studies have shown that changes in the central visual field may have already occurred in the early stage of the disease, which is consistent with the results of imaging studies. Thus, the early detection of glaucomatous VF changes is significant for the successful detection and management of glaucoma. Applying ML methods can significantly improve the detection of preperimetric glaucoma VFs from healthy VFs. Although a standard automated VF test plays a key role in diagnosing glaucoma, it consumes time and resources, as well as being a subjective test. The combination of the features mentioned above is required for the accurate diagnosis of glaucoma.

Studies using DL methods to diagnose glaucoma are few. So far, fundus images, VFs, and wide-field OCT scans have all been used to construct DL-based glaucomatous diagnostic models. Pre-perimetric open-angle glaucoma (OAG) can be detected through DL with better performance than that detected from CML techniques. Li et al. (2022) demonstrated that DL can be applied to identify referable glaucomatous optic neuropathy with high sensitivity and specificity.

DL algorithms have been trained to identify glaucoma-like disc appearance and to recognize glaucomatous nerve fibre layer damage on wide-angle OCTs, detect early visual field loss and recognize progression earlier than conventional strategies. A prediction tool that uses intraocular pressure and visual field data to project trajectories of clinical scenarios at various levels of target intra-ocular pressure (IOP) is available.

Figure 15. Acute angle closure glaucoma of the right eye (intraocular pressure was 42 in the right eye). Note the mid-sized pupil on the left that was not reactive to light and a degree of conjunctivitis.

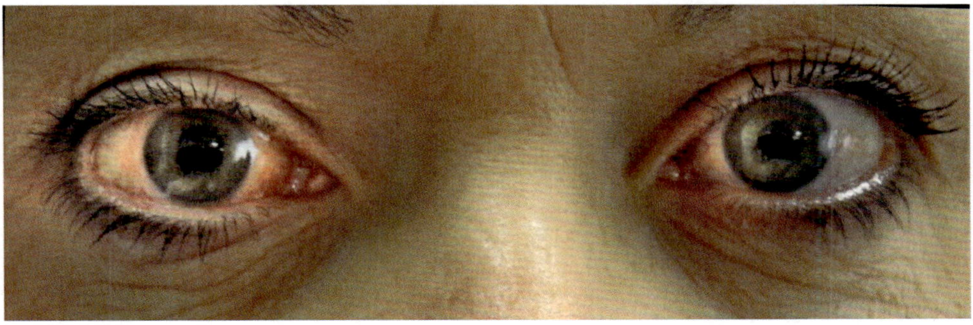

Future possibilities include the identification of optic discs associated with the potential loss of visual field and recognition of serial structural changes in the optic disc over time.

Anterior segment disorders

Investigators have explored the application of AI for cataract screening using ophthalmic imaging such as fundus photographs or slit lamp images, and to automate the selection of best-fit intraocular lens. Other studies have provided an elaborate compilation of the scope and range of anterior segment AI applications. Data from a Scheimpflug camera have been used to detect keratoconus or identify preclinical keratoconus, and to assess corneal power after refractive surgery. There have been attempts to perform AI-based eyelid and periorbital measurements, and to plan surgery for horizontal strabismus.

Other investigators have also worked on the application of AI for these conditions (Lu et al., 2018).

Cataract

Early detection and treatment can bring the light to cataract patients and improve their quality of life. ML algorithms such as RF and SVM have been applied to diagnose and grade cataracts from fundus images, ultrasounds images, and visible wavelength eye images.

Figure 16. Bilateral cataracts in an infant due to congenital rubella syndrome.

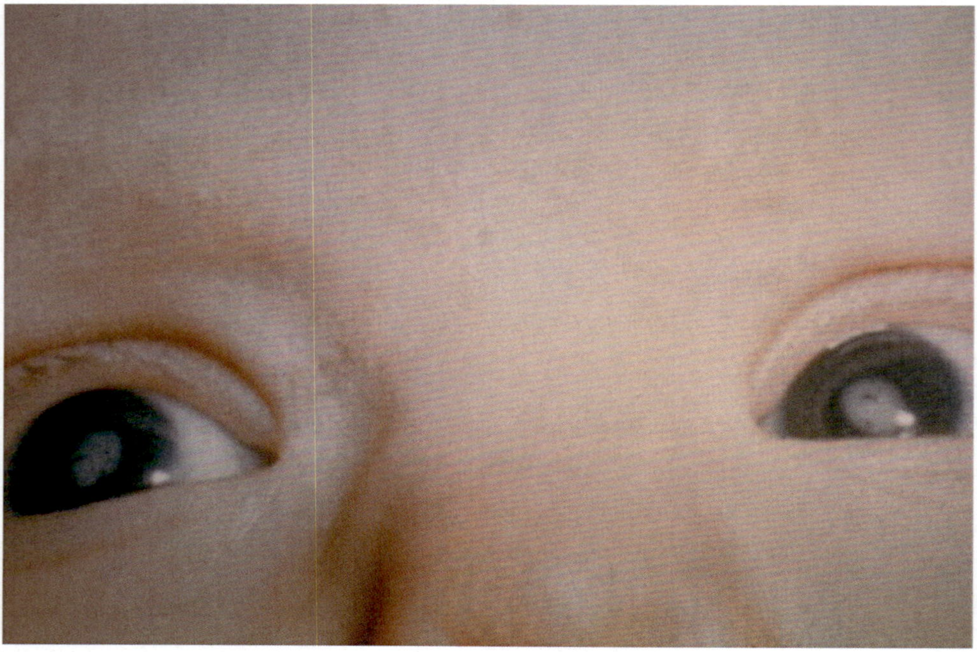

This image is by http://phil.cdc.gov/phil_images/20030724/28/PHIL_4284_lores.jpg, Public Domain, https://commons.wikimedia.org/w/index.php?curid=821959; https://en.wikipedia.org/wiki/Cataract#/media/File:Cataracts_due_to_Congenital_Rubella_Syndrome_(CRS)_PHIL_4284_lores.jpg. This image is a work of the Centers for Disease Control and Prevention, part of the United States Department of Health and Human Services, taken or made as part of an employee's official duties. As a work of the U.S. federal government, the image is in the public domain. No changes were made to this image.

Researchers can now use DL models to diagnose senile cataracts, as well as pediatric cataracts. The vlatter is one of the primary causes of childhood blindness. Long et al. (2017) constructed a CNN-based computer-aided diagnosis framework to classify and grade pediatric cataracts, as well as a cloud-based platform integrating the AI agent for multihospital collaboration. They also developed software to allow clinical application for ophthalmologists and patients.

In addition to DR, glaucoma, AMD, and cataract, AI has also been used to diagnose other eye diseases. AI algorithms can be used to detect keratoconus or identify eyes with preclinical signs of keratoconus using data from a Scheimpflug camera, to evaluate corneal power after myopic corneal refractive surgery, to make surgical plans for horizontal strabismus, and to detect pigment epithelial detachment in polypoidal choroidal vasculopathy.

Other retinal diseases

Numerous studies have found that AI could be applied to promote the automated detection of other retinal diseases including a deep-learning system to detect papilledema, lattice degeneration and retinal breaks, retinal detachment and polypoidal choroidal vasculopathy, keratitis, dry eye diseases and obstructive meibomian gland dysfunction, anterior ischemic optic neuropathy (AION), and non-arteritic anterior ischemic optic neuropathy (NAION).

Application of AI algorithms in predicting systemic diseases based on retinal images

AI has the potential to detect hidden information that clinicians are normally unable to perceive from digital health data. These breakthroughs can be attributed to the following three reasons: (1) the unique anatomy of the eye which offers an accessible "window" for the in vivo visualization of microvasculature and cerebral neurons; (2) retinal manifestations can be signs of many systemic diseases, such as diabetes and heart disease; (3) retinal changes can be recorded through non-invasive digital fundus imaging, which is low cost and widely available in different levels of medical institutions.

Cardiovascular disease (CVD)

Overt retinal vascular damage (such as retinal hemorrhages) and subtle changes (such as retinal arteriolar narrowing) are markers of CVD. One study achieved an AUC of 0.742 in predicting the presence of coronary artery calcium (a preclinical marker of atherosclerosis strongly associated with the risk of CVD) as well as systolic blood pressure, smoking status and major adverse cardiac events.

Chronic kidney disease (CKD) and type 2 diabetes

Early diagnosis and proactive management of CKD and diabetes mellitus are critical in reducing microvascular and macrovascular complications and mortality burden. As CKD and diabetes have manifestations in the retina, retinal images can be used to detect and monitor these diseases. One study was able to detect CKD and type 2 diabetes solely from retinal images or in combination with clinical metadata (e.g., age, sex, body mass index, and blood pressure) with AUCs of 0.85–0.93. The models can also be utilized to predict estimated glomerular filtration rates and blood-glucose levels. Another study established a deep-learning algorithm using 12,790 retinal images to screen for CKD. In this study, the model trained solely by retinal images achieved AUCs of 0.733–0.911 in validation and testing datasets, indicating the feasibility of employing retinal photography as an adjunctive screening tool for CKD in community and primary care settings.

Alzheimer's disease

Alzheimer's disease (AD) is the most common type of dementia worldwide and is becoming one of the most lethal, expensive, and burdensome diseases of the 21st Century. Diagnosis of AD is complex and normally involves expensive and sometimes invasive tests (such as amyloid positron emission tomography (PET) imaging. The retina offers a distinctively accessible insight into brain pathology. Research has found potentially measurable structural, vascular, and metabolic changes in the retina at the early stages of AD. One study demonstrated that a deep-learning model had the capability to identify AD using retinal images only. The model had accuracies ranging from 79.6% to 92.1% and AUCs ranging from 0.73 to 0.91 for detecting AD in testing datasets. In the datasets with PET information, the model could also distinguish between participants who were β-amyloid positive and those who were β-amyloid negative, with accuracies ranging from 80.6% to 89.3% and AUCs ranging from 0.68 to 0.86. This study showed that a retinal image-based deep-learning algorithm had high accuracy in detecting AD and this approach could be used to screen for AD in a community setting.

Figure 17. Drawing comparing how a brain of an Alzheimer disease patient is affected to a normal brain.

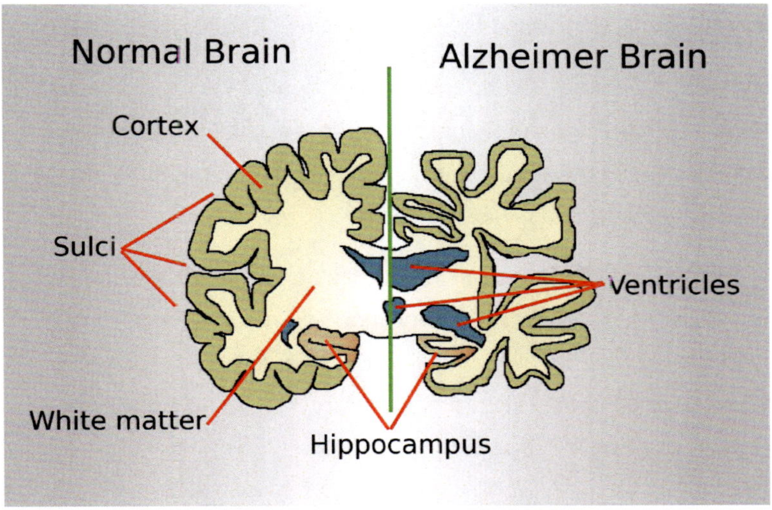

This image is by Garrondo - Own work, Public Domain, https://commons.wikimedia.org/w/index.php?curid=4387759; https://en.wikipedia.org/wiki/Alzheimer%27s_disease#/media/File:Brain-ALZH.png. The copyright holder of this work has released this work into the public domain. No changes were made to this image.

Chapter 6. How AI will improve outcomes in cardiology

AI shows considerable promise in cardiology, particularly in interpreting electrocardiograms (Attia et al., 2019) and echocardiograms (Narula et al. 2016).

The clinician's interpretation of the ECG depends on the level of their experience. The raw ECG waveform contains tens of thousands of data points, making it complex for clinicians to analyze them. AI can detect subtle and meaningful information from ECG waveforms that clinicians cannot observe.

Sophisticated ML algorithms can detect complex cardiac patterns and abnormalities, accurately predicting conditions such as atrial fibrillation and myocardial infarction. Its exponential growth in echocardiography is evident, with automated algorithms aiding in the interpretation of cardiac structure parameters, mitigating interobserver variability and enhancing diagnostic precision.

AI has considerably advanced cardiovascular imaging in recent years, enabling enhanced detection and quantification of heart diseases, comprehensive analysis of vascular abnormalities, and the integration of multi-modality imaging data. AI algorithms can efficiently interpret complex imaging data, recognising initial stages of cardiac diseases, such as coronary artery disease and congestive heart failure, through modalities like cardiac CT, MRI, or echocardiography. For example, ML models and CNNs have demonstrated the ability to automatically detect coronary artery calcification and perform automatic segmentation of the left ventricular myocardium, respectively, with strong correlation to manual analyses. AI technology has also enhanced the functional evaluation of the left ventricle in echocardiographic diagnosis by automating tasks traditionally reliant on visual observation and manual boundary tracing, such as measuring left ventricular ejection fraction using the Simpson method. Such advances promise to reduce the dependence on physician experience, increasing the repeatability and accuracy of these evaluations.

Artificial intelligence algorithms have also shown promising results in accurately diagnosing and risk stratifying patients with possible coronary artery disease, showing its potential as an initial triage tool. Other algorithms have been used in predicting patient mortality, medication effects, and adverse events following treatment for acute coronary syndrome (Wang et al., 2021).

A major breakthrough in AI-based cardiovascular imaging is the integration of data from multi-modality imaging, which combines information from CT, MRI, and echocardiography to provide a holistic representation of cardiac structure and function. This consolidated data is essential for complex assessments, such as detecting ischemia or planning interventions. For instance, ML algorithms can merge perfusion data from MRI with coronary anatomy from CT, generating sophisticated 3D heart models, thus improving the detection of cardiac ischemia and facilitating precise procedural planning (Yao et al., 2023).

Atrial fibrillation

Atrial fibrillation (AF), especially paroxysmal AF, is often asymptomatic. Patients with AF often demonstrate a normal sinus rhythm during ECG recording, which may lead to underdiagnosis. However, the structure of the heart starts to change once AF develops. Normal sinus-rhythm ECGs might undergo subtle changes that a deeply trained neural network can identify to predict AF. Attia et al. have implemented a CNN to identify patients with AF during normal sinus rhythm using a standard 12-lead ECG. The model was trained using nearly 500,000 ECGs. Applying the model in a testing set yielded an AUC of 0.87 for detecting AF from sinus-rhythm ECGs, with an overall accuracy of 79.4%. When testing the model on all the ECGs from the patients' window of interest (from 31 days before the first recorded AF ECG to that day), the AUC improved to 0.90 with improved overall accuracy of 88.3%. The results show that this algorithm can differentiate patients with AF from normal sinus-rhythm ECG.

Coronary artery disease and acute myocardial infarction

Wearables, smartphones, and internet-based technologies have also shown the ability to monitor patients' cardiac data points, expanding the amount of data and the various settings AI models can use to enable earlier detection of cardiac events occurring outside of the hospital. Taiwanese investigators found that AI can diagnose myocardial infarction more accurately than physicians in the emergency setting, reducing both low-value testing and missed diagnoses. In this study of patients in a hospital in Taiwan, artificial intelligence technology paired with electrocardiogram testing reduced the time to diagnose and transfer people with heart attacks to the cardiac catheterization laboratory for treatment by about 10 minutes. The trial evaluated patients who had ST-elevation myocardial infarction (STEMI) (a heart attack in which there is a complete blockage of a coronary artery) (Lin et al, 2023).

Figure 18. A 12 lead ECG showing an inferior and right ventricular myocardial infarct and demonstrating the raised ST segment characteristic of acute myocardial infarction.

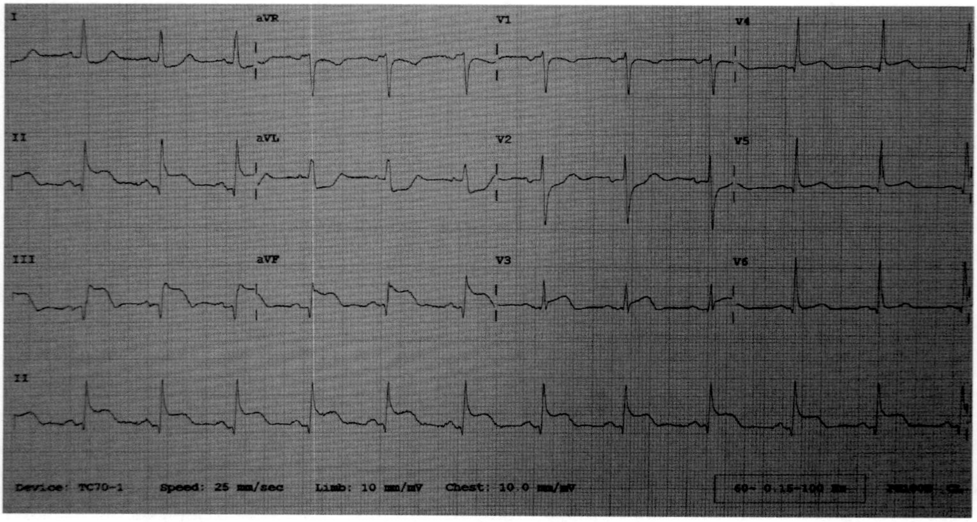

This image is by James Heilman, MD - Own work, CC BY-SA 4.0, https://commons.wikimedia.org/w/index.php?curid=40647852; https://upload.wikimedia.org/wikipedia/commons/8/8a/Inferior_and_RtV_MI_12_lead.jpg. This file is licensed under the Creative Commons Attribution-Share Alike 4.0 International license. No changes were made to this image.

Heart failure

Left ventricular ejection fraction (LVEF) is often measured by echocardiography. In the early stage of heart failure (HF), patients may demonstrate asymptomatic left ventricular dysfunction (ALVD) for a long time due to a slight decrease in LVEF. Recently, several studies showed that AI-ECG can be used for screening ALVD. Attia et al. (2019) created a large neural network using ECGs and echocardiograms of 44,959 patients to identify patients with ventricular dysfunction (ejection fraction ≤ 35%). When the network was tested on a set of 52,870 patients, it showed an AUC of 0.93, with an accuracy of 85.7%. With a median follow-up of 3.4 years, comparing those who were identified as having a normal ejection fraction (EF) by both network and echocardiography (i.e., true negative), with patients who had a positive AI-ECG but negative echocardiography (i.e., false positive), the latter group had a four-fold increase in developing left ventricular dysfunction (HR = 4.1), suggesting that the network can not only detect patients with left ventricular dysfunction but also identify abnormal ECGs before the manifestation of left ventricular dysfunction. Similarly, another group developed an AI algorithm for identifying patients with a low EF (defined as EF ≤ 50%) based on their ECG. 22,641 participants without HF and 120 primary care teams from 45 hospitals were randomly assigned to the intervention or control groups. This study found that AI-ECG improved the diagnosis of low EF by 32%, compared to the control group within 90 days after the ECG test. Furthermore, the AI-ECG improved the diagnosis of low EF more when AI-ECG was applied in the outpatient setting (OR = 1.71), demonstrating that AI-ECG may enable the early diagnosis of patients with low EF in the primary care settings and resource-scarce settings.

Investigators at the Mayo Clinic applied AI techniques to a new screening tool for people with asymptomatic left ventricular dysfunction. The AI-assisted screening tool found people at risk of this condition 93% of the time. To put that in perspective, a mammogram is accurate 85% of the time. In addition, AI developed at the Mayo Clinic used the Apple Watch to detect a low ventricular ejection fraction.

In contrast, right heart failure is often underreported in the clinical setting, which may be due to the lack of effective screening modalities to evaluate right ventricular function. However, right ventricular dysfunction is closely related to left ventricular dysfunction and total heart failure. Investigators constructed a DL model that could be used to predict left and right ventricular function from the ECG. In the internal and external database, AI-ECG performed well at detecting right ventricular systolic dysfunction (RVSD) with an AUC of 0.84 and detection of patients with LVEF ≤ 40% with an AUC of 0.94, suggesting that the DL model can extract biventricular function information from an AI-ECG.

Cardiomyopathy

Dilated cardiomyopathy (DC) is a common cause of HF with reduced LVEF. First-degree relatives of patients with DC have an increased risk of DC. Investigators built a CNN model to achieve the early diagnosis of DC using ECG. Within a cohort of 421 patients who suffered from DC and 16,025 participants with normal LVEF, the AUC of using AI-ECG to detect LVEF ≤ 45% was 0.955, with a negative predictive value of more than 99%, indicating that AI-ECG may serve as a screening tool for DC and determine the need for subsequent echocardiographic diagnosis. Cardiovascular MRI is the gold standard for diagnosing left ventricular hypertrophy (LVH), but is limited by its cost and accessibility, and cannot be used as a screening tool for LVH. One group trained a CNN model using ECGs within 32,239 individuals, aiming at predicting CMR-tested left ventricular mass based on 12-lead ECG (LVM-AI). When testing in the two independent test sets, LVM-AI predicted LVH with AUC of 0.653 and 0.621, showing that LVM-AI may have a moderate ability to discriminate LVH.

Figure 19. Gross pathology of idiopathic cardiomyopathy. Opened left ventricle of heart shows a thickened, dilated left ventricle with subendocardial fibrosis manifested as increased whiteness of endocardium. Autopsy specimen.

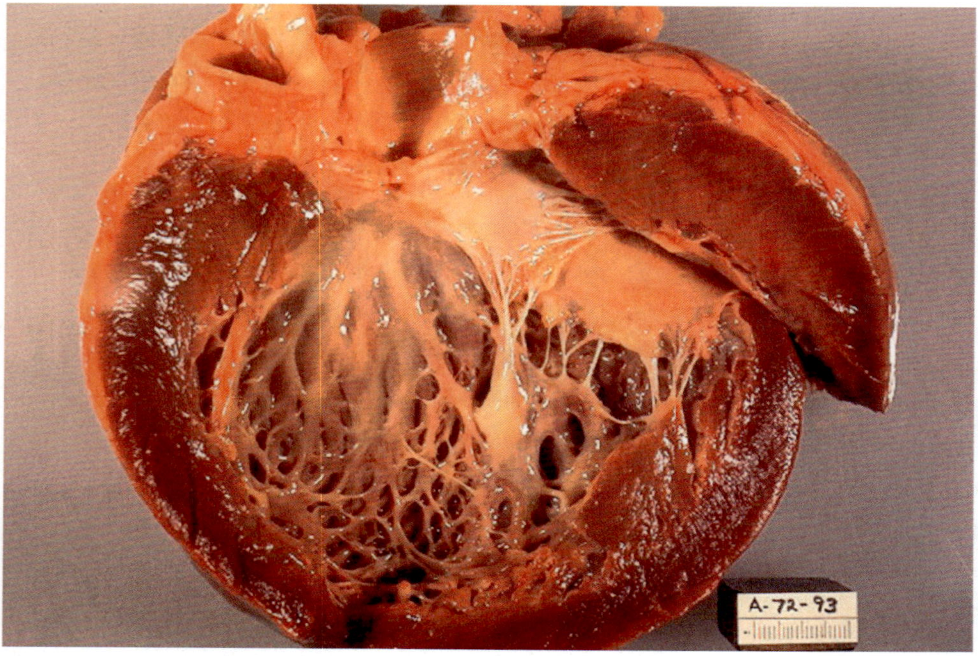

Another type of cardiomyopathy is hypertrophic cardiomyopathy (HCM). HCM is most commonly inherited in an autosomal dominant pattern. It is often due to mutations in certain genes involved with making heart muscle proteins. Other inherited causes of left ventricular hypertrophy may include Fabry disease, Friedreich's ataxia, and certain medications such as tacrolimus.

Figure 20. Asymmetric septal hypertrophy in hypertrophic cardiomyopathy

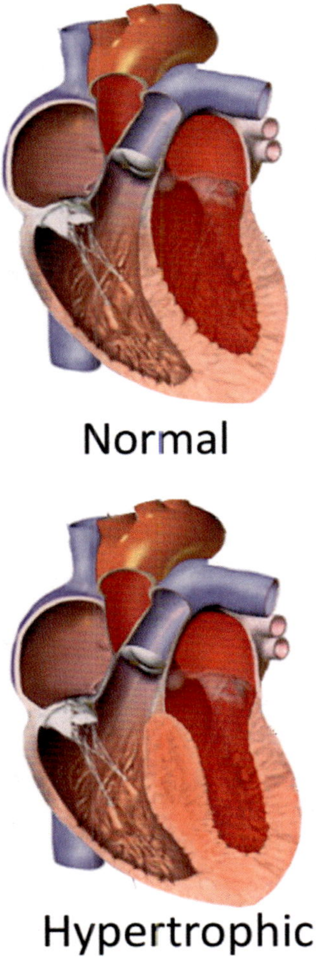

HCM is one of the leading causes of sudden cardiac death in young adults. Sudden cardiac death due to HCM is preventable if HCM can be detected early. HCM can be diagnosed with echocardiography. Although more than 90% of patients with HCM have electrocardiogram abnormalities, these are non-specific and indistinguishable from other diseases. AI-ECG may be an effective method to diagnose HCM. One group trained and validated AI-ECG with 2,448 patients with HCM and 51,153 age- and sex-matched subjects without HCM. When applying this model to diagnose HCM, the testing set, which included 612 patients with HCM and 12,788 control subjects, the AUC was up to 0.96 with the sensitivity of 87% and specificity of 90%. Surprisingly, this model performed particularly well in young individuals (age < 40), suggesting AI-ECG may be practical for screening HCM.

Congenital heart disease

Congenital heart disease (CHD) is the most common congenital disability, resulting in substantial mortality after birth. Using AI-ECG, trained models can detect abnormal image frames that are difficult for the clinician to discern. Recently, Arnaout et al. (2020) trained a neural network to distinguish normal hearts and CHD using nearly 100,000 images from echocardiographic and screening ultrasound tests performed during 18 to 24 weeks of pregnancy. In the internal test set, the model distinguished normal from abnormal hearts with an AUC of 0.99 and achieved a negative predictive value of 100%. Importantly, the model performed robustly on outside-hospital and lower-quality images, suggesting that DL-based screening ultrasound improves the fetal detection of CHD.

Cardiac valvular disease

Another growing area of cardiological research is the utility of AI in classifying heart sounds and diagnosing cardiac valvular disease (Chen et al., 2021)

Many valvular heart diseases involve long asymptomatic periods. However, once symptoms appear, mortality increases dramatically. Follow-up in asymptomatic patients and valve replacement in symptomatic patients often result in good outcomes. Echocardiography is the gold standard for confirming the diagnosis of valvular heart disease, but it is not suitable for screening tests. Therefore, it was of interest to use AI-enhanced electrocardiogram (AI-ECG) as an available tool for screening asymptomatic patients.

Figure 21. Aortic stenosis. The aorta has been removed to show thickened, fused aortic valve leaflets (autopsy specimen).

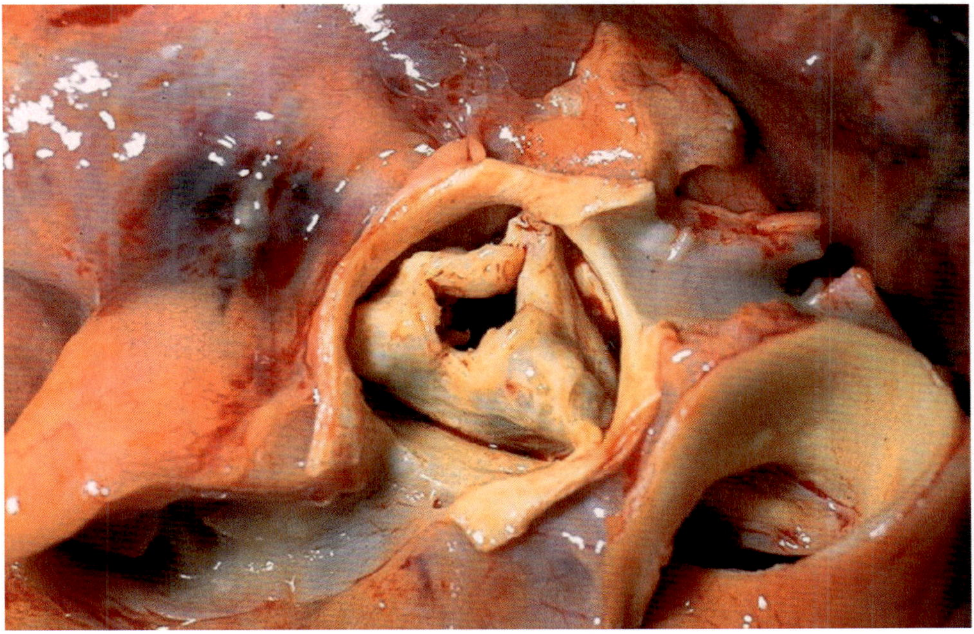

This image is by CDC/Dr. Edwin P. Ewing, Jr. - This media comes from the Centers for Disease Control and Prevention's Public Health Image Library (PHIL), with identification number #848. Public Domain, https://commons.wikimedia.org/w/index.php?curid=825654; https://en.wikipedia.org/wiki/Aortic_stenosis#/media/File:Aortic_stenosis_rheumatic,_gross_pathology_20G0014_lores.jpg. This image is a work of the Centers for Disease Control and Prevention, part of the United States Department of Health and Human Services, taken or made as part of an employee's official duties. As a work of the U.S. federal government, the image is in the public domain. No changes were made to this image.

Kwon et al. (2020) developed a DL-based algorithm combining a multilayer perceptron (MLP) and CNN, which aimed to detect moderate or severe aortic stenosis (AS) using ECGs. During internal and external validation, the AUC for identifying significant AS were 0.88 and 0.86 respectively. Sensitivity analysis showed that the algorithm focused on the T wave of the precordial lead to determine the presence of AS. This work has been confirmed by others. Cohen-Shelly et al.

(2021) developed a CNN model for screening moderate or severe AS using ECGs and echocardiograms from 129,788 adult patients. AI-ECG performed well in the testing group, including 102,926 participants with an AUC of 0.85 and an accuracy of 74%, and a negative predictive value of 98.9%. When sex and age were added to the model, the AUC was improved to 0.90. Furthermore, another group developed the Valve Net DL model: the AUC to detect moderate or severe AS, aortic regurgitation (AR), and mitral regurgitation (MR) was 0.88, 0.77 and 0.83, respectively. The AUC of the composite of any of them was 0.84. Subset analyses showed that the performance of the algorithm was equivalent with regards to gender, ethnicity, and race. These studies indicate the AI-ECG is a potential method for screening for valvular heart disease.

Chapter 7. How AI will improve outcomes in neurology

AI has proven to be indispensable in managing high-dimensional data within the realm of neuroradiology. This technology has facilitated the early detection of a different stroke subtypes, as shown by Yedavalli et al. (2021). CNNs demonstrate remarkable expertise in various tasks, including detecting infarcts or haemorrhages, segmentation, classification, and identification of large vessel occlusion. The application of CNNs in these areas has significantly influenced the approach to stroke treatment (Soun et al., 2021).

Figure 22. Anatomy of the human brain

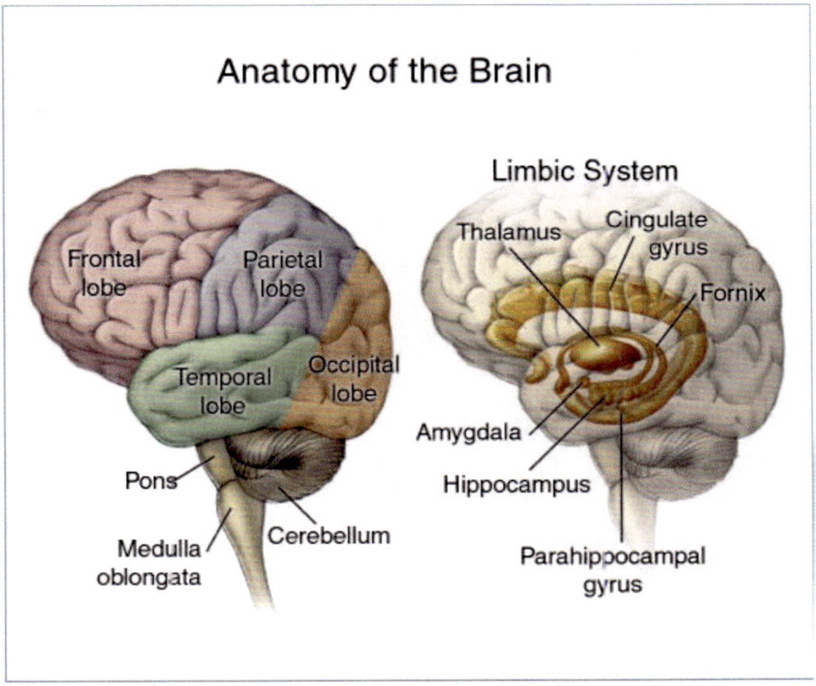

This image is by artlessstacey/artlessstacey - artlessstacey, Public Domain, https://commons.wikimedia.org/w/index.php?curid=4357054; https://en.wikipedia.org/wiki/Brain_tumor#/media/File:Brain_headBorder.jpg. The copyright holder of this work has released this work into the public domain. No changes were made to this image.

Figure 23. Illustration of an embolic stroke, showing a clot lodged in a blood vessel

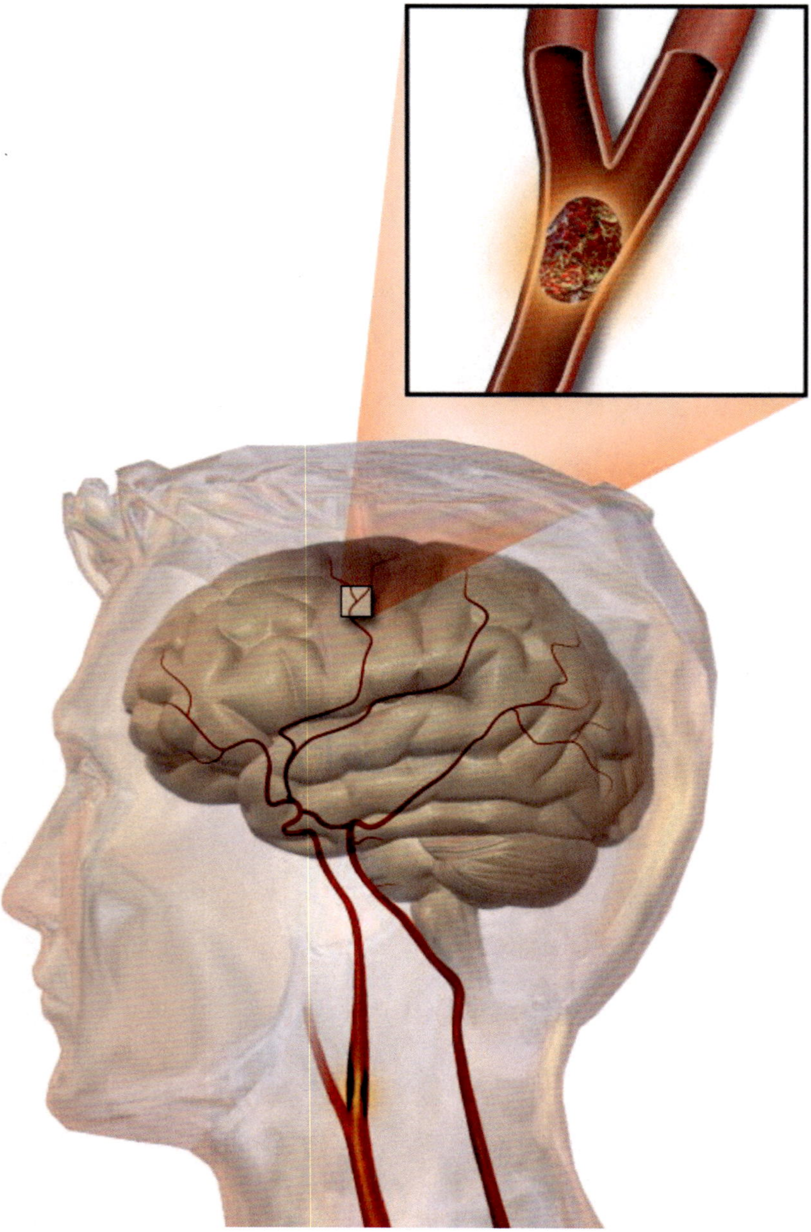

https://en.wikipedia.org/wiki/Stroke#/media/File:Blausen_0836_Stroke.png. This file is licensed under the Creative Commons Attribution 3.0 Unported license. No changes were made to this image.

.

Figure 24. CT scan of the brain with a middle cerebral artery infarct (arrow).

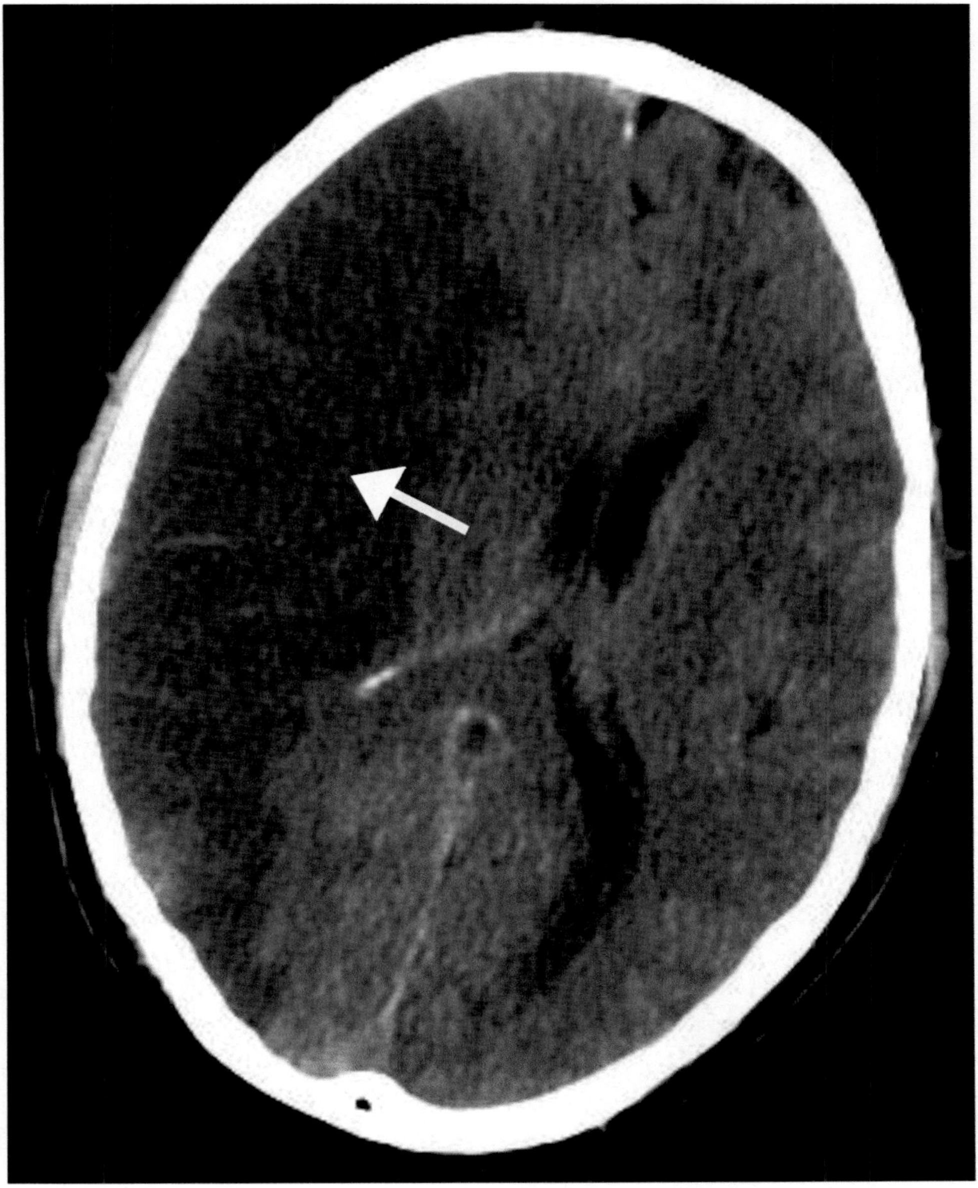

This image is by INFARCT.jpg: Lucien Monfilsderivative work: Suraj - INFARCT.jpg, CC BY-SA 3.0, https://commons.wikimedia.org/w/index.php?curid=16444670; https://en.wikipedia.org/wiki/Stroke#/media/File:MCA_Territory_Infarct.svg. This file is licensed under the Creative Commons Attribution-Share Alike 3.0 Unported, 2.5 Generic, 2.0 Generic and 1.0 Generic license. No changes were made to this image.

CNNs demonstrate remarkable expertise in various tasks, including detecting cerebral infarcts or haemorrhages, segmentation, classification, and identification of large vessel occlusion. Sophisticated AI algorithms have been designed to analyse MR images for detecting specific biomarkers or characteristic patterns associated with these conditions. The task of discerning subtle changes in brain structure or function, which is crucial in diagnosing these diseases, is made more efficient with AI due to its ability to detect refined voxel-level patterns and provide objective, quantitative assessments.

(*Voxels* are rapidly becoming the DNA of the $12 trillion manufacturing industry's digital transformation. In 3D computer graphics, a voxel represents a value on a regular grid in three-dimensional space. As with pixels in a 2D bitmap, voxels themselves do not typically have their position (i.e. coordinates) explicitly encoded with their values. Instead, rendering systems infer the position of a voxel based upon its position relative to other voxels (i.e., its position in the data structure that makes up a single volumetric image).

AI algorithms provide an objective, consistent means of assessing changes in tumour size or metabolic activity changes, automating measurements that were traditionally time-consuming and susceptible to inter-observer variability, such as those evaluated by the Response Evaluation Criteria In Solid Tumors (RECIST) criteria. AI accomplishes this by harnessing radiomic features - high-dimensional data extracted from radiological images - to build mathematical models adept at detecting subtle changes indicative of treatment response. AI also plays a key role in monitoring treatment response by quantifying tumour changes via granular analysis of medical image subunits (pixels/voxels). These smaller elements can be examined by computers to reveal objective mathematical features linked with disease behaviour or outcomes.

Traditional methods of monitoring radiation therapy response, based on visual assessment of changes in tumour size and characteristics, are often subjective and may overlook subtle indicators of treatment efficacy. AI, particularly CNNs, provide an objective means of assessing treatment response, utilising vast datasets of annotated imaging scans to accurately identify and delineate tumours. This automation streamlines the planning process, potentially enhancing treatment outcomes via precise radiation dosing. The effectiveness of this approach is often quantified by the Sørensen–Dice coefficient (DSC), facilitating early and accurate therapy efficacy assessment and timely treatment adjustments, if necessary.

Classifying brain tumors

In the USA brain cancer and other types of nervous system cancers are the 10th leading cause of death. Initially, surgeons focused on removing the brain mass. They analyzed the mass to determine the type of tumor in order to guide further treatment. Analysis tests last for 40 minutes. Introducing AI in radiology reduces the tumor classification time to three minutes.

Chapter 8. How AI will improve outcomes in kidney disease

Kidney disease is a major public health problem in part because of it is caused by diabetes, hypertension, obesity, and aging; the incidence of these conditions is increasing. According to the Global Burden of Diseases, Injuries, and Risk Factors Study 2015, 750 million people worldwide suffered from kidney disease.

In nephrology, contemporary AI applications display remarkable potential in anticipating the onset of acute kidney injury before significant biochemical changes become evident, potentially allowing for timely interventions to prevent disease progression. Additionally, AI's ability to identify modifiable risk factors for chronic kidney disease progression offers valuable insights for preventative care.

In the sphere of renal tumour detection, AI models have demonstrated proficiency - matching, or even exceeding human accuracy, in interpreting imaging studies. This impressive feat could augment prognostication and decision-making processes after renal transplantation. The heightened precision in detecting and diagnosing renal tumours fosters more effective treatment strategies, potentially leading to improved patient outcome.

Alerts for acute kidney injury (AKI) (previously known as acute renal failure)

Approximately 2 million patients die of AKI every year. At present, the diagnosis of AKI is based on serum creatinine and urine output values.

On 9 June 2014, the National Health Service (NHS) England published the national AKI algorithm for safety alert, recommending "the wide scale introduction and uptake of an automated computer software algorithm to detect AKI". In 2015 Google developed the Streams program, which could predict AKI and send warnings to doctors for early intervention.

Figure 25. Acute kidney injury showing marked pallor of the cortex (acute cortical necrosis) contrasting to the darker areas of surviving medullary tissue.

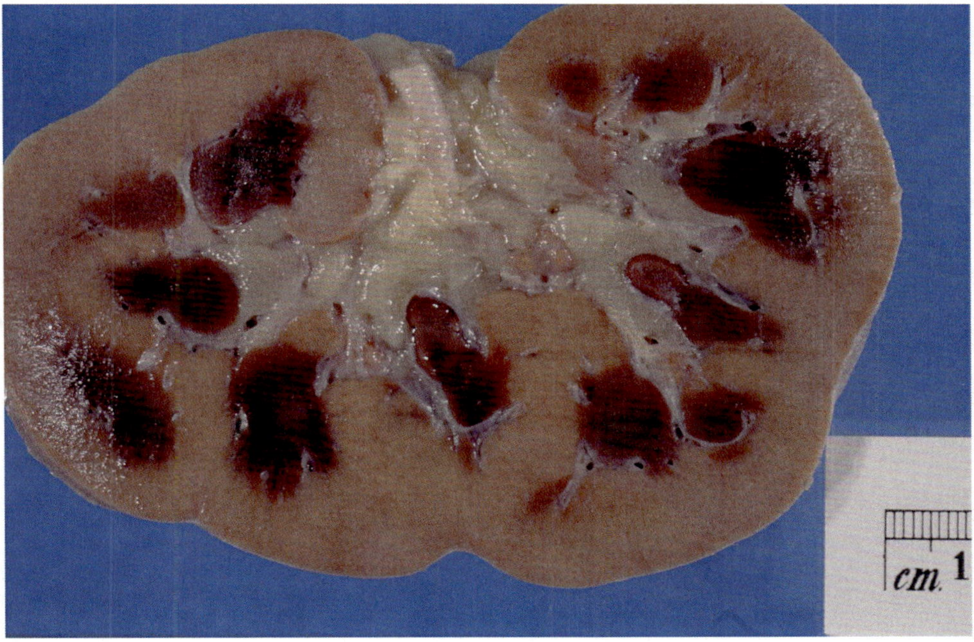

This image is by Haymanj - Self-photographed, Public Domain, https://commons.wikimedia.org/w/index.php?curid=3647869; https://en.wikipedia.org/wiki/Acute_kidney_injury#/media/File:Kidney_%E2%80%93_acute_cortical_necrosis.jpg. The copyright holder of this work, release this work into the public domain. No changes were made to this image.

Tomašev et al. (2019) built a model using data from 703,782 adult patients which could predict 55.8% of all inpatient episodes of AKI, and 90.2% of all AKI that required subsequent treatment with dialysis in. Lee et al. (2018) retrospectively reviewed 2,010 patients after cardiac surgery and used six machine learning techniques, including decision tree, random forest (RF), extreme gradient boosting, support vector machine, neural network classifier, and deep learning, to train AKI prediction models. The study demonstrated that the machine learning technique of extreme gradient boosting showed significantly better performance than the traditional logistic regression analysis or previous risk scores in predicting both AKI of all stages and stage 2 or 3 AKI after cardiac surgery.

Yin et al. (2017) retrospectively reviewed 8,800 patients undergoing contrast administration to develop the model for prediction of contrast-induced nephropathy (CIN), the third cause of all hospital-acquired renal failure, using the machine learning method of RF. The model showed good predictive ability for CIN development and might provide preventative measures for CIN. Mohamadlou et al. (2018) used boosted ensembles of decision trees to train an AKI prediction tool on retrospective data taken from more than 300,000 inpatients. The prediction tool offered useful predictive capability for detecting which patients were likely to suffer AKI.

Tang et al. (2018) built risk prediction models for AKI in 157 severely burned patients and compared the prediction performance of XGBoost machine learning and logistic regression model. The machine learning method was found to have a better prediction performance than logistic regression. Additionally, a Gradient Boosting Machine algorithm predicted serum creatinine-based kidney disease. Another study demonstrated that machine learning models (multivariate logistic regression, RF and artificial neural networks (ANN)) could predict AKI onset following admission to an intensive care unit in 23,950 patients with a competitive AUC (mean AUC 0.783).

Alerts for chronic kidney disease (CKD)

There are also reports of AI applications for alerting medical personnel to the development of CKD. A pilot program using e-technologies to detect CKD was conducted in Australia. The software was built on algorithms trained to identify at-risk patients and to order a relevant screening test for CKD.

In addition, AI has also been studied for warning of complications of CKD. Galloway et al. (2019) reported that using only 2 ECG leads, a deep-learning model detected hyperkalemia in patients with renal disease with an AUC of 0.853 to 0.883. The application of artificial intelligence to the ECG may enable screening for hyperkalemia of CKD patients. However, the study is retrospective and needs prospective testing. Additionally, the model is a screening test with low specificity, with upwards of 42% false-positive results, which may cause anxiety and inconvenience for patients. Pilia et al. (2019) also used an artificial neural network to reconstruct the extracellular ionic concentrations for both potassium and calcium with an acceptable precision in CKD patients.

Figure 26. The small irregular appearance of a human kidney affected by CKD

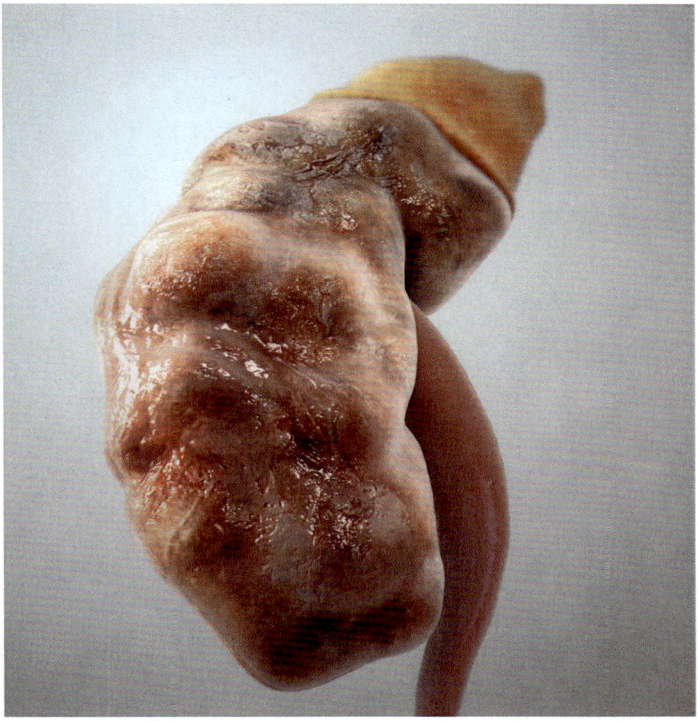

This image is by https://www.scientificanimations.com/ - http://www.scientificanimations.com/wiki-images/, CC BY-SA 4.0, https://commons.wikimedia.org/w/index.php?curid=72624073; https://en.wikipedia.org/wiki/Chronic_kidney_disease#/media/File:CKD_-_Chronic_kidney_disease.jpg. This file is licensed under the Creative Commons Attribution-Share Alike 4.0 International license. No changes were made to this image.

Several studies have identified factors for progression of CKD by using Bayesian network and artificial intelligence. Almansour et al. (2019) compared the ANN and SVM techniques in a dataset of 400 patients to predict early stage CKD. The empirical results from the experiments indicated that ANN performed better than SVM, with accuracies of 99.75% and 97.75% respectively.

The high morbidity rate associated with kidney stone disease is one of the main concerns in healthcare systems. Kazemi and Mirroshandel (2018) developed a model for the early detection of the type of kidney stone and the most influential parameters in 936 patients with nephrolithiasis. The final ensemble-based model had an accuracy of 97.1% and could be applied safely to predict the chances of developing nephrolithiasis.

Autosomal dominant polycystic kidney disease

Autosomal dominant polycystic kidney disease (ADPKD) is the most common hereditary renal disease. It is characterized by progressive enlargement of the kidneys caused by progressive development of renal cysts, often accompanied by declining renal function.

Figure 27. Gross pathologic changes in a case of polycystic kidney disease

This image is by CDC/ Dr. Edwin P. Ewing, Jr. - This media comes from the Centers for Disease Control and Prevention's Public Health Image Library (PHIL), with identification number #861. https://en.wikipedia.org/wiki/Polycystic_kidney_disease#/media/File:Polycystic_kidneys,_gross_pathology_CDC_PHIL.png. This image is a work of the Centers for Disease Control and Prevention, part of the United States Department of Health and Human Services, taken or made as part of an employee's official duties. As a work of the U.S. federal government, the image is in the public domain. No changes were made to this image.

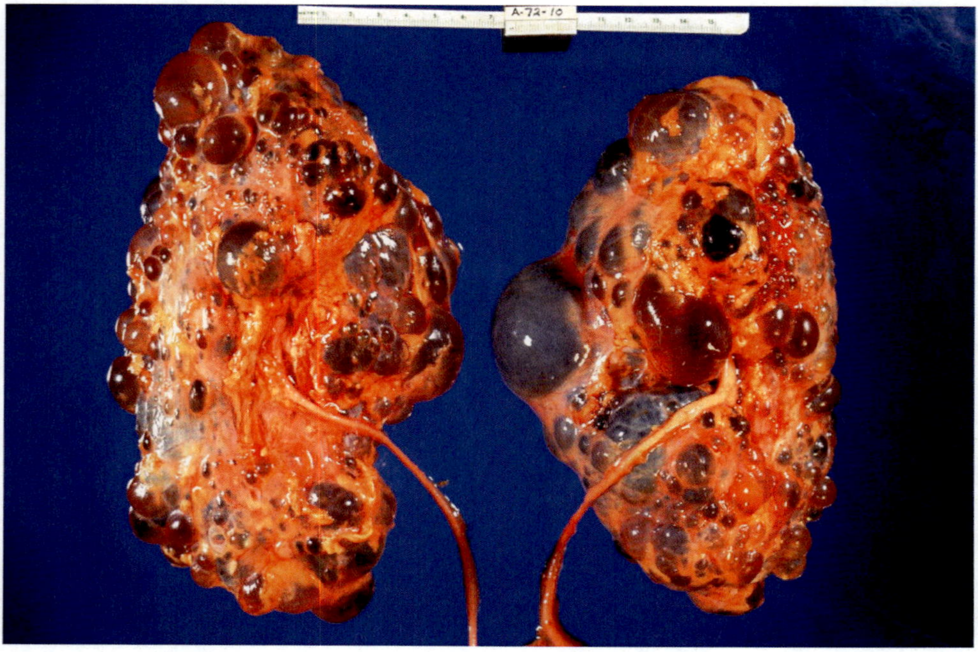

In 2017 Sharma et al. used an automated segmentation method based on deep learning for total kidney volume (TKV) computed on a CT dataset of 244 ADPKD patients. This method facilitated fast and reproducible diagnosis, and TKV measurements transmission agreed with manual segmentations from clinical experts. Most recently, van Gastel et al. (2019) successfully developed a fully automated segmentation method for TKV measurement that used a deep learning network in 540 abdominal magnetic resonance images (T2-weighted HASTE coronal sequences) from patients with ADPKD. TKV measured by the automated approach correlated highly with manually traced TKV (intraclass correlation coefficients, 0.998), with low bias and high precision (<0.1%±2.7% for TKV) 37. (HASTE is an echo-planar fast spin echo sequence trademarked by Siemens. The expanded acronym fairly completely describes what it entails: Half-Fourier Acquisition Single-shot Turbo spin Echo imaging).

Renal tumours

Figure 28. Histopathologic types of kidney tumour, with relative incidences and prognoses. Angiomyolipoma is seen at the right of the pie chart.

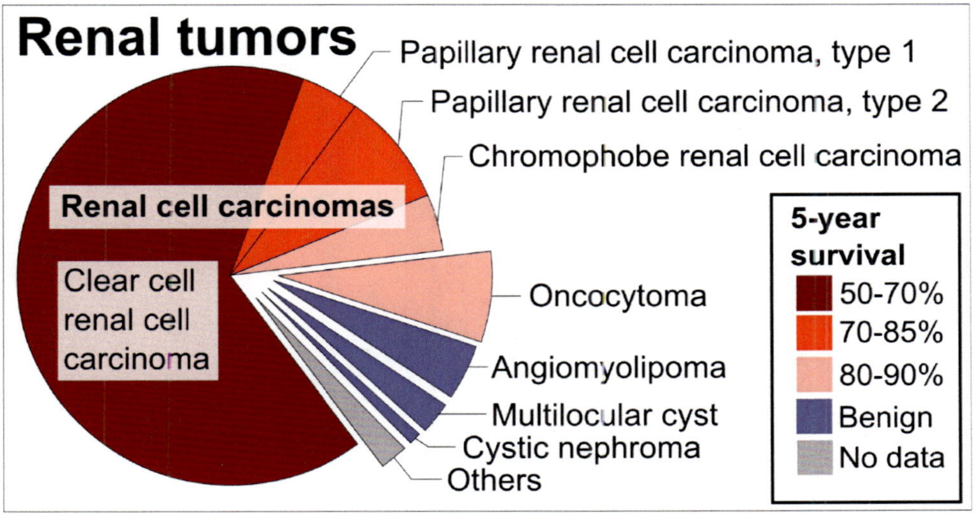

It is often difficult for physicians to achieve a preoperative differential diagnosis between renal cell carcinoma and some benign renal tumors because of factors such as adiposity angiomyolipoma. The automatic deep feature classification (DFC) method can distinguish between both benign angiomyolipoma without visible fat and oncocytoma from malignant renal cell carcinoma (RCC) using abdominal computer tomography (CT) images. (An oncocytoma is a tumor made up of oncocytes - epithelial cells characterized by an excessive amount of mitochondria, resulting in an abundant acidophilic, granular cytoplasm. The cells and the tumor that they compose are often benign but sometimes may be premalignant or malignant. Renal oncocytoma is thought to arise from the intercalated cells of collecting ducts of the kidney. It represents 5% to 15% of surgically resected renal neoplasms.

Figure 29. Gross appearance of the cut surface of a nephrectomy specimen containing a renal oncocytoma

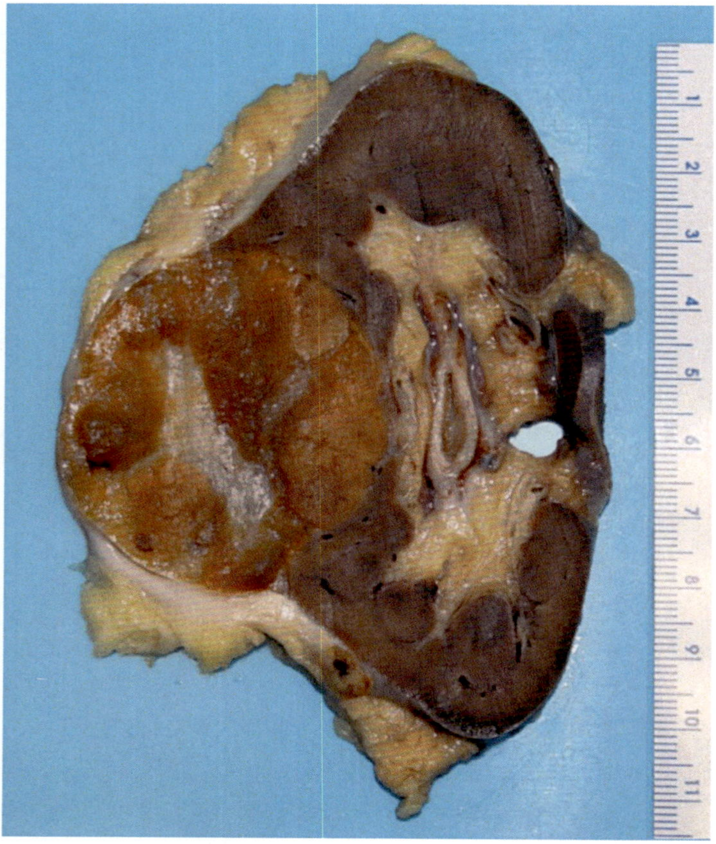

Image genomics

Image genomics can complete genomic analysis by extracting a large number of tumor image features through AI and associating the image features with the underlying mutation status of tumors, molecular markers, underlying activated biologic pathways, or clinical outcomes by developing "association maps" between them. Jamshidi et al. (2016) constructed an alternative model for multi-gene expression molecular detection of renal clear cell carcinoma based on image genomics by using CT imaging features, thus achieving the independent prediction of disease-related survival of patients without any invasive approaches.

Congenital abnormalities of the kidney and urinary tract

Congenital abnormalities of the kidney and urinary tract (CAKUT) in children are challenging. A pre-trained deep learning model (imagenet-caffe-alex) was adopted for transfer learning-based feature extraction from 3-channel feature maps computed from ultrasound images. SVM classifiers were then built upon different sets of features, including the transfer learning features, conventional imaging features, and their combination. The AUC for classifiers built on the combination features were 0.92, 0.88, and 0.92 for discriminating the left, right, and bilateral abnormal kidney scans from controls with classification rates of 84%, 81%, and 87%, specificity of 84%, 74%, and 88% and sensitivity of 85%, 88%, and 86%, respectively. It is suggested that the combination of transfer learning features and conventional imaging features yielded the best classification performance for distinguishing CAKUT patients from normal controls based on their ultrasound kidney images.

Pathological diagnosis

Renal interstitial fibrosis is an indicator of the presence and extent of chronic kidney disease. A standard quantitative method of visual evaluation is important for the diagnosis of renal diseases. The Banff schema is one of the standards used for the classification of the grade of renal allograft rejection. The visual scoring is subject to intra- and inter-observer variability and may not be repeatable or reproducible. CAD, which can reduce the workload of pathologists, has the advantages of precision and meticulousness. An automated quantification system for measuring renal interstitial fibrosis had an average error of 9%. Kannan et al. (2019) developed a deep learning framework to accurately identify and segment glomeruli from digitized images of human kidney biopsies. The segmentation model, that was based on the convolutional neural network (CNN) multilabel classifier, accurately marked the sclerosis of glomeruli on the test data. This indicated the power of deep learning for assessing complex histologic structures from digitized human kidney biopsies. A deep learning architecture has also been leveraged to better associate patient-specific histologic images with clinical phenotypes including CKD stage, serum creatinine, and nephrotic-range proteinuria at the time of biopsy, as well as 1-, 3-, and 5-year renal survival in 171 patients. AUC values for the CNN models in predicting creatinine, proteinuria and 1-, 3-, and 5-year renal survival were 0.912, 0.867, 0.878, 0.875, and 0.904.

Use of International Classification of Disease codes

International Classification of Disease (ICD) codes are important for population health and cohort discovery when clinical information is limited. Deep learning methods based on demographics, laboratory results, and medications, as well as codes from previous encounters, have been used to model coder decision making. Three test cases were investigated including acute renal failure (ARF) and CKD; the AUC of predicting ARF and CKD were 0.9194 and 0.9424 respectively.

Guiding treatment for renal diseases

Guidelines are the basis for decision-making, which are formulated through large-scale investigations. These guidelines are thus population-based and adjustments are needed using the guidelines on individual cases. Personalized and accurate treatment protocols are required. AI can analyze the association of treatment protocols and efficacy from a large number of patients, develop models based on efficacy and risk factors, guide the choice of treatment protocols, and improve clinical efficacy.

Anemia treatment

Anemia is one of the main common comorbidities in patients undergoing hemodialysis. The incidence and severity of anemia gradually increases as renal function declines. The major cause of anemia in CKD is deficiency of erythropoietin (EPO) production by the kidneys.

Substantial progress has been made in the application of computer-driven methods to provide erythropoietic dosing information for patients with anemia due to chronic kidney disease Initial solutions were computerized versions of traditional paper-based anemia management protocols. True personalization was achieved through the use of advanced modelling techniques such as artificial neural networks, physiologic models, and feedback control systems. In 2003 investigators in Spain carried out an individualized prediction of the EPO dosage to be administered to CKD patients which aided the individualization of dosage.

Robotics

Robotics are also steadily being introduced in health care, especially in surgery, with systems such as the da Vinci® Surgical System that involves a magnified 3D high-definition computer vision system (part of it aided by ML) and tiny wristed instruments that bend and rotate more complexly than the human hand

An autonomous image-guided robotic needle insertion for blood draws, intravenous insertions and tissue biopsies has also been designed that combines robotics, AI, computer vision, and image technology. It is reported that accurate needle insertion (< 3 mm error) can be achieved in common target sites including the kidneys when using a CT-guided robotic system. The proposed optical tracker based robot registration and serving method is capable of accurate three dimension needle operation for ultrasound-guided percutaneous renal access procedure with improved precision and shortened time.

Evaluating prognosis

AI can identify factors affecting prognosis by analyzing databases, and developing models that evaluate the relationship between risk factors and prognosis.

Chronic kidney disease mineral and bone metabolism disorders (CKD-MBD)

CKD-MBD is another common comorbidity in ESRD patients, which increases mortality. The serum concentrations of phosphate (P), calcium (Ca) or parathyroid hormone (PTH) were used to assess this. The three parameters, P, Ca, PTH, interplay with each other, but the relationship is non-linear. To quantify the degree of association between the three parameters, investigators developed a data analysis system using RF from 1,758 hemodialysis (HD) patients. Compared with classical statistical methods, the power of prediction of the new model was markedly increased. In 2018 investigators used RF algorithms to build a model predicting risks for development of calciphylaxis in CKD patients. With an AUC value of 0.872, the model could successfully predict calciphylaxis. (Calciphylaxis, also known as calcific uremic arteriolopathy (CUA), is a rare syndrome characterized by painful skin lesions. The pathogenesis of calciphylaxis is unclear but is believed to involve calcification of the small blood vessels located within the fatty tissue and deeper layers of the skin, blood clots, and eventual death of skin cells due to lack of blood flow. It is seen mostly in people with end-stage kidney disease but can occur in the earlier stages of chronic kidney disease and rarely in people with normally functioning kidneys. It is believed to affect 1-4% of all dialysis patients. It results in chronic non-healing skin wounds and indicates poor prognosis, with typical life expectancy of less than one year.

Figure 30. Calciphylaxis on the abdomen

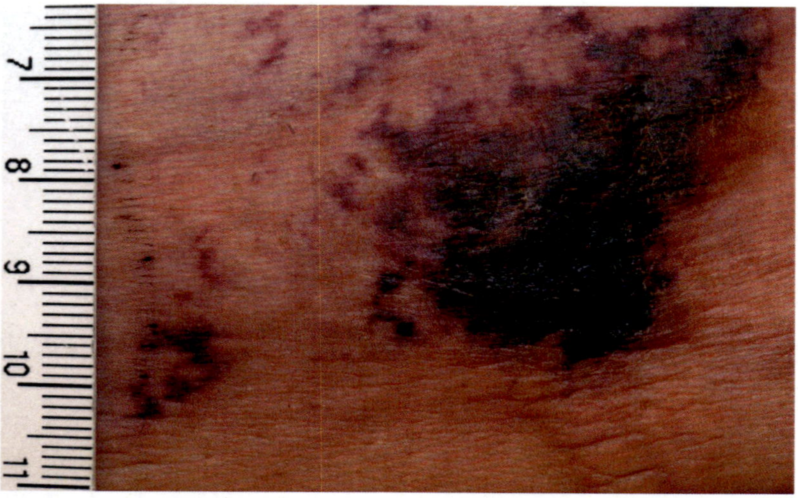

IgA nephropathy (IgAN)

IgAN is the most common primary glomerular kidney disease. About 20-40% of IgAN patients will reach ESRD within 10-20 years of diagnosis. Early prediction of ESRD is valuable. Liu et al. (2018) retrospectively reviewed 262 biopsy-proven IgAN patients, and employed artificial intelligence to predict the ESRD status in IgAN patients. The predictive model showed that Oxford-MEST scores, C3 staining and eGFR were important for ESRD prediction in Chinese IgAN patients.

Diabetic Kidney Disease (DKD)

In 2013 Leung et al. used a multi-staged strategy based on machine learning and mathematical modeling to predict genotype-phenotype risk patterns in 119 DKD patients and 554 without DKD in type 2 diabetes mellitus patients. They found out that age, age of diagnosis and lipid parameters were major clinical predictors while genetic polymorphisms related to inflammation and lipid metabolism were the most selected genetic predictors.

In 2018 Arianna et al. used machine learning to predict complications from 1,000 patients with type 2 diabetes mellitus. The Random Forest model had the highest predictive performance. The model showed that variables, such as gender, age, time from diagnosis, body mass index, glycated hemoglobin, hypertension, and smoking habit, contributed more than others. The accuracy of the model was 0.838.

Kidney transplantation

Predicting the outcome of kidney transplantation is important in order to optimize transplantation parameters and modify factors related to the recipient, donor, and transplant procedure. Lofaro et al. (2010) retrospectively analyzed 80 renal transplant patients with 5-year follow-up, using classification trees to develop two predictive models and identifying six variables that contributed significantly to patient outcomes. The AUC values of these two models are 0.847 and 0.824 respectively. In another study, 4,754 systemic lupus erythematosus patients who underwent kidney transplantation were enrolled. Predictive models were developed by 3 machine learning algorithms. The AUC of ANN (0.73) based on six variables was slightly better than that of logistic regression. The study showed that the ANN model had better predictive performance than other models. Abdeltawab et al. (2019) also developed a deep-learning based CAD system based on the fusion of both imaging markers and clinical biomarkers for the early detection of acute renal transplant rejection. The overall accuracy of the proposed system was 92.9% with 93.3% sensitivity and 92.3% specificity in distinguishing non-rejected kidney transplants from rejected ones.

CKD after AKI

Several studies between 2008 and 2017 demonstrated that, although acute kidney injury is usually reversible, some patients may experience incomplete recovery of kidney function, while others subsequently develop accelerated loss of kidney function, resulting in an increased risk of chronic kidney disease. A multivariable model was developed with 9,973 participants and was externally validated with 2,761 participants to develop a practical risk stratification approach that could be used to identify patients at high risk of chronic kidney disease after AKI. This model, using routine laboratory data, was able to predict advanced chronic kidney disease following hospitalization with acute kidney injury, but requires evaluation of its utility in a clinical setting.

CKD severity

Investigators predicted renal failure progression in 465 CKD patients by using Integrated Intelligent Fuzzy Expert System and found out that the model could accurately (>95%) predict the GFR for sequential 6-, 12-, and 18-month intervals. Xiao et al. (2019) compared nine predictive models, including logistic regression, Elastic Net, lasso regression, ridge regression, SVM, RF, XGBoost, neural network and k-nearest neighbor in prediction of CKD progression in 551 patients with proteinuria The study showed that the model with the highest sensitivity was Elastic Net (0.85), while XGBoost showed the highest specificity (0.83). Albumen, serum creatinine, low density lipoprotein and eGFR levels, showed predictive ability for CKD severity. Additionally, Zacharias et al. (2019) identified CKD patients at risk of progressing to ESRD in 4,640 patients using state-of-the-art machine learning methods. The results demonstrated that proton nuclear magnetic resonance features, such as creatinine, high-density lipoprotein, valine, acetyl groups of glycoproteins, and Ca2+-EDTA carried the highest weights as predictive factors.

Death risk and cardiovascular risk after dialysis

A study was carried out on a contemporary cohort of 27,615 US veterans with incident ESRD by implementing a random forest method on 49 variables obtained before dialysis transition to predict outcomes of 30-, 90-, 180-, and 365-day all-cause mortality after dialysis initiation. The results showed that the model provided C-statistics (95% CI) of 0.7185 (0.6994-0.7377), 0.7446 (0.7346-0.7546), 0.7504 (0.7425-0.7583), and 0.7488 (0.7421-0.7554) for predicting risk of death within the 4 different time windows.

AI plays a significant role in nephrology. Physicians are currently witnessing the development of medical practice from empirical medicine to evidence-based medicine to intelligent diagnosis and to AI-directed medicine. While AI medicine is still in its infant stage, it is clear that it will produce prediction algorithms suitable for routine clinical application in the near future.

Chapter 9. How AI will improve outcomes in lung disease

Interstitial lung diseases

Interstitial lung diseases (ILDs) comprise a heterogeneous group of diseases varying in pathophysiology, presentation, epidemiology, diagnosis, treatment and prognosis. In the majority of ILDs, imaging modalities and especially high-resolution computed tomography (CT) scans have been the cornerstone of the diagnostic approach and follow-up. The intricate nature of ILDs has led to an increasing adoption of artificial intelligence techniques, primarily on imaging data but also in genetic data, spirometry and lung diffusion, among others.

Figure 31. Interstitial lung disease affects gas flow in the alveoli

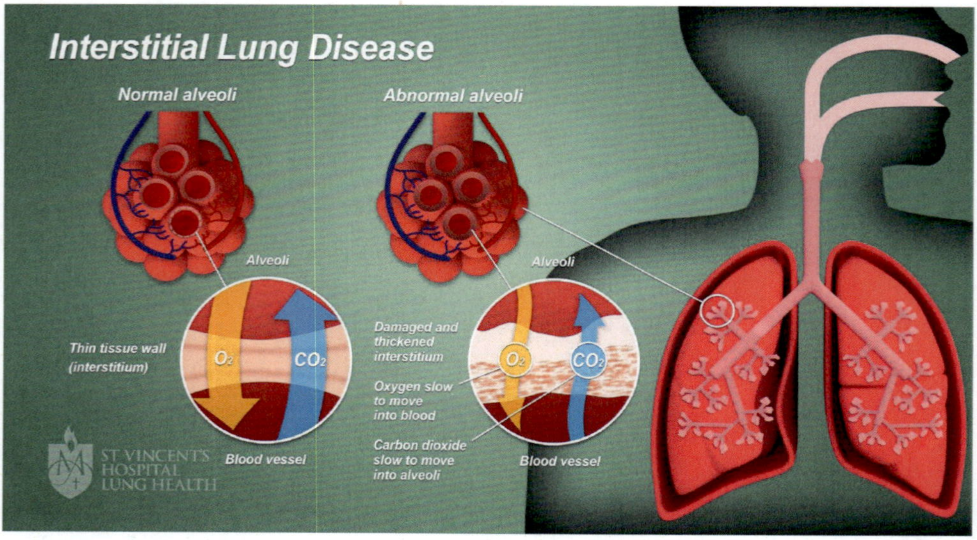

Figure 32. A chest X-ray demonstrating pulmonary fibrosis due to amiodarone

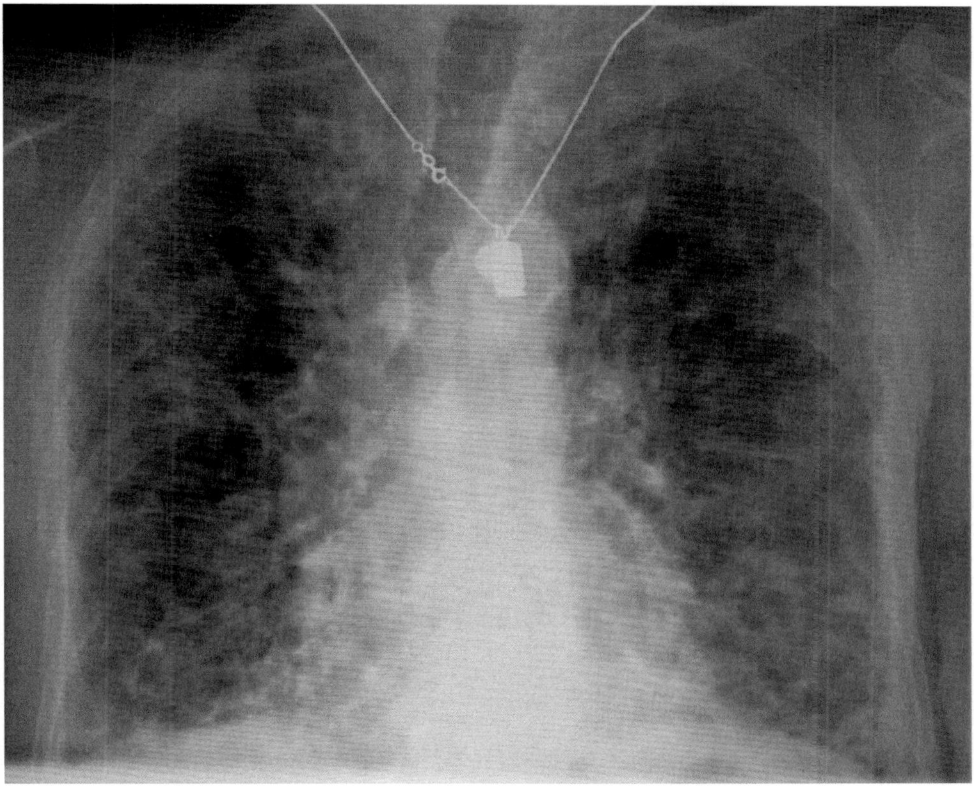

This image is by James Heilman, MD - Own work, CC BY-SA 3.0, https://commons.wikimedia.org/w/index.php?curid=11110205; https://en.wikipedia.org/wiki/Interstitial_lung_disease#/media/File:IPF_amiodarone.JPG. This file is licensed under the Creative Commons Attribution-Share Alike 3.0 Unported license. No changes were made to this image.

Interstitial lung disease (ILD), also known as diffuse parenchymal lung diseases, is an umbrella term encompassing more than 300 conditions. The term interstitial refers to the tissue surrounding the alveoli in the lung, bounded by the capillary endothelium and the alveolar epithelium. Most ILDs are often characterized by inflammation and/or fibrosis causing progressive decline in lung function and impaired gas exchange. The most common causes of ILDs include exposure to environmental toxins, viral infections and autoimmune conditions, although in many cases the cause is unknown and these cases are called “idiopathic”.

Classification of ILDs

Deep learning (DL) can analyze huge amounts of complex data. Besides imaging data, ILDs produce other sources of biomarkers that need to be analyzed in conjunction with the findings from the imaging modalities that are integral to ILDs. Recently, there is active interest in biomarkers coming from genomic, proteomic and transcriptomic investigations

Data repositories

A critical issue for the exploration of ILDs, especially with AI algorithms, is the production of high-quality data that are well characterized and annotated.

OSIC data repository

This was launched by the Open Source Imaging Consortium. It contains approximately 1500 de-identified high-resolution CT scans alongside clinical data for a wide range of interstitial lung diseases, primarily IPF. The repository contains treatment information, as well as follow-up data and mortality. It was built by a collaboration of experts in the fields of respiratory disease, radiology and AI, aiming primarily to facilitate the role of the latter in patient care with precision medicine.

ILD Database from medGIFT

This is a publicly available multimedia collection of ILD cases built from the University Hospitals of Geneva. The database contains high-resolution CT scans with annotated regions of pathological lung areas coupled with clinical parameters from patients with pathologically proven diagnoses of ILDs.

ILDgenDB

This is an integrated genetic information resource for interstitial lung diseases. This resource contains literature-curated disease candidate genes enriched with regulatory elements, as well as single nucleotide polymorphisms (SNPs) that have been associated with specific ILDs. For this propose, ILDgenDB is enriched with information from multiple popular genetic resources such as GAD (Genetic Association Database), OMIM (Online Mendelian Inheritance in Man) and GeneCards.

ILDGDB

This is a similarly oriented repository to ILDgenDB, utilizing genomic, transcriptomic, proteomic and drug information for interstitial lung diseases. ILDGDB incorporates 2018 entries for 20 ILDs and over 600 genes; its purpose is to decipher gene mechanisms that take place in ILDs.

There are also repositories, especially for genomic data, that can be exploited for ILD research. Gene Expression Omnibus (GEO) is a very popular, public repository which accommodates thousands of gene expression datasets. There is a dataset containing gene expression from lung tissue with pulmonary sarcoidosis as well as from healthy lung tissue (GSE16538). GEO also contains expression profiling of lung tissues from patients with idiopathic pulmonary fibrosis (GSE2052). Another similar repository is BioGPS, which features gene expression signatures from numerous diseases and conditions. In terms of ILDs, BioGPS contains two relevant gene sets: one for IPF (E-GEOD-24206) and another one for ILDs in general (E-GEOD-21369). The former was derived from 23 samples, while the latter was derived from 29; both contained data from healthy controls.

AI Applications in ILD Research

Screening

The most common approach in this category involves the analysis of imaging modalities for the identification of ILDs. Bermejo-Peláez et al. (2020) analyzed 208 CT scans, broken down to 37,424 radiographic tissue samples, and utilized an ensemble of deep convolutional neural networks. Their aim is to identify radiographic patterns that precede the development of ILDs and classify them into eight different parenchymal feature classes, namely: normal parenchyma, five interstitial patterns (ground-glass, reticular, nodular, linear scar, subpleural line) and two emphysematous patterns (centrilobular and paraseptal). The authors reported very good performance with an average sensitivity of 91.41% and average specificity of 98.18%. Another study employed 168 CT scans and used a convolutional neural network (CNN) to identify three radiographic patterns (consolidation, emphysema and fibrosis), yielding acceptable performance,

Figure 33. End-stage pulmonary fibrosis (sometimes known as honeycomb lung)

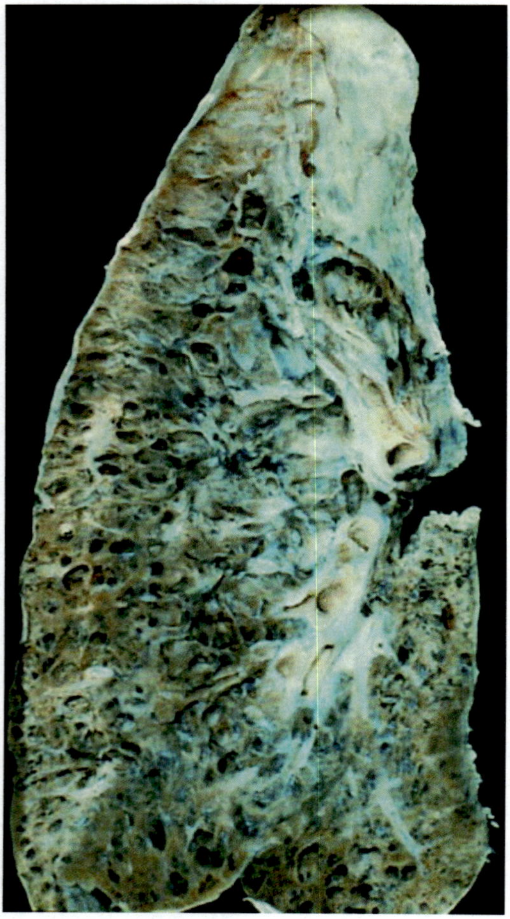

This image is by http://web2.airmail.net/uthman/specimens/index.html, Public Domain, https://commons.wikimedia.org/w/index.php?curid=841015; https://commons.wikimedia.org/wiki/File:End-stage_interstitial_lung_disease_(honeycomb_lung).jpgThis work has been released into the public domain by its author, Ed Uthman. No changes were made to this image.

A methodologically different approach was proposed by Onishchenko et al. (2022) who systematically searched electronic health records for comorbidity patterns that were potentially associated with the development of IPF. Interestingly, the proposed non-invasive methodology can predict IPF from 1 to 4 years prior to definite diagnosis, with Area under the ROC Curve (AUC) > 0.84. The proposed algorithm can be applied to large cohorts, including in primary care, thus enabling early diagnosis with potentially better outcomes.

Another interesting approach was presented by Axelsson et al. (2022), who aimed to identify proteins in circulating blood that are associated with ILDs. More than 4,700 protein analytes from two major databases with more than 10,000 patients combined were searched for potential association with the incidence and progression of ILDs. The extracted protein markers were subsequently coupled with machine learning algorithms in order to identify interstitial lung disease early and predict its progression.

Diagnosis and classification

Some of the first articles to use AI in ILD research were in this category. The majority utilized machine learning algorithms, primarily deep-learning-based ones, in order to analyze CT scans and identify regions pertaining to interstitial lung diseases. Pawar and Talbar (2022) proposed a two-stage approach: the first was for segmenting HRCT images and the second was for classifying segmented images into six ILD classes (normal, emphysema, fibrosis, ground glass, micronodules and consolidation). The proposed classifier yielded an overall accuracy of 89.39%.

AI based approaches have been used for segmenting and classifying images. Three studies utilized deep learning algorithms and were developed with 1,068, 105 and 1,239 patients reporting overall accuracy 83.6%, 81%, and 0.87 respectively. Yang et al. (2021) focused on another popular ILD entity, i.e., pneumoconiosis, and analyzed 1,760 chest X-rays with a deep learning algorithm in order to discriminate between patients with pneumoconiosis and normal controls. The best performing algorithm resulted in 92.46% accuracy, which is significantly higher compared to other machine learning algorithms such as support vector machines, artificial neural networks, random forests, k-nearest neighbours) that were used in the same study.

A totally different approach was presented by Horimasu et al. (2021), who developed a machine learning algorithm in order to discriminate fine crackles from other auscultatory sounds and subsequently associate them with respective regions of pulmonary fibrosis. In total, 60 patients underwent chest X-ray and HRCT, and respiratory findings were recorded in six positions. An interesting finding was that the identification of fine crackles indicated a higher sensitivity compared to a chest-X-ray-based determination of the presence or absence of ILD.

Li et al. (2023) identified a six-gene subset whose expression was significantly different in patients with IPF compared to healthy controls. A random forest algorithm was used on a set of more than 600 patients, yielding an AUC of 0.856.

Prognosis

One study proposed that the use of imaging features of quantitative lung fibrosis scores in patients with early stages IPF can predict the progressive fibrosis status later on. New software such as the artificial-intelligence-based quantitative CT image analysis software (AIQCT) of Handa et al. (2022) quantified parenchymal lesions and airway volumes; they suggested that lung volume on HRCT imaging of the chest may provide additional prognostic information on the gender/age/lung physiology stage of IPF.

Since patients with idiopathic pulmonary fibrosis are at a higher risk of developing lung cancer, radiomics could be an early prognostic indicator. Budzikowski et al. (2021) correlated image features with patients' genetic mutations. They stated that the combination of radiomic features and genetic mutations might serve as prognostic indicators.

Another domain that AI is applied to is the investigation of the proteomic signature of ILD. The exact correspondence of cell state changes in diseased organs to peripheral protein signatures currently remains unknown. Certain plasma biomarkers in patients with progressive fibrosing ILD have been identified, and consistent associations across ILD subtypes have been reported. In a recent research study, a proteomic signature comprising 12 biomarkers was derived via machine learning, and suggested that approximately 10% of patients with a low-risk proteomic signature would experience ILD progression in the year after. Mayr et al. (2021), using cross-modal analysis and machine learning, identified the cellular source of biomarkers. They demonstrated that information transfer between modalities predicts disease status, thus also suggesting the feasibility of clinical cell state monitoring.

From an algorithmic point of view, primarily deep learning algorithms are employed, especially in most recent articles. Since the majority of studies in the field of ILDs utilize imaging data, deep learning algorithms are a very appealing choice. Deep learning algorithms have been extensively used in several fields with promising results, especially in the case of image analysis in which they have proven particularly effective.

Future directions

The use of AI and especially deep learning in the analysis of imaging modalities in interstitial lung diseases has been on the rise during the last few years and is far from being saturated. Imaging biomarkers are being identified and correlated with disease outcomes. Also, advanced AI techniques are being utilized with increased generalization capability. Another important factor affecting the acceptance of AI techniques in ILD research, and medicine in general, is the explainability of the reported outcomes, which is gradually becoming available for many algorithms. Nevertheless, the complex nature of ILDs' pathobiology, which encompasses both environmental and genetic interactions, makes the utilization of AI algorithms ideal for this elusive purpose. Another interesting prospect for the use of AI in ILD research is the exploration and characterization of interstitial lung abnormalities.

The use of AI in other lung diseases

Air trapping

One study applied AI to approach the quantification of air trapping on CT scans, an important finding with diagnostic and patient management implications. It is observed in obstructive lung diseases such as asthma, bronchiolitis obliterans syndrome and chronic obstructive pulmonary diseases such as emphysema and chronic bronchitis. While radiologists can easily identify air trapping as areas of persistent hypoattenuation on expiratory images compared with inspiratory images, the evaluation is subjective and changes on serial examinations are difficult to detect. Retson et al. (2021) showed that the use of an AI algorithm improved inter-reader consistency and correlation with pulmonary function testing.

Figure 34. High resolution computed tomography scan of lung showing extensive fibrosis, a large emphysematous bulla and several smaller bullae.

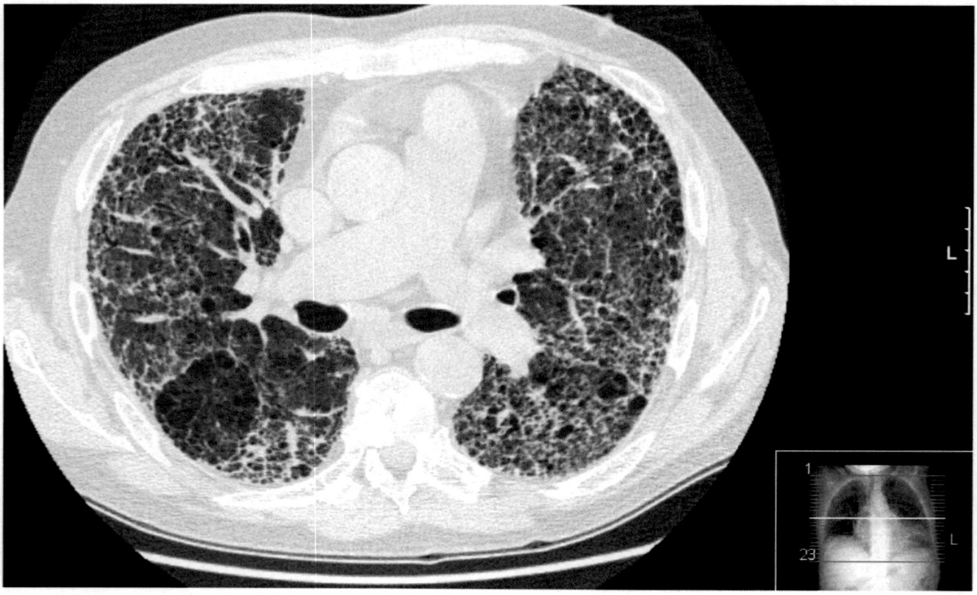

Mesothelioma

DL can be useful for diagnosing lesions with ambiguous histomorphologic features, such as for sarcomatoid mesotheliomas. and for distinguishing cholangiocarcinomas from hepatocellular carcinomas. DL has also been applied to site of origin classification for metastatic cancers of unknown primaries. DL can detect subtle histomorphologic features corresponding to underlying genomic alterations in tumors.

Figure 35. Diffuse pleural mesothelioma with extensive involvement of the pericardium.

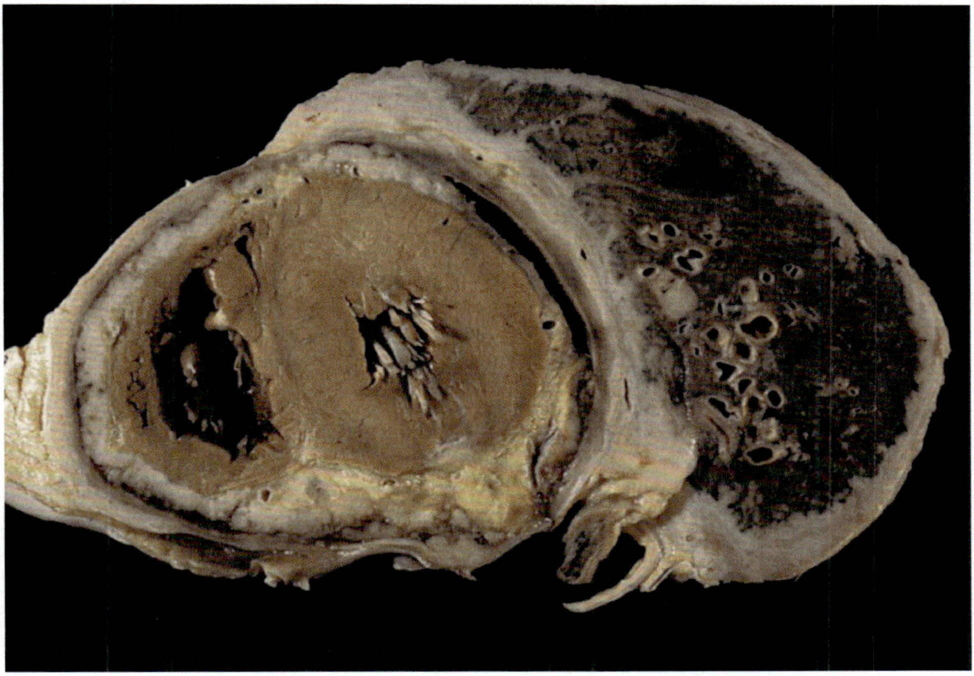

Chapter 10. How AI will improve outcomes in diabetes mellitus

Type 1 diabetes mellitus (T1D)

Type 1 diabetes (T1D) is characterized by pancreatic beta cell dysfunction and insulin depletion. Over 40% of people with T1D manage their glucose through multiple injections of long-acting basal and short-acting bolus insulin, so-called multiple daily injections (MDI). Errors in dosing can lead to life-threatening hypoglycaemia events (<70 mg dl-1) or hyperglycaemia (>180 mg dl-1), as well as an increase in the risk of retinopathy, neuropathy, and nephropathy.

The main current challenge in the treatment of type 1 diabetes is the complete automation of blood glucose control coupled with the automatic infusion of insulin, alone or together with glucagon. This is the so-called "artificial pancreas" - the technological replacement of the pancreatic beta cell destroyed by the autoimmune process. More properly, as the current state of technological advances, it is more correct to define the artificial pancreas as an automated insulin delivery (AID) system, considering that only hybrid AIDs are currently available; hybrid AIDs are insulin pump systems that automatically increase or decrease basal insulin delivery in response to sensor glucose values but also have the capacity to deliver automatic correction boluses. However, the user still needs to dose prandial insulin manually.

Significant advances have been made in the management of T1D including wearable sensors that are positioned on the skin of the abdomen. The sensor samples the blood glucose level continuously and sends a signal to an insulin pump, implanted subcutaneously, to adjust the insulin dose accordingly. Dexcom G6 is an example. No finger pricks are needed and the system has been proven to lower blood HbA1c levels.

As a result of advances in Machine Learning (ML) and Artificial Intelligence (AI), the disease detection and diagnosis of T1D at an initial stage by an automated program was found to be more probable and efficient than manual DM recognition method. Benefits included a decreased workload for medical practitioners and a smaller risk of fault caused by humans. An automated device is capable of identifying DM and handling anomalies with greater simplicity and reliability compared to manual detection and diagnosis.

Tyler et al (2020) described an algorithm that provides weekly insulin dosage recommendations to adults with T1D using MDI therapy. They employed a unique virtual platform to generate over 50,000 glucose observations to train a k-nearest neighbours decision support system (KNN-DSS) to identify causes of hyperglycaemia or hypoglycaemia and determine necessary insulin adjustments from a set of 12 potential recommendations. The KNN-DSS algorithm achieved an overall agreement with board-certified endocrinologists of 67.9% when validated on real-world human data. It delivers safe recommendations.

In silico benchmarking using a platform accepted by the United States Food and Drug Administration for evaluation of artificial pancreas technologies indicated substantial improvement in glycaemic outcomes after 12 weeks of KNN-DSS use. These data indicate that the KNN-DSS allows for early identification of dangerous insulin regimens and may be used to improve glycaemic outcomes and prevent life-threatening complications in people with T1D.

The investigators observed that over 99% of recommendations delivered across 100 weeks of data by the KNN-DSS passed a safety review in which the endocrinologists reviewed each recommendation for the potential to cause hypoglycaemia episodes.

Castle and colleagues (2022) described a decision support system, using an iphone app, designed to provide real-time dosing advice and weekly insulin dose adjustments for adults living with type 1 diabetes using multiple daily insulin injections. They named the system DailyDose. In their trial twenty-five adults were enrolled in a single-arm study. All participants used Dexcom G6 for continuous glucose monitoring, InPen for short-acting insulin doses, and Clipsulin to track long-acting insulin doses. Participants used DailyDose on an iPhone for 8 weeks. The primary endpoint was % time in range (TIR) comparing the 2-week baseline to the final 2-week period of DailyDose use.

They found that there were no significant differences between TIR or other glycemic metrics between the baseline period compared to final 2-week period of DailyDose use. TIR significantly improved by 6.3% when more than half of recommendations were followed compared with 50% or fewer recommendations (95% CI 2.5%–10.1%, P = 0.001). They concluded that the use of DailyDose did not improve glycemic outcomes compared to the baseline period. However, in a post hoc analysis, accepting and following recommendations from DailyDose was associated with improved TIR.

Type 2 diabetes (T2D)

Type 2 diabetes is often diagnosed through blood glucose tests long after the onset of symptoms. Early detection of risk factors, however, could help a patient avoid the disease. Machine learning is a useful tool for scanning vast databases of patient data to extract the most predictive risk factors, but if applied incorrectly can give misleading results.

Ismail and colleagues (2022) first classified risk factors into five categories - lifestyle, medical condition, heredity, psychology and demography - to enable an analysis of which category of risk factors contributed most significantly to the prediction of type 2 diabetes in an individual patient. They then compared the predictive performance of the different models. They found that machine learning methods could identify patterns in patient data to extract correlations between risk factors and the incidence of diabetes. These investigators are currently building an AI-based automated end-to-end patient-centric system for the prediction and management of type 2 diabetes.

Chapter 11. How AI will improve outcomes in gastroenterology

The development of artificial intelligence (AI) has increased dramatically in the last 20 years, with clinical applications progressively being explored for most medical specialties. The fields of gastroenterology, hepatology and pancreatic disease, which are substantially reliant on vast amounts of imaging studies, are not an exception. The clinical applications of AI systems in this field include the identification of premalignant or malignant lesions (e.g., identification of dysplasia or oesophageal adenocarcinoma in Barrett's oesophagus, pancreatic malignancies), detection of lesions (e.g., polyp identification and classification), small bowel bleeding lesion on capsule endoscopy, and pancreatic cystic lesions, development of objective scoring systems for risk stratification, predicting disease prognosis or treatment response (e.g., determining survival in patients following resection of hepatocellular carcinoma), determining which patients with inflammatory bowel disease (IBD) will benefit from biologic therapy), and evaluation of metrics such as bowel preparation score or quality of endoscopic examination.

AI has fostered unprecedented advances in abdominal and pelvic imaging, particularly within the domain of gastrointestinal imaging. AI's contributions have been pivotal in improving detection, diagnosis, and staging of liver and pancreatic diseases. The conceptualisation of diverse AI-based predictive models has broadened the diagnostic spectrum, encompassing gastrointestinal and inflammatory diseases, non-malignant conditions, and the detection of bowel bleeding using cutting-edge technology such as wireless capsule endoscopy.

AI has been instrumental in optimising image quality, accelerating image acquisition, and predicting patient prognosis as well as their response to treatments.

AI has reshaped abdominal and pelvic imaging through its ability to deliver precise and reproducible imaging diagnoses. The technology facilitates automated or semi-automated segmentation and registration of the liver and pancreas, along with their associated lesions.

Special interest has already been devoted to several areas, including the detection of gastrointestinal neoplastic lesions to assist with rapid diagnosis, reduction of misdiagnosis, improvement in quality of imaging, reduction of interobserver variability in visual classifications, and radiologic and histopathologic interpretation.

The central motivation of AI/ML is to use large datasets to recognize patterns of interactions between variables, often in a way that allows the learned function to be applied to new data. ML is composed of both “supervised” and “unsupervised” learning methods. The goal of supervised learning is to predict a labelled output focusing primarily on classifying data input into specific subgroups, or alternately for prediction of quantitative outcomes. An example of supervised learning is training a system to assist in identifying gastric intestinal metaplasia (GIM) using a large database of lesions that have previously been identified by an operator as corresponding to GIM. In comparison, unsupervised learning does not have an output to predict. It relies on attempting to identify naturally occurring patterns from within the input, and to then group them accordingly (e.g., tissue sample clustering based on similar gene expression values). DL autonomously utilizes the data input to learn, identify, and leverage predictive factors of an outcome, which can use multi-layered systems (i.e., convolutional neural networks [CNN]) to process complex information. With increased recognition of the importance of AI in gastroenterology, the first global summit on AI in gastroenterology and endoscopy was held in Washington D.C. in late 2019, and included multiple experts in the domains of academia, industry and regulatory institutions. The consortium anticipated that in the next 10 years the clinical applications of AI in gastroenterology will positively influence patient care and clinical workflow. The consortium recognized the importance of a close multidisciplinary collaboration between gastroenterologists, industry, and regulatory institutions in the development and application of new technologies in the clinical setting.

Upper gastrointestinal tract

Detection of premalignant and malignant lesions

The upper gastrointestinal tract has several areas of interest for detection of premalignant and malignant lesions, including identification of dysplasia and early neoplasia in Barrett’s oesophagus (BE), oesophageal squamous cell carcinoma (SCC), and gastric cancer.

Figure 36. Endoscopic image of Barrett's oesophagus

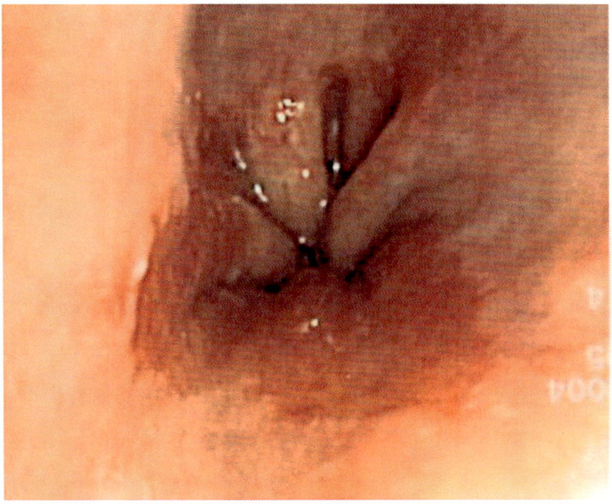

Figure 37. Endoscopic image of patient with oesophageal carcinoma seen at gastro-oesophageal junction.

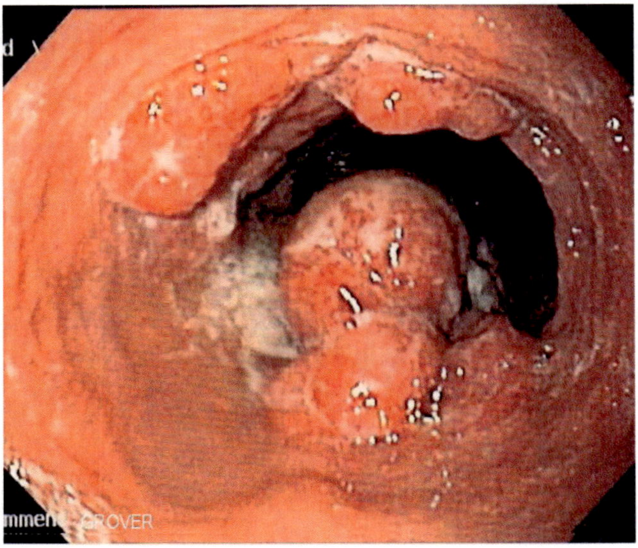

Despite the fact that histopathologic analysis is the gold standard for establishing the diagnosis of BE and determining the presence of dysplasia, it is important for endoscopists to obtain targeted biopsies from specific locations that harbor the actual lesion. By identifying areas that may harbor BE with or without dysplasia, AI can orient the clinician in performing directed biopsies instead of relying on random sampling. Importantly, detection of early esophageal neoplasia with conventional white light imaging (WLI) and digital chromoendoscopy (i.e., narrow band imaging [NBI]) represents a challenge, an issue for which AI has been proposed as a possible solution.

A study by Kröner et al (2021) included evaluation of 8 studies that examined BE, all of which addressed the detection of dysplasia or early esophageal adenocarcinoma (EAC) based on endoscopic imaging or laser endomicroscopy. The most popular analytic models were CNNs and support vector machines (SVMs), while cross-validation techniques were the primary basis of validation methods. In general, the models were able to discern between normal and dysplastic/neoplastic images with an accuracy of at least 89.9%, performing better than nonexpert endoscopists. One study developed a DL algorithm based on a hybrid ResNet-UNet model using 4-fold per-patient cross-validation to detect early neoplasia in BE. The model was trained in a stepwise fashion, using a database with over 490,000 endoscopic still images of the gastrointestinal tract for training, out of which 1,247 corresponded to early BE neoplasia. This model achieved higher level of accuracy than non-expert endoscopists and could also detect the optimal biopsy site in up to 97% of patients. Another study developed a computer-aided diagnosis model based on ResNet that differentiated between normal BE and early EAC, with 89.9% accuracy, 83.7 sensitivity and 100% specificity.

Figure 38. Gastric cancer in a subtotal gastrectomy specimen

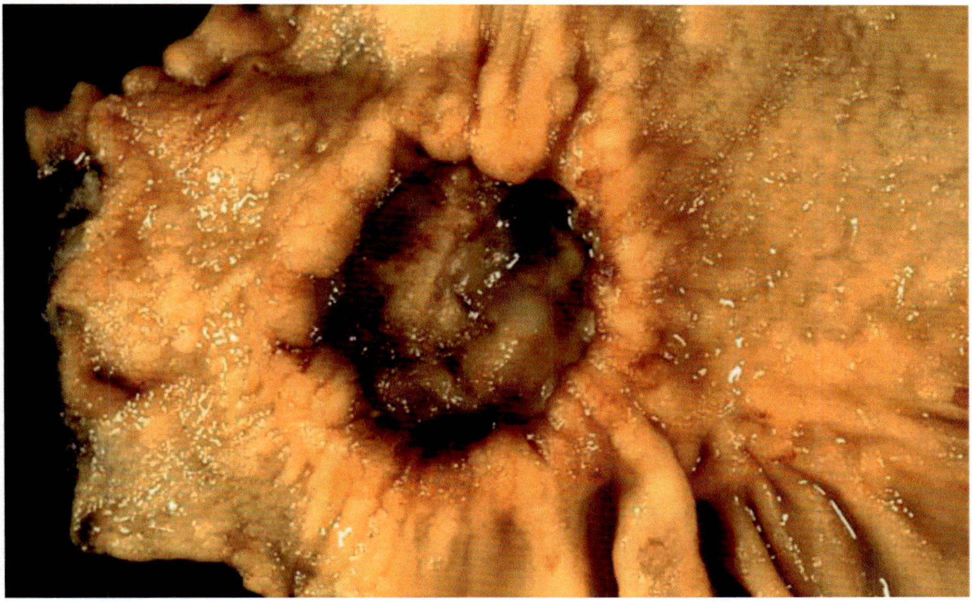

This image is by http://web2.airmail.net/uthman/specimens/index.html, Public Domain, https://commons.wikimedia.org/w/index.php?curid=840055; https://en.wikipedia.org/wiki/Stomach_cancer#/media/File:Adenocarcinoma_of_the_stomach.jpg. This work has been released into the public domain by its author, Ed Uthman. No changes were made to this image.

Identification of gastric cancer poses a similar clinical challenge, because traditional diagnostic techniques have relatively low specificity. As complex novel methods that rely heavily on endoscopic imaging such as endocytoscopy or volumetric laser endomicroscopy have been progressively implemented in clinical practice, the interpretation of large volumes of images is a challenging and time-consuming issue. AI-assisted image interpretation has also found a use in identifying abnormalities in the image inputs of gastric neoplasms.

Kröner's paper also commented on thirteen studies of oesophageal cancer, of which 11 has squamous cell carcinoma (SCC). Nine of the studies targeted DL models for malignancy detection, while two studies aimed to develop models that predicted malignancy depth of invasion using DL models. Most studies were based on CNN models, while others used joint diagonalization principal component analysis (JDPCA), VGG16 Net, or GoogLeNet as classifiers. Although the values of accuracy, sensitivity and specificity in oesophageal cancer detection varied between the studies, all models performed at least as well as endoscopists in lesion detection and characterization or substantially improved the endoscopists' lesion detection. Another study developed a DL model aimed at detecting suspicious lesions and characterizing SCC using more than 28,000 NBI-enhanced images in the construction of the model. The model achieved a higher sensitivity for SCC detection and higher accuracy for SCC characterization from normal tissue than endoscopic experts. Two other studies aimed at developing models that predicted oesophageal malignancy depth utilizing a DL model based on a CNN with a belief-propagation decoder using independent validation datasets. These models achieved an accuracy of 89.2% and 91% in predicting invasion depth, with sensitivities of 70.8% and 90.1%, and specificities of 94.4% and 95.8%, respectively.

Gastric cancer (GC) is the fourth most common cause of cancer-related deaths globally. Identification of premalignant lesions or early gastric neoplasia is of great importance. Unfortunately, as with oesophageal diseases, several studies have shown that conventional endoscopic imaging or other advanced endoscopic modalities (e.g., magnifying endoscopy, blue laser imaging) have relatively low sensitivity and specificity in identifying premalignant or early neoplastic gastric lesions.

Twenty-four studies examined gastric malignancy or premalignant conditions. Eleven (46%) studies directly addressed early GC detection, of which eight models used DL, two used SVM and one used joint diagonalization principal component analysis (JDPCA). The sample size in the training and validation datasets varied from less than 100 million to 1.03 million. The accuracy in early GC detection of all models ranged from 86.5%-98.7%, with sensitivity of 80.0%-96.7% and specificity of 89.2%-100%. Specifically, one study developed a CNN-based model using over 9,000 images to train the algorithm, which not only detected early GC lesions with a 92.5% accuracy, 94.0% sensitivity and 91.0% specificity but also performed significantly better than expert endoscopists. Two studies, one based on faster region-based CNNs and another one based on quantum neural networks, used biomarkers, histology and computed tomography (CT) images to predict metastasis to the liver or lymph nodes. These models predicted metastasis to liver and lymph nodes with sensitivity of 66.7%, specificity 97.1% and an area under the curve (AUC) of 0.95.

Four studies developed models predicting survival in GC or stratification of risk of developing GC. While one model based on SVM achieved higher accuracy than the tumor, nodes, metastasis (TNM) cancer staging system to predict overall survival and disease-free survival, another model based on a preoperative ANN was not superior in predicting survival compared to the TNM system. Other investigators developed a ResNet50-based computer-aided detection and diagnosis (CAD) model to predict GC invasion depth, based on endoscopic images. The model achieved an accuracy of 89.16% in identifying GC invasion depth, compared to 71.49% by endoscopists.

Non-malignant conditions

Helicibacter pylori infection

Currently, the diagnosis of *Helicobacter pylori (H. pylori)* infection, which is a known risk factor for the development of peptic ulcer disease and GC, relies on stool or breath testing and histopathology. Endoscopic identification of *H. pylori* has been a target for AI-assisted systems. For *H. pylori* detection and classification, 4 of 4 studies used a CNN model. One study using gastric biopsy histopathology images as an input with small number of samples (n = 210 in the training dataset and 90-106 in 2 test datasets) had a diagnostic accuracy of 98.9%-99.1% for detecting current *H. pylori* infection. This result was higher than the accuracy achieved in 2 studies using oesophagogastroduodenoscopy images as an input with a higher number of samples (98.9%-99.1% vs 77.5%-87.7%). The mean accuracy of endoscopists for detecting *H. pylori* in 2 studies was around 79.0%-79.4%. Another study found that the average *H. pylori* diagnostic time for the AI model was 194 seconds, while it was 230 ± 65 minutes for endoscopists. The AI model also had a significantly higher accuracy than the endoscopists by 5.3%, demonstrating that AI algorithms had significantly better accuracy and faster diagnostic time for *H. pylori* than the endoscopists. More recently, another study developed a CAD system based on linked color imaging combined with DL, which achieved 82.5% accuracy, demonstrating comparable diagnostic accuracy of *H. pylori* to that of experienced endoscopists.

Figure 39. Micrograph of H. pylori colonizing the stomach lining.

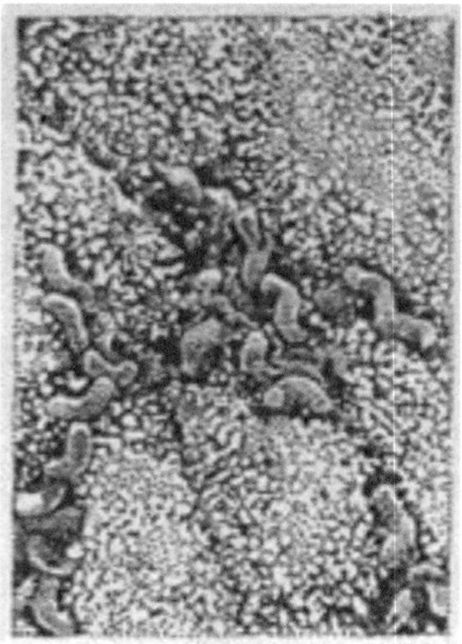

This image is by Helicobacter_pylori.jpg: USGov-HHS-NIHderivative work: F. Lamiot (talk) - Helicobacter_pylori.jpg, Public Domain, https://commons.wikimedia.org/w/index.php?curid=9580156; https://en.wikipedia.org/wiki/Helicobacter_pylori#/media/File:Helicobacter_pylori2.jpgThis image is a work of the National Institutes of Health, part of the United States Department of Health and Human Services, taken or made as part of an employee's official duties. As a work of the U.S. federal government, the image is in the public domain. No changes were made to this image. No changes were made to this image.

Gastro-intestinal bleeding

In the area of gastrointestinal bleeding (GIB), risk stratification is of great importance, not only in identifying high-risk patients and as a guide in clinical decision-making, but to also identify areas where relatively scarce resources require allocation. In general, risk-stratification tools examine risk factors that are associated with a condition to predict one or several outcomes (such as survival, length of hospitalization, rebleeding rates, need for endoscopic therapy, and response to treatment). With regard to upper GIB, studies have focused on developing prognostic models that predict rebleeding or the need for endoscopic/surgical therapy.

Seven studies examining outcome measures in GIB were included, all of which were developed by reviewing medical record parameters to construct ML algorithms, which were primarily based on ANN. Half of the studies had both internal and external validation cohorts, and patient sample sizes varied from 147 to over 22,800.

One study developed a gradient-boosting ML model that identified patients with upper GIB who met a composite endpoint with superior AUC, sensitivity and specificity to that of the Glasgow-Blatchford (GBS), Rockall and AIMS-65 scores. Another study developed 4 different ML algorithms in patients with nonvariceal upper GIB that achieved superior AUC for mortality, rebleeding and hypotension than that of the GBS, particularly with the use of the random forest (RF) analytic model. However, for rebleeding prediction, a gradient-boosting model showed a higher accuracy compared to the previously mentioned study (88% vs 78.5%). Another study developed a predictive ML model for lower GIB and compared it in internal and external validation cohorts to the validated BLEED score. (The BLEED score is a validated scoring system for predicting the risk of bleeding). Both internal and external validation cohorts reached accuracies, sensitivities, and specificities that were superior to the bleeding risk score.

Lower gastrointestinal tract

Direct endoscopic visualization of the colon continues to be the gold standard for detection and resection of colonic premalignant lesions. In addition, patient- and polyp-specific characteristics have also been identified as predictors of missed colorectal cancer (CRC). Therefore, quality measures such as cecal intubation time, withdrawal time, bowel preparation quality and adenoma detection rates (ADR) have been instituted to attempt and standardize practice and mitigate the rates of missed CRC. Since colonoscopy is an operator-dependent procedure, this may lead to variability in polyp detection rates, polyp characterization and estimation of depth of invasion of malignant lesions between endoscopists. CAD has been studied to address these shortcomings, as well as to improve ADR and reduce CRC risk and colon cancer-related deaths.

Detection of premalignant and malignant lesions

Polyp detection during colonoscopy is the cornerstone of CRC prevention. It is estimated that CRC develops in 2%-6% of cases after colonoscopy but before the next scheduled surveillance and, therefore, could represent missed or new CRC. A large number of research studies have been devoted to identifying factors that play a role in the detection of premalignant lesions during colonoscopy, as well as factors that are associated with missed CRC. An observation that has gained considerable attention is that the presence of experienced endoscopy nurses, fellows or any trained second observer during the procedure itself improves ADR. Therefore, and answering the call for improved polyp detection measures during colonoscopy, AI has become a promising technology serving the role of a more standardized "second observer," appropriately termed "computer-aided detection" (CADe).

Figure 40. Gross appearance of a colectomy specimen containing two colorectal polyps and one invasive colorectal carcinoma

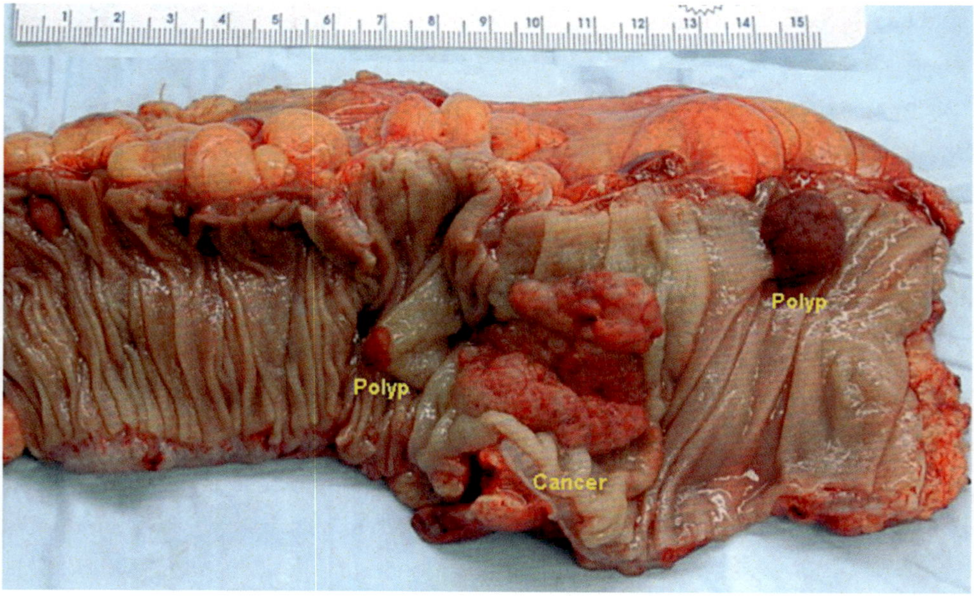

Eighteen studies that evaluated polyp detection were included in the review by Kröner and colleagues, thirteen of which employed DL models, while five used other ML models. Nearly all the studies were limited to having internal validation only. The training datasets in these studies utilized still images from colonoscopy videos ranging from 176 to more than 8,600 images. Seven studies calculated the ADR of the developed model and compared it to that of endoscopists, most of which found that the AI had a significantly higher ADR than endoscopists, while the remaining studies showed an equivalent ADR. A further multicenter study showing that the ADR was 40.4% by the study's participating endoscopists alone, while it was 54.8% in the group using the CADe-based GI-Genius (®Medtronic, Minneapolis, MN) module. Similarly, other investigators conducted a study that evaluated over 520 colonoscopies, examining the use of a CADe model, and found that the ADR increased from 20.34% by endoscopists alone to 29.12% in the CADe-assisted group. Other studies explored the accuracy, sensitivity and specificity of polyp-detection AI models, displaying accuracies of up to 96.4%, sensitivity of up to 99.7% and specificity of up to 93.7%. A study used an SVM-based model using real-time images with NBI and magnification enhancement to detect colon polyps, achieving an accuracy, sensitivity, and specificity of 93.2%, 93.0%, and 93.3%, respectively.

Three studies addressed subjects in the realm of CRC, specifically detecting malignancy on colonoscopy with chromoendoscopy and NBI enhancement, hematoxylin-eosin histopathology slides, or estimating invasion depth on regular WLI colonoscopy images. One study developed a DL model based on CNN to detect deeply invasive CRC based on WLI colonoscopy, which utilized over 9,900 images from 41 patients to train the model. Furthermore, over 5,000 images were used in the testing cohort, achieving an accuracy, sensitivity and specificity in differentiating invasion depth of 81.2%, 67.5%, and 89.0%, respectively. A second study developed a model based on EndoBRAIN (®Cybernet Systems Co., Tokyo, Japan) using colonoscopy with chromoendoscopy and NBI enhancement to detect malignant lesions in the colon. The training sample used over 69,000 images and achieved accuracies of 98.0% and 96.0% for chromoendoscopy and NBI enhancement, respectively. These diagnostic parameters were higher than those of expert and nonexpert endoscopists.

In an attempt to morphologically classify polyps according to their malignant potential, numerous classification systems have been developed. As an example, the Paris classification classifies polyps according to whether they are pedunculated, sessile, slightly raised, or excavated. These visual characteristics are then used to predict whether the polyp has invasive potential or lymph node involvement and potentially contribute to clinical decision-making, such as determining whether the polyp is resectable endoscopically. Unfortunately, research has shown that interobserver variability with this classification is moderately high, suggesting that this visual classification should not be routinely used in research or practice. In addition, considering that most resected polyps during colonoscopy are diminutive and that histopathologic analysis of resected polyps is costly, optical diagnosis has been proposed in this subset of polyps and termed “optical biopsy”. The concept of optical biopsy has been proposed to support cost-effective strategies in CRC screening such as resecting-and-discarding, as well as diagnosing-and-leaving this subset of polyps. However, the concept of optical biopsy has the same limitations as endoscopic polyp characterization does: relatively high interobserver variability. Hence, computer-aided diagnosis has been proposed as a potential solution to standardization of interpretation of endoscopic images.

Nine studies pertaining to colonic polyp classification or differentiation were included in this review. While some studies did not report on validation methods, others had cross-validation, internal, and external methods. Most studies relied on ML-based algorithms to assess colonoscopy with enhancement measures (such as magnification, narrow band imaging (NBI), endocytoscopy), while deep CNN models were used in studies evaluating real-time polyp differentiation. A third study developed an SVM-based model to predict polyp histologic classification using high-definition WLI from 225 colonoscopies, achieving accuracy, sensitivity, and specificity of 91.1%, 92.3%, and 89.2%, respectively. Another study evaluated the performance of EndoBRAIN (®Cybernet Systems Co., Tokyo) in analyzing endocytoscopic images obtained during colonoscopy to characterize polyps as neoplastic vs non-neoplastic with an accuracy, sensitivity, and specificity of 96.9%, 97.6%, and 95.8%, respectively. These findings hold promise in determining screening and surveillance schedules, and in instituting cost-effective strategies such as “resect-and-leave”.

Knowledge on the depth of invasion of early CRC is important for determining resection modality. Intramucosal and submucosal cancerous lesions can be resected with endoscopic techniques such as endoscopic mucosal resection or endoscopic submucosal dissection. However, lesions that invade the deeper layers have a higher association with lymph node metastasis and, hence, may require a combined surgical and medical oncologic approach. Several features on direct endoscopic visualization have been associated with deep invasion of a lesion, including lesion depression, fold convergence, and significantly irregular and heterogeneous surface capillary pattern. As with any image-based field, a significant degree of interobserver variability exists in characterizing lesions and determining their depth or invasion, for which CAD represents an attractive option to standardize the approach of estimating lesion invasion depth.

Finally, 6 studies assessed other subjects within the realm of the lower gastrointestinal tract, including developing models that predict outcomes in patients with CRC, models examining quality of colonoscopy performance, and studies estimating cost reductions of the use of AI. Of 4 studies examining prediction of outcomes, 2 were based on DL (CNN-based) models, using a wide numerical range of histopathologic images: from 300 million to 12 million. One study developed a DL model using over 12 million histopathological images to develop a biomarker for automatic prediction of cancer-specific survival, which outperformed existing markers. The authors concluded that this strategy can potentially be utilized in the treatment selection process by identifying high-risk groups. Another study recently developed a DL model aimed at automatically quantifying quality metrics during colonoscopy, providing intra-procedural feedback to the performing endoscopist.

Non-malignant conditions

Video capsule endoscopy

Owing to its ease of use and noninvasiveness, video capsule endoscopy (VCE) is the current diagnostic method of choice to assess the small bowel for conditions such as occult GIB and Crohn's disease (CD). However, since the capsule lacks self-locomotion, it relies on the motility of the bowel to advance down the gastrointestinal tract. Therefore, it requires a very large number of images (up to 60,000 per examination) to be automatically obtained, rendering the process of interpretation lengthy and tedious. VCE has been an area of focus for AI since its early stages, using AI classifying methods such as SVM and multilayer perceptron network. With faster processors, increased computational power with improved graphics processing units and evolving CNNs, DL algorithms have become the modality of choice for image analysis in VCE. As with the lower gastrointestinal tract, the same principles of CADe and computer-aided diagnosis could be applied to deep balloon-assisted or motorized enteroscopy systems.

Figures 41. Side view of a wireless video capsule

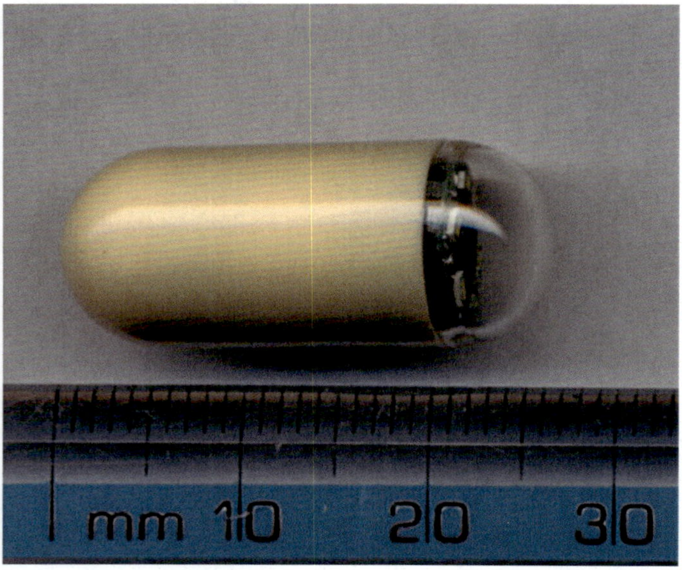

Figure 41. Front end view of a wireless video capsule showing 6 LEDs and the camera lens

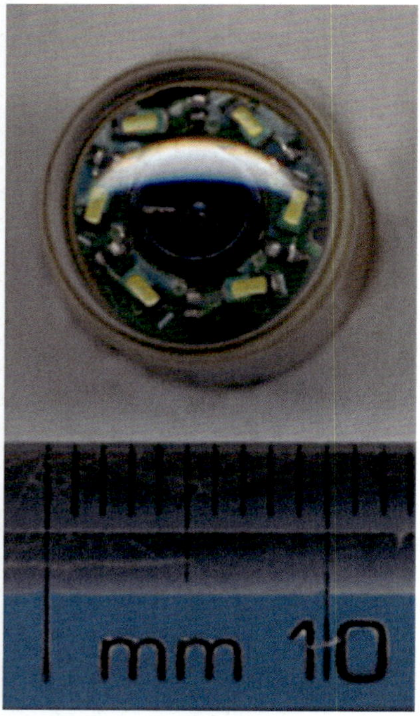

Figure 41 is by No machine-readable author provided. Euchiasmus assumed (based on copyright claims). - No machine-readable source provided. Own work assumed (based on copyright claims)., Public Domain, https://commons.wikimedia.org/w/index.php?curid=819900; https://en.wikipedia.org/wiki/Capsule_endoscopy#/media/File:CapsuleEndoscope.jpg. The copyright holder of this work has released this work into the public domain. No changes were made to this image.

Figure 42 is by No machine-readable author provided. Euchiasmus assumed (based on copyright claims). - No machine-readable source provided. Own work assumed (based on copyright claims)., Public Domain, https://commons.wikimedia.org/w/index.php?curid=819900; https://en.wikipedia.org/wiki/Capsule_endoscopy#/media/File:CapsuleEndoscopeEnd.jpg. The copyright holder of this work has released this work into the public domain. No changes were made to this image.

A total of 31 studies pertaining to VCE were identified. Fifteen studies (48%) developed models to assist in detection of active GIB or angioectasia. Four studies used CNN, five used SVM, and the remaining ones used ML-based analytic models. Five studies reported cross-validation methods. All studies reported accuracy ranging from 94% to 98% in identifying GIB and angioectasias, with a sensitivity of 92.0%-100% and specificity of 82.9%-99.9%. Specifically, one study developed a DL model based on CNN for angioectasia detection, which achieved an AUC of 0.998, with a sensitivity and specificity of 98.8% and 98.4%, respectively.

(Angioectasia is an acquired vascular malformation associated with advanced age. Pathogenesis of colonic angioectasia formation is multifactorial and commonly attributed to mild chronic venous obstruction and to chronic mucosal hypoxemia resulting in increased vascular endothelial growth factor (VEGF) expression).

Six studies assessed for the presence of small intestinal ulcers, of which five used DL models based on CNN and one used SVM. One group conducted 2 studies in testing DL models to detect ulcerations, yielding a sensitivity of 88.2%, a specificity of 90.9%, and an AUC of 0.958, respectively. Two more studies evaluated the detection of small-bowel CD by identifying ulcers on VCE. One of these developed a DL model based on CNN that used over 17,000 VCE images to identify CD ulcers, achieving an AUC of 0.99. Two studies examined small intestinal polyp detection using NN-based models, both achieving an accuracy of at least 98%, with sensitivity and specificity of up to 95.5% and 98.5%, respectively.

Celiac disease

Regarding celiac disease (CeD) detection, 4 studies were evaluated, 3 of which used CNN and 1 that used a clinical decision support system. One study reported 100% sensitivity and specificity in detecting CeD using GoogLeNet as classifier. Another study using AlexNet, VGGf net, and VGG-16 net as classifiers obtained an optimal accuracy of 92.5% using VGG-16, although the report did not include sample size.

(VGG Image Annotator is a simple and standalone manual annotation software for image, audio and video).

More recently, other investigators developed a DL model using the CNN-based InceptionV3 as well as the SVM-based ResNet50 that was 95.94% accurate, 97.20% sensitive and 95.63% specific in identifying common elements of data (CED) in video capsule endoscopy (VCE) images.

Figure 43. Duodenum of a person with coeliac disease showing scalloping of folds and "cracked-mud" appearance to mucosa

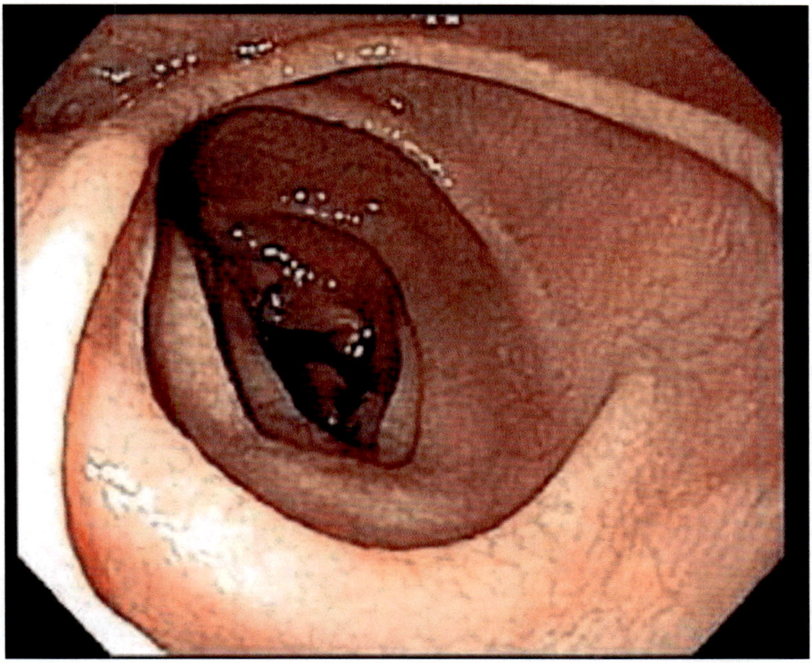

Hookworm infection

Hookworm infection represents a significant healthcare issue in low income countries, with an estimated 600 million people having this infection. As this helminth typically dwells in the small bowel, it may occasionally be a finding in VCE. Three studies evaluated hookworm detection, of which two used CNN and one used SVM with all using cross-validation. Specifically, one study developed a DL model based on deep CNN, which was trained on a large VCE dataset consisting of more than 44,0000 images. The model outperformed other handcrafted, feature-based methods, reaching an accuracy of 88.5% and a sensitivity of 84.6% in detecting hookworm in the small bowel.

Figure 44. Hookworms on intestinal mucosa

This image is by transferred from en.wikipedia to Commons. This media comes from the Centers for Disease Control and Prevention's Public Health Image Library (PHIL), with identification number #5205., Public Domain, https://commons.wikimedia.org/w/index.php?curid=1877700; https://en.wikipedia.org/wiki/Hookworm#/media/File:Hookworms.JPG. This image is a work of the Centers for Disease Control and Prevention, part of the United States Department of Health and

Human Services, taken or made as part of an employee's official duties. As a work of the U.S. federal government, the image is in the public domain. No changes were made to this image.

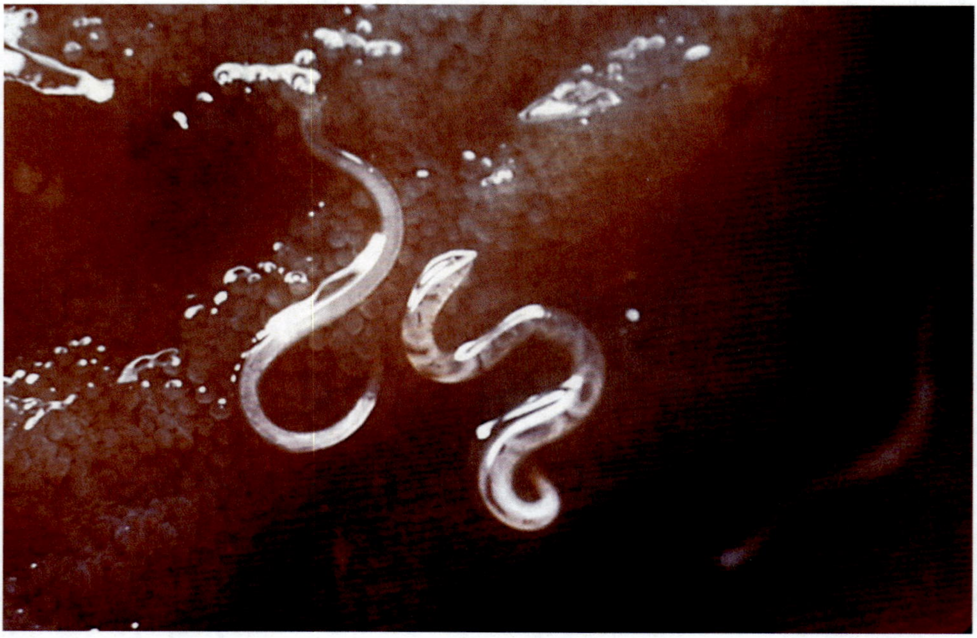

Bowel preparation

To assess quality of bowel preparation during VCE, two studies developed a DL model based on CNN. Both models achieved accuracy of over 95%, with sensitivity and specificity of 94.7%-96.18% and 94.0%-94.33%, respectively. A DL model based on CNN to identify and categorize all small bowel ulcers, polyps, bleeding, lymphangiectasia, follicular hyperplasia, protruding lesions, diverticula or inflammation used over 100 million VCE images. The model achieved an impressive 99.90% overall sensitivity and 99.88% specificity, whereas gastroenterologists identified lesions with a 74.57% sensitivity in the per-patient analysis and 76.89% sensitivity in the per-lesion analysis. Furthermore, the reading time per patient was 5.9 min by the CNN model, compared to 96.6 min by conventional reading.

Inflammatory bowel disease

The complex interplay of pathophysiological factors in inflammatory bowel disease (IBD) has led to the realization that differences in patients' biology may confer differences in disease activity and response to therapy- an example of the use of "precision medicine". Integration of AI algorithms into the IBD realm brings promise not only in diagnosis or in reducing interobserver variability in severity grading, but also opens up the possibility of analysing large databases to identify complex or occult patterns of disease.

Figure 45. Resected ileum from a person with Crohn's disease

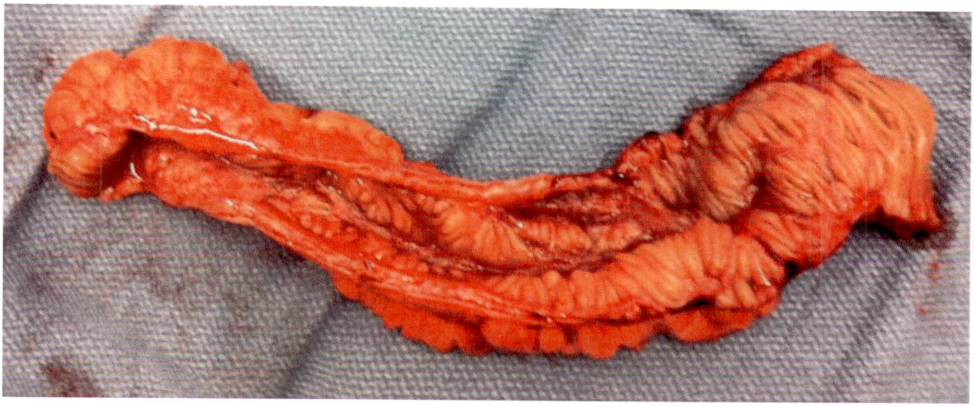

Figure 46. Normal colon on the left side of the image and severe ulcerative colitis on the right side of the image showing pseudopolyps

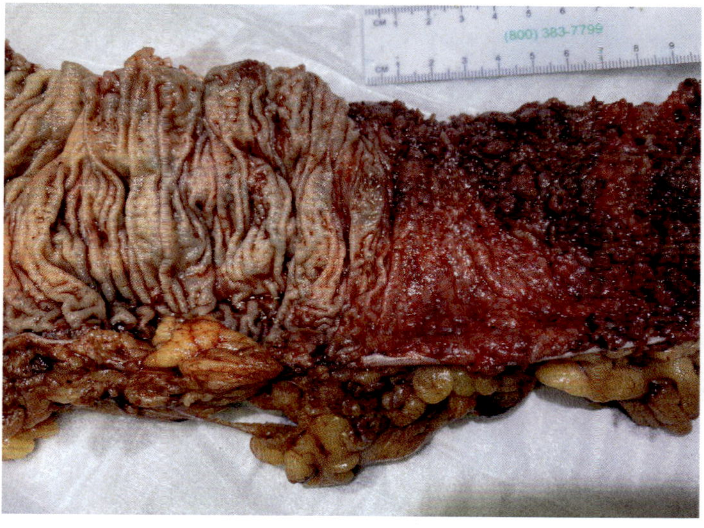

A total of 25 studies pertaining to IBD were included in the review by Kröner and colleagues, of which 9 dealt with Crohn's disease (CD), 6 studied ulcerative colitis (UC,) and 10 investigated both. Five studies aimed to detect CD, UC, or IBD in general from VCE images, endoscopic images, histology, magnetic resonance imaging (MRI) images, and genetics. Most of the studies used cross-validated ML methods, of which SVM was the method of choice; while another study used DL-based CNN. These studies displayed high levels of accuracy in detecting IBD, from 83.3%-90.8%. One group developed a DL model based on CNN that used more than 10,000 VCE images in the validation dataset to detect CD ulcers in the small bowel, achieving an accuracy, sensitivity and specificity of 90.8%, 88.2% and 90.9%, respectively.

Nine studies that addressed predicting disease severity were primarily based on endoscopic imaging. Five studies utilized ML-based analytic models, while the remaining four utilized DL-based models, of which CNNs were the preferred ones. Five studies reported internal validation, and two studies had external validation cohorts, while two studies did not report validation. The size of patient cohorts varied greatly, from 87 to over 3,000, with studies reporting up to 40,000 images in the validation datasets. One study designed a DL model based on CNN to grade the severity of UC using colonoscopy images, which was constructed with over 16,000 images from 3,000 patients. The reported accuracy, sensitivity, and specificity was 87.6%, 90.2%, and 87.0%, respectively. The authors concluded that these results supported the use of AI in UC severity grading, since they approximated the scores of experienced human reviewers. Another study designed a ML model with CAD to detect histologic inflammation based on colonoscopy images enhanced with endocytoscopy. The model achieved an accuracy, sensitivity and specificity of 90.0%, 74.0%, and 91.0%, respectively, using over 9,900 images from 100 patients in the validation cohort.

To predict therapeutic response in patients with IBD treated with thiopurines or biologics, seven studies constructed internally validated ML algorithms, based on RF analytic models. All models achieved an accuracy of 80.0%-89.8% or an AUC of 0.73-0.846 in identifying patients who would respond at 6-8 weeks to therapeutic regimens. One study designed a model using only demographic and laboratory data from 401 patients to predict response at 8 weeks in patients receiving ustekinumab with an AUC of 0.78, potentially laying the foundation to avoid costly therapeutic drug monitoring. (Ustekinumab is a monoclonal antibody developed for the treatment of Crohn's disease, ulcerative colitis, plaque psoriasis and psoriatic arthritis, targeting both IL-12 and IL-23).

Another study also constructed a model based on laboratory values and demographics with a validation dataset of over 6,100 patients to predict IBD-related hospitalization and outpatient steroid use, achieving an AUC of 0.87, suggesting such AI models could be used to identify patients at risk of an IBD flare and enable precision medicine-based therapeutic approaches.

A further 2 internally validated ML models using SVM and RF were developed to predict the risk of IBD based on a genomic datasets. One developed a gene prioritization model using 4 combined analytic models (RF, SVM GB, and an elastic net regularized generalized linear model) to identify genes related to IBD, achieving an accuracy of 80.8%. An internally validated natural language processing (NLP) model used histopathology reports to identify surveillance vs nonsurveillance colonoscopy in patients with IBD, with an accuracy of 80.0%. Lastly, a study developed an internally validated model based on Waikato Environment for Knowledge Analysis which identified, with an accuracy of up to 89.8%, patients with IBD who required a bone mineral density scan, using electronic health record data.

The latest advances in AI in gastroenterology are promising for many fields of clinical care, from detection of neoplastic lesions on endoscopic assessment and improving current survival models to predicting treatment response. The application of AI to large and complex datasets may assist in the identification of new associations between variables, potentially leading to changes in clinical practice. Furthermore, the use of AI-assisted technologies has the potential to dramatically improve the quality of care. Finally, the time for assisted precision medicine is at hand, with the AI being able to tailor a treatment regimen or potentially predict the response to treatment in a specific patient based on extensive amounts of clinical data from large patient datasets. It is important to realize that, while AI currently does not substitute for human clinical reasoning, it has a bright future in the improvement of patient care.

Chapter 12. How AI will improve outcomes in disease of the liver

Liver diseases range from asymptomatic elevation of liver function on blood tests to life-threatening conditions such as acute liver failure or orthotopic liver transplantation (OLT). Hepatology is a fertile ground for applying AI in survival models (e.g., model for end-stage liver disease), disease detection models (e.g., early detection of non-alcoholic fatty liver disease [NAFLD]), disease severity models (e.g., alcoholic hepatitis discriminant function) as well as for pattern recognition in radiological images, histopathology and even selection of liver transplant candidates.

Christou and Tsoulfas (2021) reviewed the application of AI to liver disease.

Fatty liver/steatosis

In one study multiple AI/ML models were developed as a basis for a non-invasive tool for assessing the level of fibrosis progression in NAFLD patients. Notably, the Random Forest (RF) model demonstrated the best performance. A different study developed an ML model for patients at high risk of developing NAFLD to classify patients with non-alcoholic fatty liver (NAFL) and non-alcoholic steatohepatitis (NASH). In another study, four different AI/ML-based models were developed utilizing data from biochemical and enzyme-linked immunosorbent assays to classify patients with NAFLD and alcoholic liver disease with or without cirrhosis.

Figure 47. The progression of fatty liver disease to cirrhosis

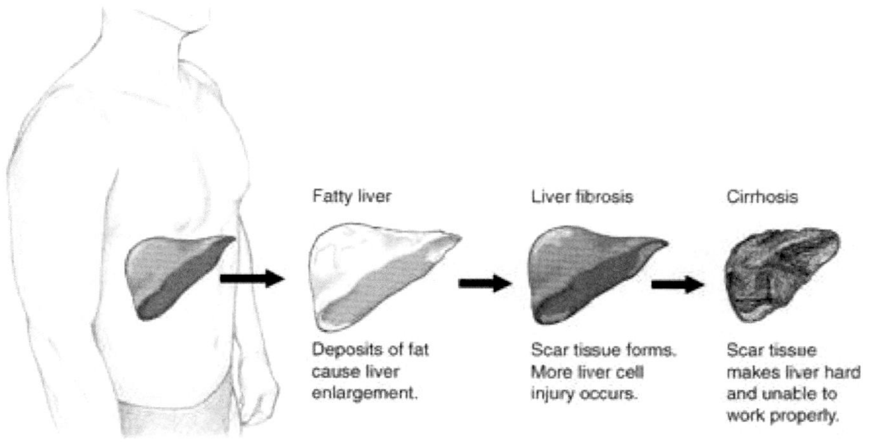

The original uploader of this image was Countincr at English Wikipedia.(Original text: National Digestive Diseases Information Clearinghouse) - https://catalog.niddk.nih.gov/catalog/ImageLibrary/detail.cfm?id=154, Public Domain, https://commons.wikimedia.org/w/index.php?curid=2310132; https://en.wikipedia.org/wiki/Fatty_liver_disease#/media/File:Stage_of_liver_damage.JPG. This work is in the public domain in the United States because it is a work prepared by an officer or employee of the United States Government as part of that person's official duties under the terms of Title 17, Chapter 1, Section 105 of the US Code. No changes were made to this image.

Hepatitis

AI/ML models that utilize data directly from the electronic health records from patients infected with hepatitis B (HBV) and hepatitis C (HCV) could be used as the basis for targeted screening tools for liver carcinomas. A gradient boost (GB) model was developed in a study using only serum markers aiming to predict fibrosis and classify the stage of fibrosis in two cohorts of patients with HBV and HCV. An ANN model was developed in another study that employed only routine clinical data to predict significant fibrosis for patients with HBV. In a similar study, an ANN model was developed by employing only routine laboratory data from HBV patients to identify patients with a cirrhotic liver. A different study developed an ANN model employing only non-invasive data to predict advanced liver fibrosis in HCV patients. A similar study developed several AI/ML-based models to develop a non-invasive tool for identifying HCV patients with advanced fibrosis. Among the developed models, a model based on alternating decision trees (DTs) demonstrated the best performance. These studies demonstrate how AI/ML models using routine clinical data can be used to identify patients who will benefit from a sustained virological response (SVR) to delay chronic liver disease progression.

In HBV management, one study developed several AI/ML-based models that used soluble immune markers to predict early virological relapse after discontinuation of nucleoside analog treatment. The model could be used to exclude patients at high risk of virological relapse from treatment cessation.

In HCV management, a study utilized data from full-length HCV genome sequencing of variants of HCV to develop multiple AI/ML-based models that classify HCV anti-viral resistance variants. Notably, the SVM model demonstrated the highest performance.

Figure 48. This electron micrograph shows the presence of hepatitis-B virus (HBV) "Dane particles", or virions. These particles measure 42nm in their overall diameter, and contain a DNA-based core that is 27nm in diameter.

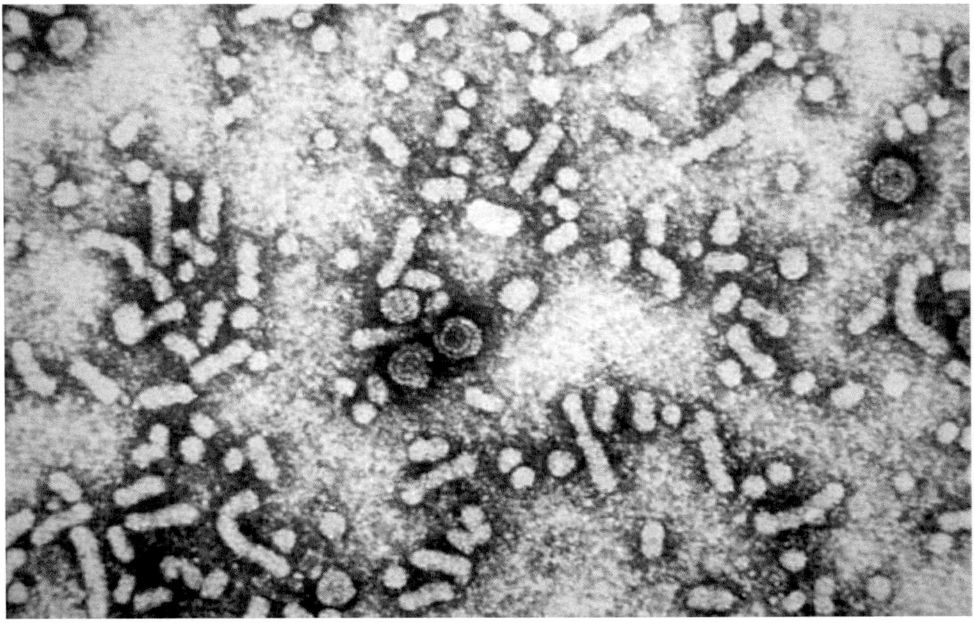

This image is by CDC - This media comes from the Centers for Disease Control and Prevention's Public Health Image Library (PHIL), with identification number #5631. Public Domain, https://commons.wikimedia.org/w/index.php?curid=9023749; https://en.wikipedia.org/wiki/Hepatitis_B#/media/File:Hepatitis-B_virions.jpg. This image is a work of the Centers for Disease Control and Prevention, part of the United States Department of Health and Human Services, taken or made as part of an employee's official duties. As a work of the U.S. federal government, the image is in the public domain. No changes were made to this image.

Figure 49. Electron micrographs of hepatitis C virus purified from cell culture. Scale bar is 50 nanometers.

This image is by HCV_pictures.png: Maria Teresa Catanese, Martina Kopp, Kunihiro Uryu , and Charles Rice derivative work: TimVickers (talk) - HCV_pictures.png, Public Domain, https://commons.wikimedia.org/w/index.php?curid=10903740. Electron micrographs of hepatitis C virus purified from cell culture. Scale bar is 50 nanometers. Public Domain, https://commons.wikimedia.org/w/index.php?curid=10903740; https://en.wikipedia.org/wiki/Hepatitis_C#/media/File:HCV_EM_picture_2.png. This work has been released into the public domain by its author, Charles Rice. No changes were made to this image.

Figure 49. Electron micrographs of hepatitis C virus purified from cell culture. Scale bar is 50 nanometers.

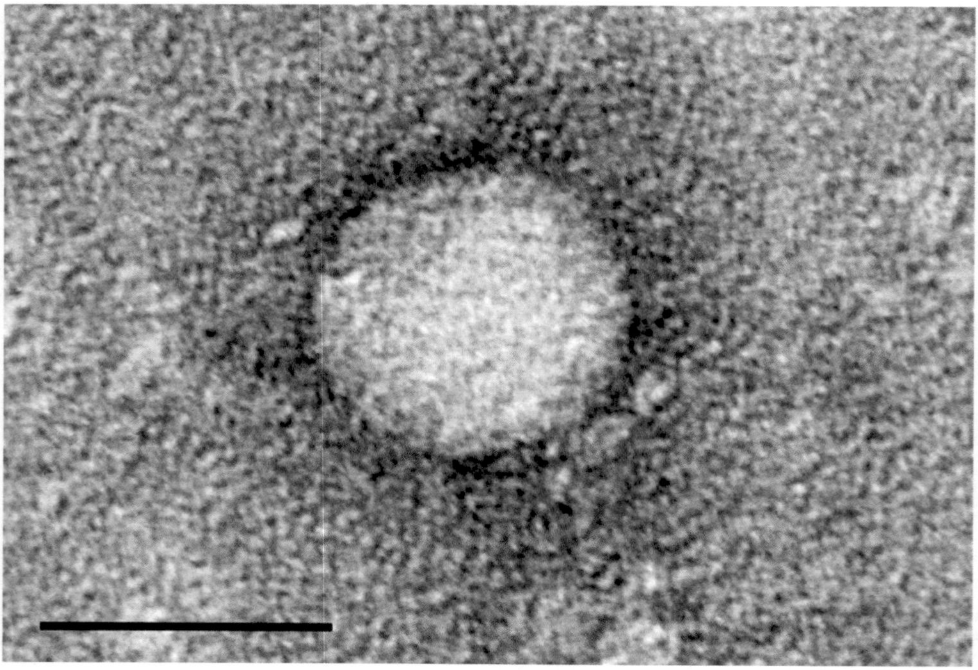

One study using variables including demographic, laboratory results, and clinical findings, developed RF, DNN, and LR models to reliably predict the stage of liver cirrhosis in patients infected with HCV. Accurately predicting patients with HCV prone to develop HCC could help identify patients who would benefit from targeted screening and who are in a greater need of antiviral treatment to achieve a sustained virological response (SVR).

Hepatocellular carcinoma (HCC)

CT imaging was employed to develop an ANN model that differentiates between hepatocellular carcinoma (HCC), intrahepatic peripheral cholangiocarcinoma (CCA), hemangioma, and metastasis. Interestingly, when radiologists evaluated the images, their performance significantly increased when they considered the ANN's output, from an AUROC of 0.888 to one of 0.934.

A retrospective study developed a CNN that employed MRI images of patients with HCC. The model was trained with a combination of images that met the Liver Imaging Reporting and Data System (typical) and with images that did not (atypical). In a multicenter, retrospective study, a CNN was developed that employed MRI scans to identify HCC lesions. Notably, the model surpassed the performance of less experienced radiologists in the diagnosis of small HCC lesions. The model was able to analyze 100 images in just 3.4 seconds. Finally, a different study aimed to develop a non-invasive ANN model that predicts the presence of microscopic vascular invasion and the tumor grade of HCC.

Figure 50. Hepatocellular carcinoma This specimen is from a 50ish woman who presented to the hospital with abdominal pain and ascites.

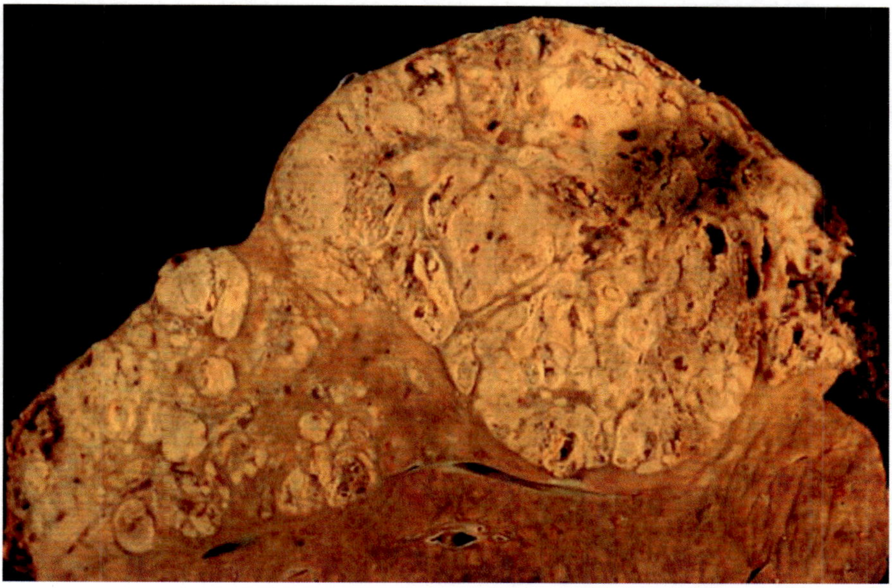

This image is by http://web2.airmail.net/uthman/specimens/index.html, Public Domain, https://commons.wikimedia.org/w/index.php?curid=841059; https://en.wikipedia.org/wiki/Hepatocellular_carcinoma#/media/File:Hepatocellular_carcinoma_1.jpg. This work has been released into the public domain by its author, Ed Uthman. No changes were made to this image.

Cholangiocarcinoma (CAA)

Regarding diagnosis of CCA and pancreatic adenocarcinoma, one study developed an ANN model using data generated by metabolomic and proteomic analyses of bile from patients undergoing endoscopic retrograde cholangiopancreatography aiming to classify patients with and without cancer. A different study used data from the plasma levels of bile acids to develop six different AI/ML-based models to classify patients as having CCA or a benign biliary disease. Among the six developed models, a model based on the Naive Bayes classifier demonstrated the best performance. Finally, in another study, an ANN model was designed to analyze images from magnetic resonance cholangiopancreatography to diagnose CCA with a reported accuracy of 92.8%.

Figure 51. Cholangiocarcinoma in human liver

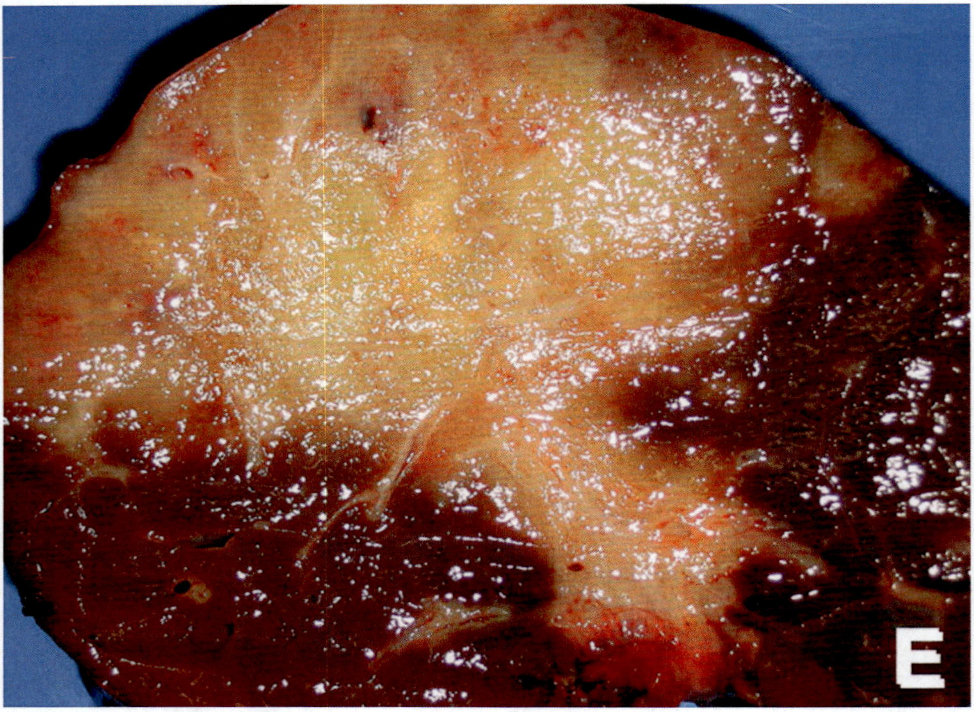

Figure 52. Immunohistochemistry for CK19 in metastatic cholangiocarcinoma to the liver. The positive staining supports the diagnosis, in contrast to hepatocellular carcinoma which is typically CK19 negative. (CK19 is also known as Keratin, type I cytoskeletal 19).

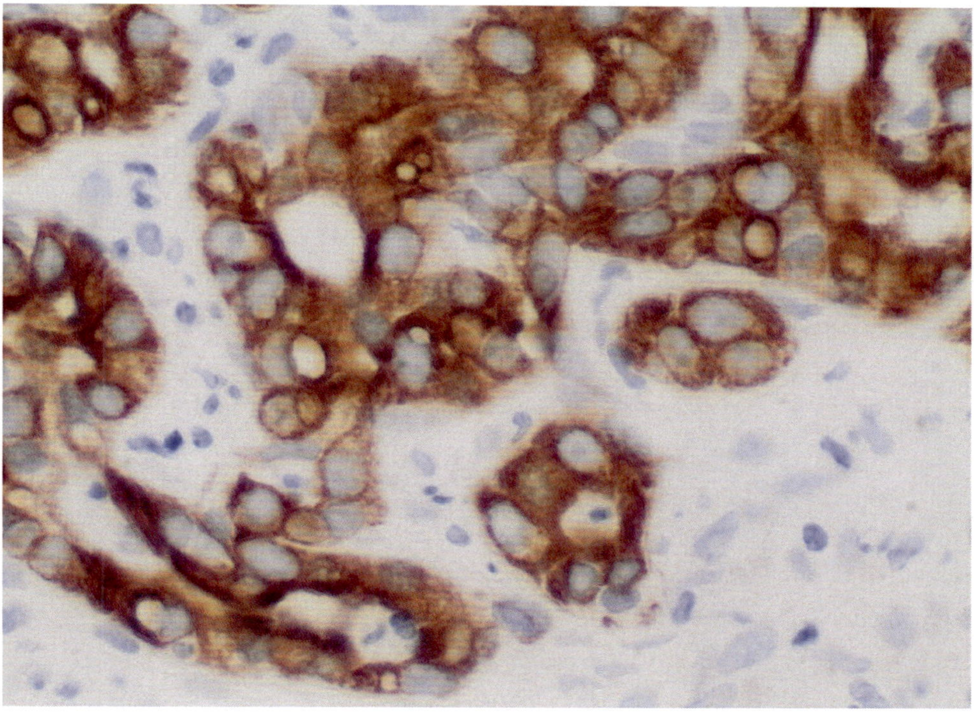

Primary sclerosing cholangitis

A team of researchers derived and validated a risk estimate tool based on GB algorithms to predict the outcomes of the disease. In a different study, an ML model was developed to predict survival curves for patients with primary sclerosing cholangitis following liver transplantation. The P value of the $\chi 2$ test of the distributional calibration was 1, indicating excellent calibration of the model.

Figure 53. Cholangiogram of primary sclerosing cholangitis

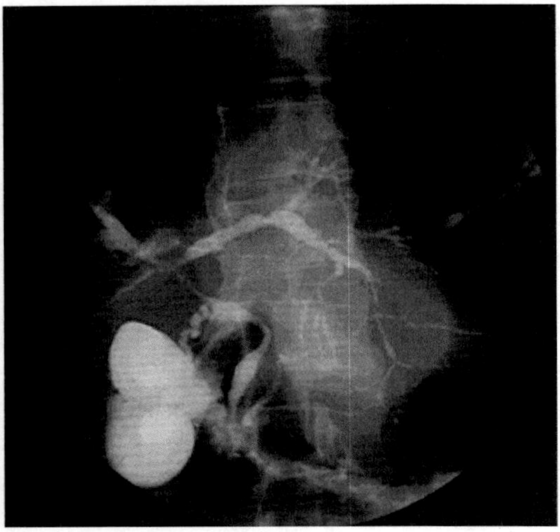

Liver transplantation

A team developed an ANN model combined with genotyping for microsatellite mutations/deletion to predict HCC recurrence in a cohort of patients receiving a liver transplant. Several other studies have focused on the survival of individual liver transplant recipients. In a multi-centre study, the authors developed an ANN model to predict the 3-month graft survival and loss rate. Interestingly, their model outperformed all extensively validated scores, including the model for end-stage liver disease (MELD), the donor risk index (DRI), the survival outcome following liver transplantation, and the balance of risk. In a different study, an RF model was developed to predict the 30 day graft failure rate. Notably, this model too outperformed MELD and DRI.

Figure 54. Human liver

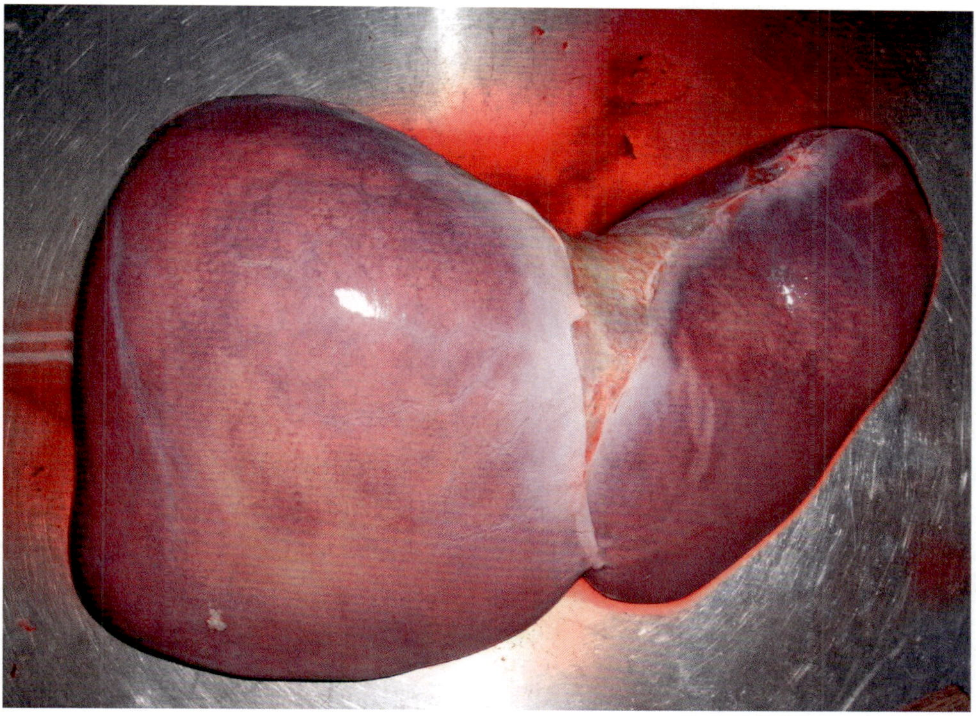

Disease management

With the guidance of AI/ML-based software trained by data generated from gene mutation biomarkers, serum markers, imaging, and the clinical setting, high-quality, evidence-based, and individualized treatments could be employed including chemotherapy, radiotherapy, and immunotherapy.

In HCC management a recent study used data from DNA methylation profiling to develop an RF-based model that predicted 6-month progression-free survival. Such models could be used to personalize patient surveillance. In an international, multi-institutional study, a CART model was developed that aimed to create a framework beyond the Barcelona-Clinic-Liver-Cancer (BCLC) staging system, which is currently endorsed by guidelines for treatment allocation. The model defined six distinct prognostic groups of patients based on predictive factors of overall survival that could be used as a framework for treatment allocation. Notably, the radiologic tumor burden score, which is not integrated into the BCLC staging system, was found as the best predictor of long-term outcome for BCLC stage B patients. These findings could help re-evaluate HCC management into a multidisciplinary, individualized approach that goes beyond the BCLC criteria.

In the management of patients with CCA, in an international study, a CART model was developed with solely preoperative variables to identify patients who would be more likely to benefit from surgery. The model managed to isolate four distinct prognostic groups of patients with similar patient outcomes. The authors concluded that this model could be used to inform presurgical decisions - for example, the use of neoadjuvant therapy for patients with poor prognoses. In a different study researchers developed a DNN model to establish an AI framework through which specific prognostic groups could be used to identify which patients were more likely to benefit from different treatment modalities such as neoadjuvant chemotherapy or transarterial chemoembolization. The framework was found to be significantly more accurate than the current guidelines of the American Joint Committee of Cancer. Finally, a study developed an ANN to predict which patients with inoperable hilar CCA will develop early occlusion following a bilateral plastic stent placement.

Diagnosis

AI/ML models provide the opportunity for increased diagnostic accuracy of various hepatic diseases and with multiple diagnostic modalities (such as US/CT/MRI imaging and histologic images). Current efforts include CAD models for the diagnosis of chronic liver disease, HCC and CCA. Deep learning techniques are useful for distinguishing cholangiocarcinomas from hepatocellular carcinomas.

AI/ML models that accurately and reliably predict the response to specific treatments could be used to tailor evidence-based frameworks for individualized treatment allocation. Current efforts include the development of frameworks for the management of HCC and CCA.

Prognosis

An ANN model was developed in a study to identify patients with HBV cirrhosis at a high risk of developing oesophageal varices. In a different study, two different RF models were created using clinical data, the first to identify oesophageal varices and the second to classify patients with oesophageal varices that required treatment.

Regarding HCC, several studies have focused on developing AI/ML-based models that would reliably predict patient outcomes (survival and recurrence). A retrospective study compared the performance of an ANN, an LR model, and a DT to predict the 1-, 3-, and 5-year disease-free survival in patients with HCC following resection. A similar study used a nationwide database to compare an ANN and an LR model in predicting the 5-year survival of patients with HCC following hepatic resection and concluded that the ANN model surpassed the performance of the LR model. In a different study by the same group, an ANN model and an LR model were compared, but instead, the outcome was in-hospital mortality, and the ANN was found superior to the LR model. Regarding predictors, a different study comparing ANN and LR models reported that the ANN model identified a greater number of significant predictors than the LR model. In a prospective study that aimed to compare an ANN model's performance to the performance of traditional staging systems in predicting survival for patients with early HCC, the ANN model outperformed the Hepato-Pancreato-Biliary Association's system, the TNM system, and the BCLC staging system with higher reported AUROCs in all training, internal validation, and external validation cohorts. In another study, a gradient boosting (GB) survival classifier-based model was developed to stratify the risk of an HCC-related death into three distinct categories. Finally, in another study, an ANN identified albumin-bilirubin grade as the most important prognostic factor for the survival of patients with HCC treated with the combination of transarterial chemoembolization and sorafenib as initial treatment. A systematic review aimed at comparing the performance of AI/ML-based software and that of traditional linear prediction models in predicting survival for patients with HCC concluded that AI/ML models provided enhanced accuracy.

Apart from survival, other studies have developed AI/ML models to predict the recurrence of HCC following treatment. An interesting study employed several AI/ML methods, including Artificial Plant Optimization, SVM, and RF to predict HCC recurrence following radiofrequency ablation. Another study developed a CNN employing histopathologic images to predict recurrence in operated HCC patients. A different study developed an SVM model to predict the recurrence in a group of patients who underwent radiofrequency ablation.

Chapter 13. How AI will improve outcomes in diseases of the pancreas

AI can be effectively applied to pancreatic diseases. Of primary interest is the use of AI in improving existing disease severity scoring systems or prognostic models in complicated acute pancreatitis (AP) or chronic pancreatitis (CP), based on clinical and radiological data, detection and differentiation of pancreas cystic neoplasms (PCN) with prediction of malignant potential, radiologic early detection of pancreatic ductal adenocarcinoma (PDAC), radiologic differentiation between PDAC and benign pancreatic conditions (for example, autoimmune pancreatitis (AIP), and histopathologic interpretation of tissue samples. A total of 59 studies pertaining to the pancreas were reviewed. Of these, 20 (34%) addressed prediction of outcomes in patients with pancreatic diseases ranging from acute pancreatitis (AP) to neoplasia.

Figure 55. Axial CT in a patient with acute exudative pancreatitis showing extensive fluid collections (black areas) surrounding the pancreas

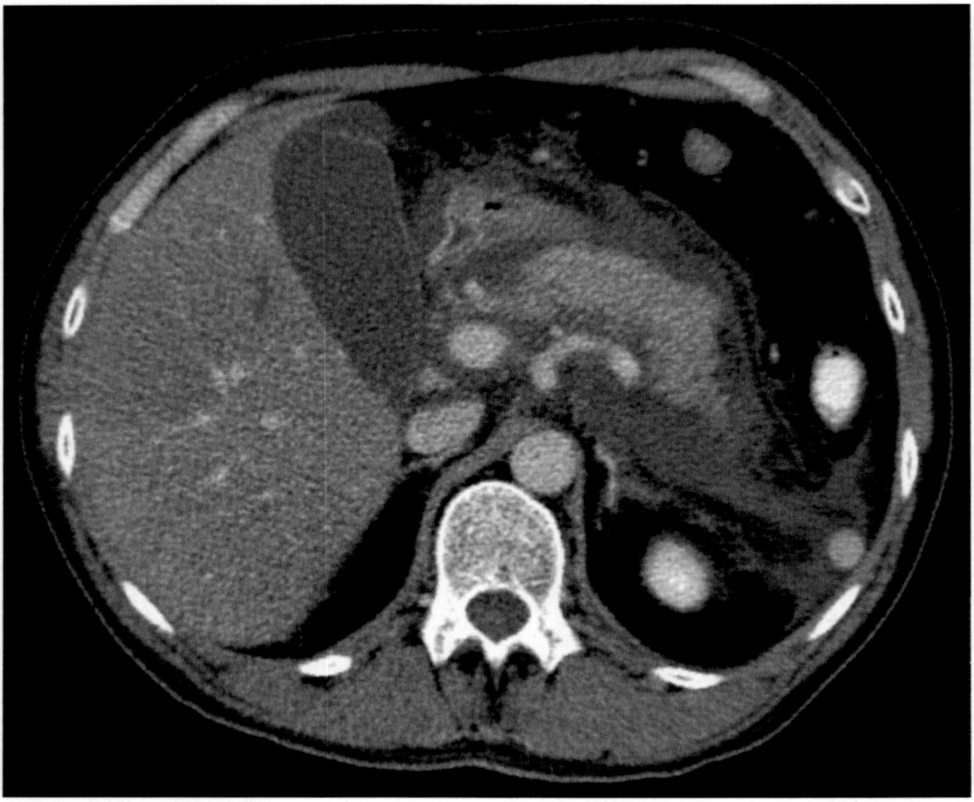

Figure 56. Axial CT showing multiple calcifications (arrow) in the pancreas in a patient with chronic pancreatitis

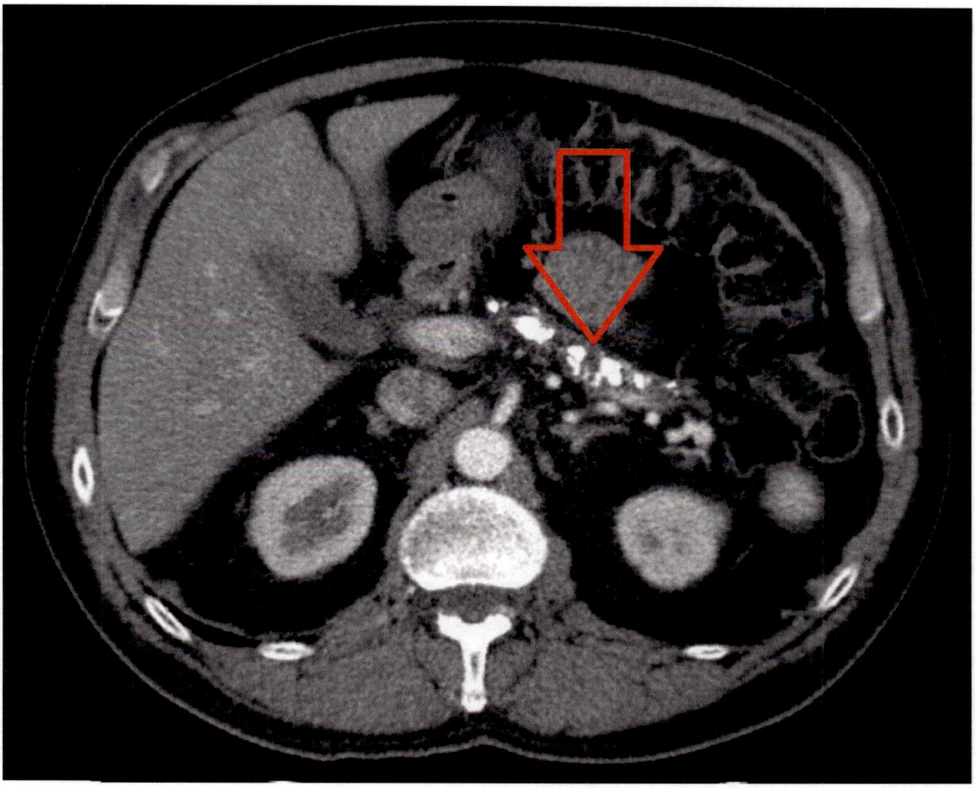

Eleven of these studies examined outcome prediction in AP. All the ANN models outperformed logistic regression models, Glasgow, and APACHE-II scoring systems in predicting AP severity, while requiring a lower number of parameters. Another study compared the performance of SVM, logistic regression analysis, and ANN models to predict multiorgan failure in AP. All 3 models predicted multiorgan failure, with AUC of 0.840, 0.832, and 0.834, respectively, with ANN requiring a lesser number of parameters.

Seven studies used AI algorithms to construct clinical registries, segment the pancreas based on imaging, or differentiate between certain pancreatic diseases based on cross-sectional imaging or endoscopic ultrasound (EUS). Another study constructed a DL station classification model and a segmentation model to reduce the difficulty in EUS interpretation for trainees. The trainee station recognition accuracy improved from 67.2% to 78.4% in the crossover study. Inter-observer agreement between endoscopists and deep CNN with Cohen's kappa coefficient was substantial, ranging from 0.826-0.879.

Figure 57. Cross-section of a human liver, at autopsy, showing many large pale tumor deposits that are metastatic tumours from pancreatic cancer

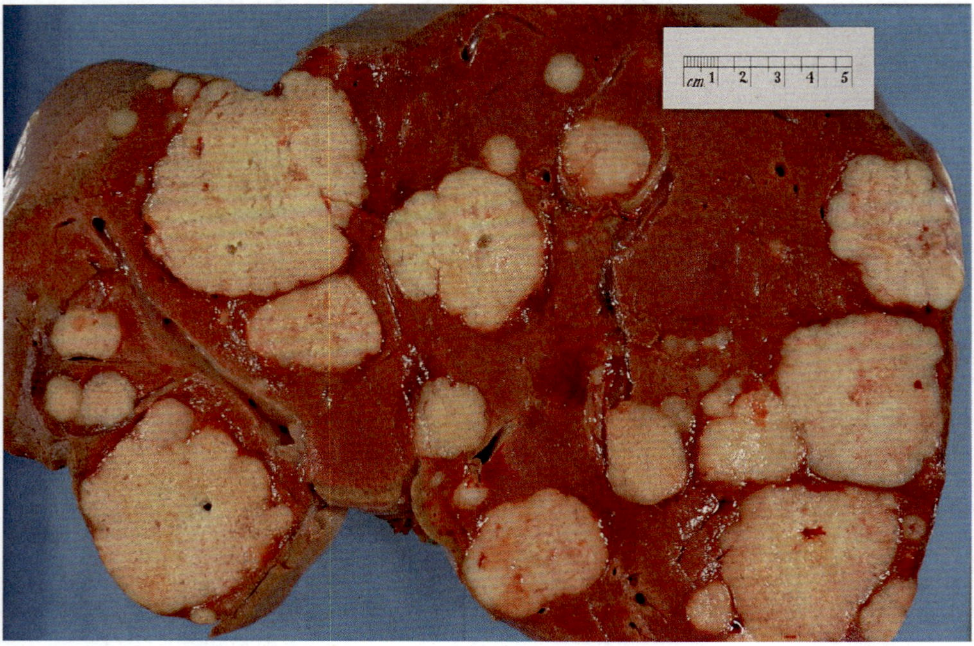

Fifteen studies addressed prediction of malignancy based on imaging findings, or differentiation of benign from malignant pancreatic conditions. Investigators developed an EUS-based CNN model that distinguished AIP from normal pancreas with 99% sensitivity and 98% specificity, AIP from CP with 94% sensitivity and 71% specificity, and AIP from PDAC with 90% sensitivity and 93% specificity. A study was conducted a utilizing CT radiomics features to differentiate PDAC from normal pancreas tissue. The accuracy of the RF binary classification was 99.2%, with an AUC of 99.9%. All cases of PDAC were correctly identified, with a sensitivity of 100% and specificity of 98.5%.

Other studies evaluated differentiation of pancreatic cystic neoplasms (PCNs) by classifying them into their respective subtypes based on their characteristics on imaging. One study developed a multimodality ML model that integrated clinical, radiological and genetic/biochemical markers data to determine whether patients with a pancreatic cyst should undergo surgery, monitoring, or no further surveillance. The model correctly identified serous cystic neoplasms in 65% of the cases with 99% specificity, clearly outperforming the current standard of care of clinical identification in only 18% of cases. The authors concluded that these systems may serve an adjunct role in clinical practice, enabling the clinician to make better informed clinical decisions.

Eight studies addressed pancreatic ductal adenocarcinoma (PDAC), from developing risk scores for development of PDAC based on urinary biomarkers, predicting clinical performance and response to celiac plexus neurolysis, to prediction of survival time. AI models performed at least as well as the logistic regression models in predicting the selected outcome.

Six studies directly examined early pancreatic cancer detection in PDAC or PCN by examining the imaging characteristics or identifying high-risk patients on electronic health records based on factors such as a family history of pancreatic cancer. One developed NLP-based algorithms based on common terminology used by physicians in describing pancreatic cysts and applied them to automatically conduct searches in electronic health records. The algorithm tracked patients with cysts with a 99.9% sensitivity and 98.8% specificity, demonstrating its utility in capturing the diagnosis swiftly and with more ease than manual review. Another study developed a CAD image-processing system using EUS images to diagnose PDAC, taking patient age into consideration. The accuracy of the model was 87.5, with sensitivity and specificity of 83.3% and 93.3%, respectively.

Thus, AI's fusion with endoscopic ultrasound technology has substantially improved both the accuracy and speed of diagnosing pancreatic carcinoma, consequently enhancing patient management strategies (Najjar et al., 2023).

Chapter 14. How AI will improve outcomes in cancer

The four commonest cancers are lung cancer, breast cancer, colo-rectal cancer and prostate cancer.

In precision oncology the synergy between AI, markedly increased computing power, and deep learning strategies, coupled with the integration of multi-omics data, has streamlined cancer diagnosis, prognosis, and treatment. In tumour detection and classification, AI is increasingly being used to discern between benign and malignant lesions and various tumour types, particularly in the diagnosis for breast, lung, and prostate cancers, with AI-based devices already being introduced into clinical practice. Studies have revealed that deep learning models and CNNs can classify lung nodules on CT scans and differentiate renal cell carcinoma subtypes on MRI with high accuracy, often rivalling the expertise of experienced radiologists.

By computing the image pixel-by-pixel, radiomics expands the definition of image features from a computer perspective. By computing the image texture and density using different mathematical techniques, the region of interest area can be converted to higher dimension data and expressed as a huge matrix. Because the principle of radiomics is mathematics, the various image qualities of CXRs give the computer another task. To obtain accurate radiomics data, image augmentation is an important procedure before nodule detection, including pre-processing, lung segmentation, and rib suppression.

AI algorithms such as those used in machine learning, deep learning, and radiomics have shown remarkable capabilities in the detection and characterization of lung nodules, thereby aiding in accurate lung cancer screening and diagnosis. These systems can analyse various imaging modalities, such as low-dose CT scans, PET-CT imaging, and chest radiographs, accurately identifying suspicious nodules and facilitating timely intervention. AI models have exhibited promise in utilizing biomarkers and tumor markers as supplementary screening tools, effectively enhancing the specificity and accuracy of early detection. These models can accurately distinguish between benign and malignant lung nodules, assisting radiologists in making more accurate and informed diagnostic decisions.

Additionally, AI algorithms hold the potential to integrate multiple imaging modalities and clinical data, providing a more comprehensive diagnostic assessment. By utilizing high-quality data, including patient demographics, clinical history, and genetic profiles, AI models can predict treatment responses and guide the selection of optimal therapies. Notably, these models have shown considerable success in predicting the likelihood of response and recurrence following targeted therapies and optimizing radiation therapy for lung cancer patients. Implementing these AI tools in clinical practice can aid in the early diagnosis and timely management of lung cancer and potentially improve outcomes, including a decrease in mortality and morbidity.

Lung cancer

Worldwide, lung cancer is the commonest type of cancer, and the leading cause of cancer death. In 2020, 2.2 million new cases were diagnosed, and 1.8 million people died from lung cancer, representing 18% of all cancer deaths. Lung cancer deaths are expected to rise globally to nearly 3 million annual deaths by 2035, due to high rates of tobacco use and aging populations. Lung cancer is divided into two types – the very aggressive small cell lung cancer in 15% of cases and non-small cell lung cancer in the rest.

Although experts were shown to detect more pulmonary nodules on CXRs, approximately 20% of lung nodules <3 cm are missed by radiologists. In the 21st Century, the prediction accuracy of pulmonary nodules on CXRs has improved with computer-aided diagnosis systems or AI-based programs. The sensitivity of radiologists improved from 65.1% to 70.3% with the assistance of AI and the false negative rate decreased from 0.2 to 0.18, changing the diagnosis in 6.7% of the cases. In CT images, more than 90% of lung nodules were detected by AI-based programs.

CheXNet, a radiologist-level deep learning algorithm trained on Chest-Xray14, one of the largest CXR databases in the world, exceeds radiologist performance in the detection of 14 pulmonary diseases, including lung nodules and lung masses with an area under the receiver operating curve (AUROC, AUC) of 0.78 and 0.87, respectively. Further deep learning models increased the sensitivity to 0.83 with a false-positive rate of 0.2 per CXR.

Figure 58. Lung cancer seen on CXR (red arrow)

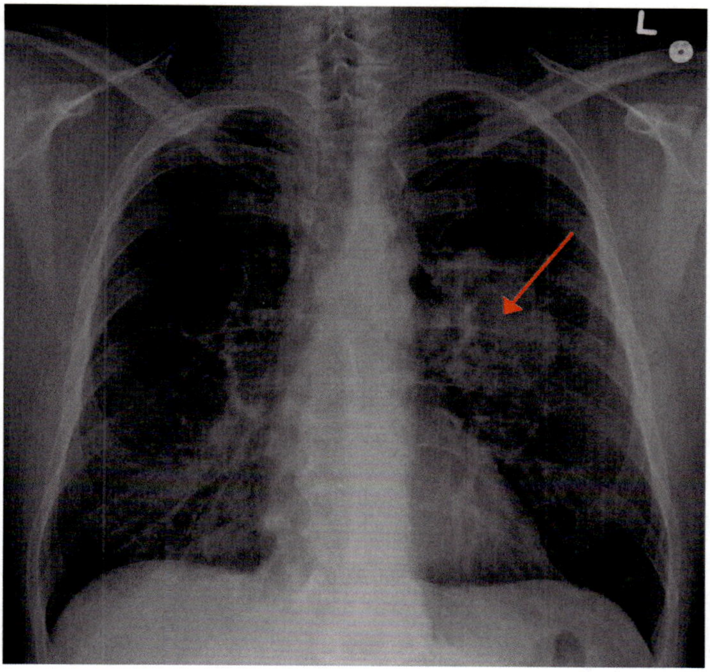

Chiu and colleagues (2022) reviewed the applications of AI to the management of lung cancer. They concluded that AI has the potential to help to treat lung cancer from detection, diagnosis and decision making to prognosis prediction. AI could reduce the labor involved in radiological tests such as CT scanning and chest radiographs, and in the reading of pathology slides. AI as a second reader in radiology reduces the effort of radiologists and increases the accuracy of nodule detection. The addition of AI helps to predict molecular phenotypes with radiomics and H&E staining. By extracting radiomics from image data and whole slide images (WSI) from the histopathology field, clinicians could use AI to predict tumor properties such as gene mutation and programmed death ligand (PD-L1) expression. Furthermore, AI could help clinicians in decision-making by predicting treatment response, side effects, and prognosis prediction in medical treatment, surgery, and radiotherapy.

The FDA has approved several AI programs in CXR and chest CT reading, which enables AI systems to take part in lung cancer detection. Following the success of AI application in the radiology field, AI was applied to digitalized whole slide imaging (WSI) annotation. Integrating with more information, such as demographics and clinical data, AI systems can play a role in decision-making by classifying epithelial growth factor receptor (EGFR) mutations and PD-L1 expression. AI systems also help clinicians to estimate the patient's prognosis by predicting drug response, the tumor recurrence rate after surgery, radiotherapy response, and side effects.

Lung nodule

When a lung nodule is detected, clinicians need to know the properties of the lung nodule. The gold standard is to acquire tissue samples via either biopsy or surgery. Aside from imaging features, the histopathological features also determine further treatment. Whole slide imaging (WSI) has digitized digital histopathology. With digitalized WSI data, AI can help pathologists with tasks ranging from tumor cell recognition and segmentation, histological subtype classification, PD-L1 scoring, and tumor-infiltrating lymphocyte (TIL) count. Each WSI digital slide is a large image. It may contain more than 4 billion pixels and may exceed 15 GB when scanned with a resolution of 0.25 micrometers/pixel.

Researchers used logistic regression of radiomics and clinical features to distinguish small cell lung cancer from non-small cell lung cancer with an AUC of 0.94 and an accuracy of 86.2%. The LASSO logistic regression model was used to classify adenocarcinomas and squamous cell carcinomas in the NSCLC group. Further molecular features such as Ki-67, epidermal growth factor receptor (EGFR), anaplastic lymphoma kinase (ALK), and programmed cell death 1 ligand, (PD-L1) were also shown to be predictable with AI-analyzed radiomics - a non-invasive and simple method.

Several studies were conducted to find the benchmark model of nodule detection using CT scanning. The best algorithm achieved a sensitivity of 97.2% at one false-positive rate per scan. AI has also been proven to help radiologists increase the sensitivity of nodule detection. Many studies have used AI algorithms to detect lung nodules in chest CT images.

Lung nodule classification and malignancy prediction are important tasks in nodule detection. Nodules are classified according to their texture as solid, part-solid, or non-solid, and their size. An AI model trained on the Multicentric Italian Lung Detection (MILD) trial dataset and externally validated on the Danish Lung Cancer Screening Trial (DLCST) showed that AI performed equivalently to a human expert on six different textures (sold, part-solid, non-solid, calcified, peri-fissural, and speculated). The classification was then used to predict the malignancy probability as recommended by the Lung CT Screening Reporting and Data System (LUNG-RADS) and the Fleischner guideline.

Similar to nodule detection on CT scanning, studies were conducted to compare the prediction models. In 2015 the LUNGx Challenge for computerized lung nodule classification was established. Ten teams sent their reports with AUC between 0.50 and 0.68, and only three of them performed statistically better than a random guess, while radiologists performed with AUC between 0.70–0.85. The technology advanced rapidly in the ISBI 2018 Lung Nodule Malignancy Prediction Challenge, and 11 participants completed the challenge with an AUC between 0.70–0.91. The top five participants used deep learning models with AUC between 0.87–0.91 without significant differences from each other. The accuracy was 93% with a sensitivity of 82% and precision of 84% based on the weighted voting method of the autoencoder, ResNet and 96% with deep convolutional network learning.

Genomics

Genomics is currently one of the most popular topics in oncology. With the polymerase chain reaction (PCR) amplification method and related technology, scientists can now analyze the whole genome, exome, transcriptome, and epigenome of cancers and produce large sets of information about patients and their tumors. By analyzing whole-genome and whole-transcriptome sequencing data from treatment-naïve patients in The Cancer Genome Atlas (TCGA), the machine learning model successfully discriminated cancer-free healthy controls from patients with cancer.

To handle the extremely large number of variables produced by proteomics, researchers have used machine learning methods to reduce dimensionality and feature selection. In 2003 machine learning methods were applied to analyse 1,676 original and 124 prescreened mass spectra data from 24 diseased and 17 healthy specimens, and researchers successfully built predictive models to discriminate lung cancer specimens from healthy specimens. However, the most accurate predictions were obtained using less interpretable models. Following this idea, the urine proteome combined with machine learning analysis successfully established models that can discriminate lung cancer samples not only from healthy ones, but also from samples from other cancers.

Histopathology and genetic markers

It is difficult to perform histological subtyping of lung cancer without special immunohistochemistry (IHC) staining. In the detection of lymph node metastasis, a well-trained AI model can help reduce human workload and prevent errors. It performs better than a pathologist in a limited time and has a greater detection rate of single-cell metastasis or micro-metastasis.

Although WSI with H&E-stained slides is designed to view the morphology of tissues, with the aid of AI, researchers have designed methods to predict specific gene mutations, PD-L1 expression level, treatment response, and the prognosis of patients. Focusing on lung adenocarcinoma, one study developed an AI application using Inception-V3 for the prediction of frequently appearing gene mutations including STK11, EGFR, FAT1, SETBP1, KRAS, and TP53. The AUC of this prediction reached 0.754 for EGFR and 0.814 for KRAS which can be treated with effective targeted agents. Another study used ResNet-18 as the backbone to predict the PD-L1 status in NSCLC. Their model showed an AUC between 0.67 and 0.81, when different PD-L1 cutoff levels were chosen.

Next-generation sequencing (NGS) plays an important role in modern lung cancer treatment. Successful NGS testing depends on a sufficient number of tumor cells and tumor DNA. AI can assist in determining tumor cellularity. In addition, a trained AI can help count immune cells, when the tissue specimen is adequately stained for specific surface markers. Since the PD-L1 expression level is the key predictor for immunotherapy in lung cancer, AI has been trained to count the proportion score for PD-L1 expression. When properly stained, computer-aided PD-L1 scoring and quantitative tumor microenvironment analysis may meet the requests of pathologists, eliminate inter-observer variations and achieve precise lung cancer treatment.

The identification of driver mutations, expression of PD-L1 and oncogenes significantly affects the treatment of choice in lung cancer. Using WSI and radiomics, AI could help to identify EGFR mutations, ALK expression, and PD-L1 expression. EGFR mutation subtypes have also been classified using radiomic features.

Medication selection

A retrospective analysis of data from prospective clinical trials found that an AI model based on the random forest algorithm and CT-based radiomic features predicted the treatment sensitivity of nivolumab with an AUC of 0.77, docetaxel with an AUC of 0.67, and gefitinib with an AUC of 0.82.

Surgery

The gold standard for the treatment of early-stage lung cancer is surgical resection. AI was applied to pre-surgical evaluation, and prognosis prediction after surgery, and helped identify patients who were suitable candidates to receive adjuvant chemotherapy after surgery.

In pre-surgical evaluation, radiologist-level AI could help predict visceral pleural invasion and identify early stage lung adenocarcinomas suitable for sub-lobar resection. After surgery, AI could play a role in predicting prognosis. The model based on radiomic feature nomograms could identify high-risk groups whose postsurgical tumor recurrence risk was 16-fold higher than that of low-risk group.

A CNN model pre-trained with the radiotherapy dataset successfully predicted a 2-year overall survival after surgery. The model integrating genomic and clinicopathological features was able to identify patients at risk for recurrence and who were suitable to receive adjuvant therapy.

Radiotherapy

Stereotactic body radiotherapy (SBRT) is currently the standard of care for treating early-stage lung cancer and/or provide local control for patients who are medically inoperable or who refuse surgery. Radiomics-based models have been reported to successfully predict 1-year tumour recurrence using CT scans performed after 3 and 6 months of SBRT. Lewis and Kemp also developed a model trained on the Cancer Genome Atlas (TCGA) dataset to predict cancer resistance to radiation. As a well-known side effect of radiotherapy, radiation pneumonitis can be lethal. An AI model based on pretreatment CT radiomics was superior to the traditional model using dosimetric and clinical features in predicting radiation pneumonitis. Another ANN algorithm trained with radiomics extracted from a 3D dose map of radiotherapy was shown to predict the acute and late pulmonary toxicities of radiotherapy with an accuracy of 0.69.

Breast cancer

The incidence of breast cancer has been increasing, with breast cancer surpassing lung cancer as the most commonly diagnosed cancer in women. Despite advances in diagnostic modalities, the current workflow for breast cancer diagnosis is not without errors. In breast pathology, AI algorithms have been applied to tasks such as cancer detection, classification, histological grading, lymph node (LN) metastasis detection, biomarker quantification, and genetic abnormality prediction, such as the BRCA mutation (Ahn et al., 2023).

Screening

Breast imaging has played a pivotal role in reshaping early cancer detection and reducing mortality in breast cancer since the first mammogram was developed in 1913. The introduction of imaging modalities, such as mammography (MMG), has significantly improved the initial detection of cancer, precise segmentation and characterization of cancerous lesions, as well as monitoring treatment response and post-treatment follow-up. Consequently, two-dimensional (2D) MMG has been widely adopted as the gold standard screening test for women in many countries worldwide, offering cost-effective and scalable approaches. However, there is inherent difficulty in detecting cancers using 2D MMG because of overlapping structures in pathological regions. In particular, the difficulty in interpreting mammograms increases with breast density. Dense breasts have a higher proportion of glandular and fibrous tissues, which can mask potential tumors and make them appear similar to normal breast tissue on mammograms. Because breast cancer may be missed or diagnosed at a later stage in women with dense breasts (characterized by ≥ 75% density on MMG), they are at a higher risk of breast cancer.

In regions, such as the USA, alternative forms of MMG, such as digital breast tomosynthesis (DBT), are being explored. DBT, also known as three-dimensional

MMG, provides a more detailed and clearer view of breast tissues. Thus, the chances of detecting cancerous lesions are increased, while reducing false-positive findings and recall rates compared to 2D MMG. Nonetheless, the drawback of the added three-dimensional information is that it requires radiologists to review multiple image slices, leading to an increased reading time.

Figure 59. Mammograms showing a normal breast (left) and a breast with cancer (right)

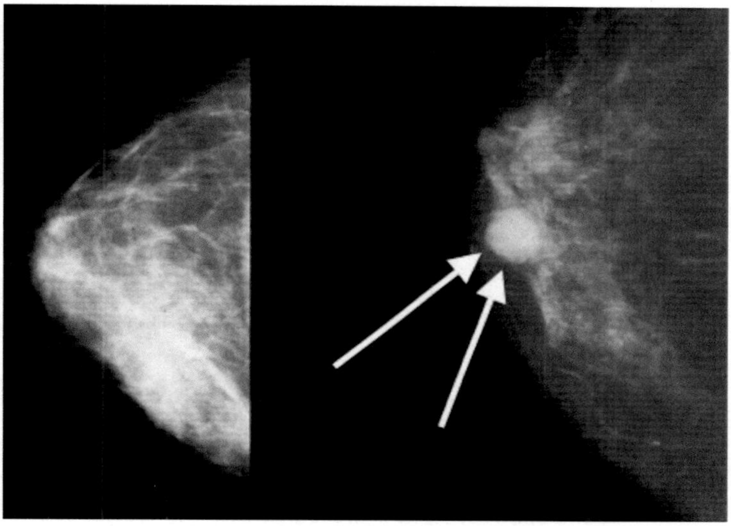

CAD systems

The introduction of digital imaging has significantly increased data availability, prompting the development of computer-aided detection (CAD) algorithms to assist with data interpretation. The first CAD algorithm that obtained a USA Food and Drug Administration (FDA) clearance in 1998, showed improved cancer detection in 2D MMG by presenting regions of interest (ROIs) to radiologists, thereby aiding focused reviews. Traditional CAD approaches rely on rule-based methodologies that incorporate domain knowledge to extract handcrafted radiologic features from abnormal tissues, such as pixel values, surrounding pixels, texture, and shape. These features are utilized to make a final decision by comparing them with all detected lesions, thereby enhancing the specificity of lesion detection. Feature engineering plays a crucial role in these systems, with support vector machine classifiers frequently employed. The traditional CAD system demonstrated promising results and was considered effective, with the potential to replace a human reader in a double-reading screening workflow when used as an aid alongside a single human reader. However, this was at the cost of an incremental increase in recall rates. Despite the limitations of traditional CAD systems, the growing volume of medical scans, shortage of radiologists, and imperative need for early and accurate cancer detection have underscored the need for an improved CAD system. Rapid advancements in AI and DL techniques have provided opportunities for the development of sophisticated CAD systems that can detect subtle signs and features that may not be readily apparent to the human eye – known as AI-CAD.

AI-CAD systems

An AI-CAD system can achieve high cancer detection rates while maintaining high specificity and performs significantly better than the traditional CAD. Numerous studies have demonstrated that AI can perform equivalently or even better than humans. In a systematic review and meta-analysis of 16 studies, standalone AI performed equally well or better than individual radiologists in digital MMG interpretation, based on sensitivity, specificity, and AUC metrics. A large study from Sweden that included over 55,000 women showed that a strategy of double reading of mammograms by one radiologist plus AI resulted in an increased cancer detection rate compared with double reading by two radiologists. Two combined reasons contributed to the results: the ability of AI to detect cancer with sufficient sensitivity, and the ability of consensus readers to increase specificity by dismissing AI false positives.

Interval cancer

Interval breast cancers are those that are diagnosed after a normal mammogram but before the next screening examination. They have a different tumour biology than screening-detected breast cancers, and thus are not detected on mammography. AI algorithms have shown promise in detecting ICs. Hickman et al. demonstrated that a standalone AI can detect 23.7% of ICs (referenced in Ahn et al., 2023).

Figure 60. An extreme example of an advanced recurrent breast cancer with an ulcerating axillary mass.

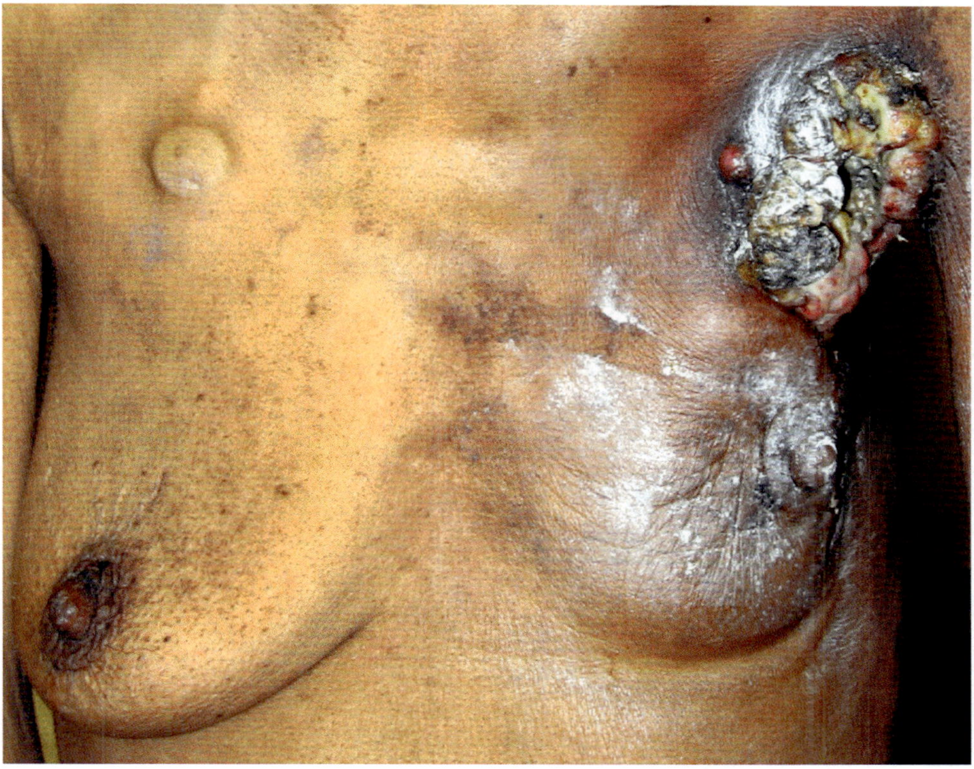

Detection of breast cancer in women with dense breasts

Supplemental imaging techniques, such as DBT, MRI, handheld ultrasound, and automated breast ultrasound, are commonly used as additional tools to traditional MMG to enhance cancer detection in women with dense breasts. Attempts have also been made to apply AI to these modalities to enhance their performance, as has been demonstrated by adding ultrasound examination to mammography: one study demonstrated that implementing an AI system was beneficial to the radiologists' diagnostic process for identifying breast cancer using ultrasound. The use of AI led to a significant reduction in false-positive rates by 37.3% and biopsy requests by 27.8%, while maintaining sensitivity. Moreover, a standalone AI system outperformed an average of ten board-certified BRs, with an AUROC improvement of 0.038 (95% CI, 0.028–0.052; $p < 0.001$). This suggested that the AI system can not only assist radiologists in improving the accuracy, consistency, and efficiency of breast ultrasound diagnosis but also performs better than human experts. In the case of MRI, DL-based CAD systems have shown a significantly higher average sensitivity in early phase scans.

Figure X. Breast cancer prediction by artificial intelligence on a whole-slide image

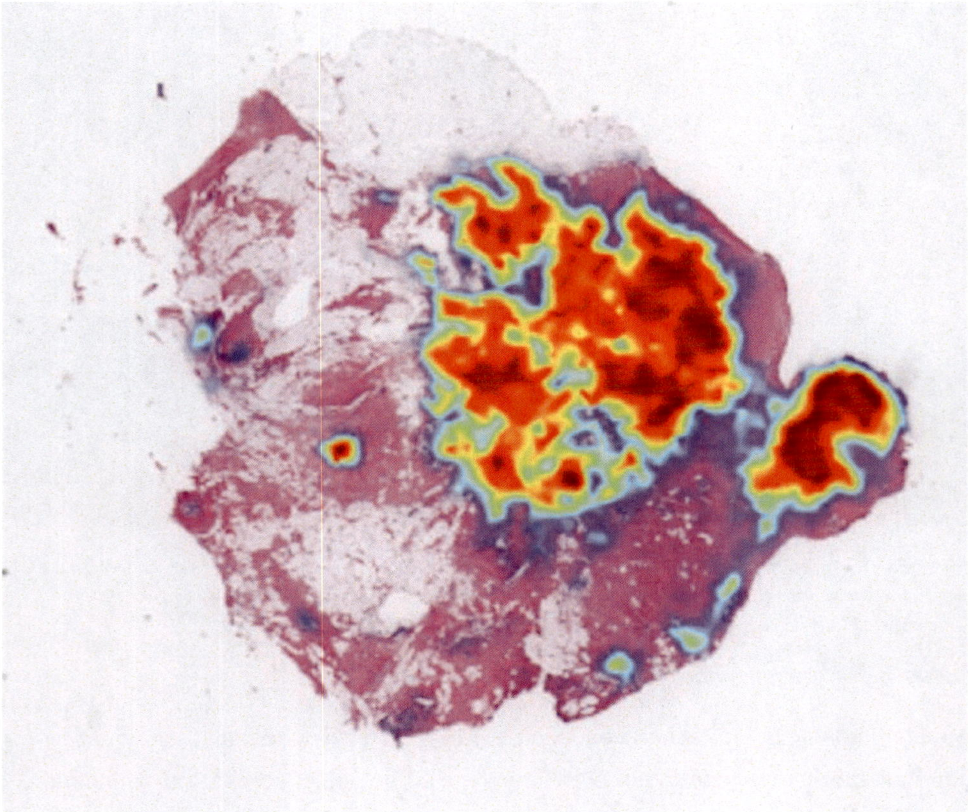

This image is by Cruz-Roa A,et al. (2017). "Accurate and reproducible invasive breast cancer detection in whole-slide images: A Deep Learning approach for quantifying tumor extent.". Sci Rep 7: 46450. DOI:10.1038/srep46450. PMID 28418027. PMC: 5394452."This work is licensed under a Creative Commons Attribution 4.0 International License.", CC BY 4.0, https://commons.wikimedia.org/w/index.php?curid=145735262; https://en.wikipedia.org/wiki/Breast_cancer#/media/File:Histopathology_of_tumor_identification_by_AI.png. This file is licensed under the Creative Commons Attribution 4.0 International license. No changes were made to this image.

Diagnosis

One study developed a CNN model that can classify patches containing invasive ductal carcinoma from the whole slide image (WSI) of breast cancer and estimated the degree of infiltration and extent of invasive foci from the WSI using the ConvNet classifier. Another study reported a DL model with an average accuracy of 93.2% across eight classes (four benign and four malignant) in a test dataset.

A commercially available AI algorithm is the GALEN Breast. This AI model utilizes breast biopsy specimens to detect cancer cells and classifies them into different breast cancer subtypes. The AUC values of this model based on a large-scale, multi-institutional dataset were reported as 0.99 and 0.98 for the detection of invasive carcinoma and ductal carcinoma in situ (DCIS), respectively.

Histological grading

Investigators developed a DL model capable of detecting tubule nuclei in WSI obtained from patients with estrogen receptor (ER)-positive breast cancer by introducing a tubule formation indicator (TFI) based on tubule nuclei to total nuclei ratio. Notably, the TFI correlated with the corresponding risk categories from Oncotype Dx (ODX). (Oncotype Dx [ODx] is a genomic assay which estimates the risk of distant recurrence and predicts adjuvant treatment benefit in early stage breast cancer patients).

Another study showed that an ML classifier utilizing quantitative features related to nuclear shape, texture, and architecture could predict ODx risk categories for early stage ER-positive breast cancer patients (accuracy between 75%–86%). In another study conducted on H&E tissue microarray cohorts of early stage LN-negative, ER-positive breast cancer patients, a model using nuclear shape and orientation stratified short- and long-term survival outcomes, indicating high-risk group outcomes independent of tumour stage, histologic grade, and nuclear grade.

Similar to the approaches used for tubule formation and nuclear pleomorphism, a study demonstrated a DL model capable of counting mitotic figures from H&E-stained slides of early stage ER-positive breast tumors. This model achieved an accuracy of 83.19% in distinguishing ODx risk groups. A specific DL algorithm utilizing Faster R-CNN with a ResNet-101 backbone network exhibited not only high accuracy in mitosis counting tasks but also the potential to decrease pathologists' reading time by 27.8%. Another study introduced a fully automated system that encompassed regions of interest (ROI) identification, mitosis counting from WSI, and prediction of tumor proliferation scores. When evaluated using the TUPAC-16 dataset, this system outperformed all previous methods in these tasks.

Preoperative breast cancer evaluation

AI may also play a significant role in preoperative breast cancer evaluation, including the prediction of lymph node (LN) metastasis. One study demonstrated that LN metastasis could be predicted with an AUROC accuracy of 0.90 based on primary breast cancer ultrasound images. AI has also been used to predict occult invasive disease and improve the prediction of ductal carcinoma in situ (DCIS) upstaging, thereby aiding decision-making and appropriate treatment planning. Other preoperative uses of AI include the prediction of molecular subtypes based on radiomic features. This prediction is important because of the heterogeneous nature of breast cancer, in which single biopsy specimens may not accurately represent the disease, especially when immunohistochemistry (IHC) test results are uncertain. Radiomic features can provide a better overall representation of cancer, enabling more accurate classification and treatment. For example, previous studies have shown that combining MMG and ultrasound images to extract features has high accuracy in discriminating luminal and non-luminal diseases.

Staging

The widely used tumour/node/metastasis (TNM) staging system serves as an important determinant of treatment decisions and prognosis. Sentinel LN (SLN) evaluation plays a critical role in breast cancer clinical staging and subsequent treatment planning. SLN biopsy (SLNB) is a widely used procedure in breast cancer staging for assessing whether cancer cells have spread to regional LNs, particularly to the ipsilateral axilla. However, the false-negative rates of SLNB are almost 10%, indicating that additional imaging modalities, such as ultrasound, MRI, or positron emission tomography/CT, need to be considered to improve the accuracy of nodal staging and identify cases where SLNB alone may be insufficient.

LN metastasis detection in histologic slides

One study demonstrated state-of-the-art performance and significantly reduced false-negative results for predicting the pathologic nodal status on the CAMELYON17 dataset by combining a patch-level CNN-based metastasis detection model and slide-level LN classifier.

Biomarkers

Breast cancer management involves the use of key tissue biomarkers, including estrogen receptor (ER), progesterone receptor (PgR), human epidermal growth factor receptor 2 (HER2), and Ki-67. Despite the importance of biomarker assessment, several studies have demonstrated intra- and inter-laboratory variability in the assessment of ER, PgR, HER2, and Ki-67. This could influence treatment decisions regarding hormonal and anti-HER2 targeted therapies.

Assessing hormone receptor (HR) status via IHC can help identify patients who are likely to benefit from endocrine therapies, such as tamoxifen or aromatase inhibitors. Several studies have explored automated quantitative digital imaging analysis (DIA) techniques. Although manual interpretation of IHC staining is inherently subjective and time-consuming, studies have shown a strong correlation between manual and DIA-based scoring of ER and PgR immunohistochemistry (IHC) staining in breast cancer. Notably, the utilization of DIA has demonstrated improved reproducibility compared with manual scoring methods. Efforts have been made to integrate DIA algorithms into routine digital pathology workflows and ensure the robustness of AI models. Some AI models show promise in predicting ER and PgR status using only H&E-stained slides, thereby eliminating the need for specific IHC staining.

HER2 status, determined by IHC with or without in situ hybridization (ISH), is essential for identifying candidates for anti-HER2 therapies, such as trastuzumab. Levels of HER2 are classified based on the proportion and intensity of stained tumor cells. One study demonstrated the potential of an AI-powered HER2 analyzer to mitigate interobserver variability and aid pathologists in achieving a consistent evaluation of HER2 expression levels. Several studies have used AI models to predict the amplification state of HER2 by analysing digitized fluorescence in situ hybridisation (FISH) images.

Several AI models have been developed to exclusively predict the HER2 status using H&E-stained slides. 21 international teams presented their AI models, and the best-performing model exhibited a classification accuracy of 0.68 in terms of F1 score. Beyond simply predicting the HER2 status, some studies have shown associations between AI models and therapeutic responses. One study developed a CNN classifier, achieving an AUC of 0.80 in predicting the response to trastuzumab therapy based on HER2 status. Another intriguing application of AI was observed in patients who achieved a pathologic complete response (pCR) with anti-HER2 agents, revealing a notably higher proportion of tumor cells with intense HER2 staining. This insight suggests that AI models may be pivotal in providing nuanced information for predicting responses in patients with HER2-positive early breast cancer.

Ki-67 (a marker of cell proliferation) has also been evaluated using IHC and several digital imaging analysis (DIA) platforms with promising results. A comparative study revealed excellent reproducibility among three DIA platforms and reference standards, with the platforms demonstrating indistinguishable capabilities for predicting patient outcomes in breast cancer. Another study revealed that incorporating AI support in the evaluation of Ki-67, ER, and PgR expression led to a slight improvement in pathologist agreement, with 95.8% of the AI analysis results for Ki-67 confirmed by most of the pathologists.

Recently, immunotherapy combined with chemotherapy has demonstrated efficacy in specific breast cancer subsets, necessitating the use of predictive biomarkers like PD-L1. Validation of PD-L1 IHC expression was provided by the KEYNOTE-355 trial, revealing improved survival outcomes in patients with metastatic triple-negative breast cancer (TNBC) exhibiting a PD-L1 combined positive score ≥ 10.

In terms of applying AI, a study utilizing a digital pathology platform for PD-L1 scoring in breast cancer showed that an AI algorithm could predict chemotherapy outcomes in patients with TNBC, as well as in those with HER2-positive and ER-negative breast cancer. The potential utility of AI as an aid to pathologists was highlighted in a multi-institutional ring study that showed that the degree of agreement among pathologists when assessing PD-L1 expression levels could be improved with AI assistance. Moreover, the DL model was able to predict PD-L1 status from H&E-stained images, indicating the potential role of AI in clinical practice for decision support and quality assurance.

Prediction of clinical outcome and treatment response

By analysing the imaging features and patterns, AI can assist in predicting treatment responses and optimizing treatment strategies to improve patient outcomes. AI has emerged as a potential tool for assessing the response to chemotherapy in post-treatment MRIs and predicting recurrence risk.

In pathology, the wealth of information extracted from pathological slides is of great value for predicting treatment responses and broader clinical outcomes. In a comparative study of ML models utilizing clinical and pathological data, the random forest model demonstrated the highest performance, with an AUC of 0.88, for predicting pCR following treatment in patients with locally advanced or high-risk early breast cancer. A CNN-based model trained on H&E-stained WSIs from core biopsies of TNBC patients was reported to have a positive predictive value of 73.7% for pCR. Other investigators developed an AI-based automatic WSI feature extraction pipeline, named IMPRESS, using WSIs stained with both H&E and multiplex IHC (PD-L1, CD8+, and CD163+). ML models using features from IMPRESS and clinical variables accurately predicted the treatment response in patients with HER2+ or TNBC, surpassing a model trained with manually generated pathological features, suggesting that it may be a preferred method for developing algorithms to predict treatment responses in the future. A multi-omics ML model, trained on a combination of clinical, DNA, RNA, digital pathology, and treatment features, showed an AUC of 0.87 in predicting pCR following treatment, with or without HER2-targeted therapy.

Conclusions

The innovative intersection of AI and breast cancer care promises to revolutionize disease screening, disease diagnosis, biomarker evaluation, prognostication, and treatment strategies by overcoming human limitations and achieving remarkable precision and efficiency.

Colo-rectal cancer

Colorectal cancer (CRC) is the third most fatal cancer and is becoming commoner due to unhealthy diets, heavy consumption of alcohol, smoking, and genetic and environmental conditions. The applications of AI to CRC include detection, diagnosis, grading, characterization, drug discovery, treatment, and prevention.

Screening and diagnosis

The bioinformatics tools embedded in AI can help screen and identify CRC biomarkers. AI assisted pathology recognition technology can help pathologists improve efficiency, reduce workload, and lower the rate of misdiagnosis and missed diagnosis. ML can greatly improve the readability of medical images, reduce empirical errors, objectively provide reliable and comprehensive reference opinions, and help in making more accurate clinical decisions.

Colonoscopy has long been regarded as the gold standard procedure for diagnosing colorectal diseases and is widely used as an early screening test. Due to high variability of operator quality, challenging and sometimes inadequate preparation, , the detection rate of polyps and adenomas in early colorectal screening often varies significantly.

Researchers have used computer-aided detection (CADe) systems and AI, based primarily on DL algorithms, to improve the speed and accuracy of clinical detection of CRC and reduce the detection of missed lesions. The adenoma detection rate (ADR) is a reliable indicator for CRC detection. A higher ADR is often linked to a lower incidence and mortality in CRC patients. The combination of AI and colonoscopy can effectively improve ADR. It not only reduces the risk of CRC but also contributes to accurate resection. A large number of studies support AI-assisted colonoscopy in the diagnosis of CRC.

Another colonoscopy index is the adenoma miss rate (AMR). One group established a CADe system that uses a CNN algorithm to aid in the detection of adenomas. This demonstrated that the AMR of the CADe-assisted group was 22.9%, which was lower than that of the standard colonoscopy group. These results showed that the AMR was greatly decreased due to the assistance of AI.

Figure 62. Longitudinally opened freshly resected colon segment showing a cancer and four polyps and a schematic diagram indicating a likely field defect (a region of tissue that precedes and predisposes to the development of cancer) in this colon segment. The diagram indicates sub-clones and sub-sub-clones that were precursors to the tumors.

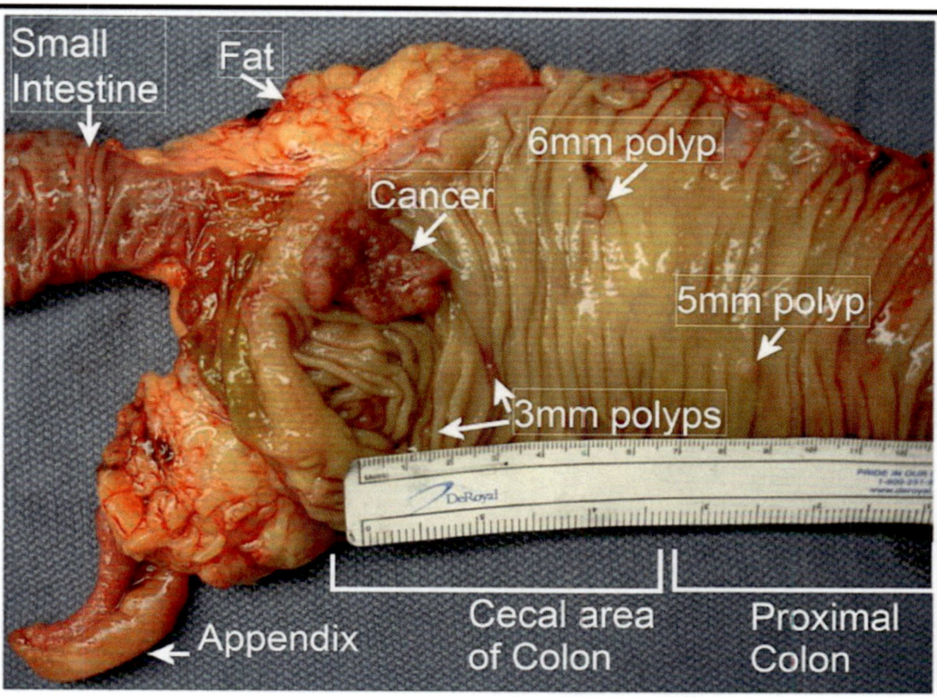

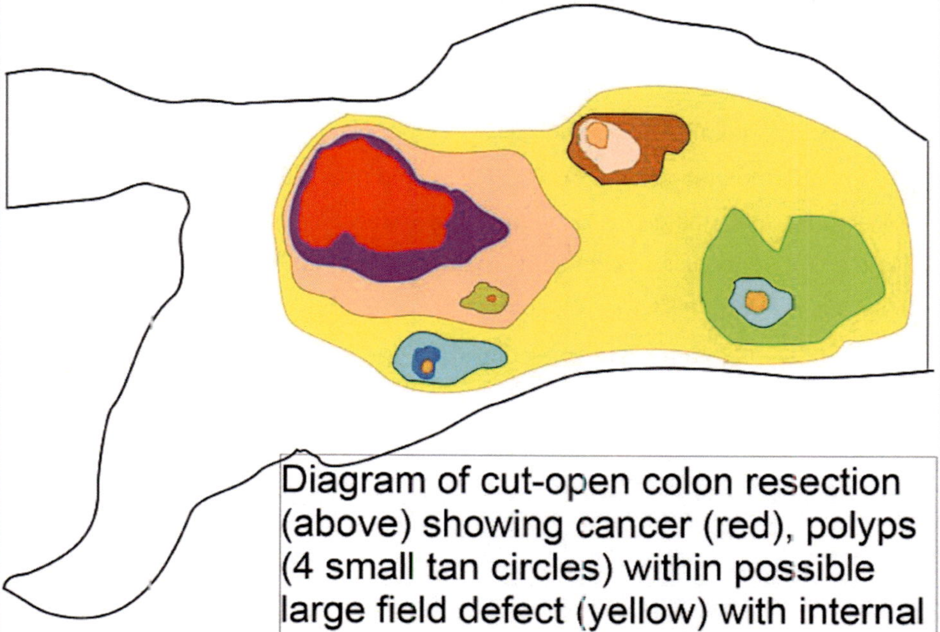

Diagram of cut-open colon resection (above) showing cancer (red), polyps (4 small tan circles) within possible large field defect (yellow) with internal sub-clones and sub-sub-clones (other colors)

Endoscopic tools including magnifying endoscopy, chromoendoscopy, confocal laser endomicroscopy, and autofluorescence endoscopy, continue to be developed and will likely improve further the results of colonoscopy. Using narrow-band imaging (NBI) combined with magnification endoscopy, investigators calculated the difference between microvessel density in colorectal lesions; this was used as the differential point for the diagnosis of CRC and adenoma. Investigators in the USA developed CADe algorithms to distinguish tumor polyps from non-tumor polyps based on probe confocal laser endoscopy. The sensitivity, specificity and sensitivity were more than 90%.

Biomarkers

One hundred and five differentially expressed genes (DEGs) and 10 hub genes in colon cancers were identified through bioinformatic analysis of gene expression microarray data in the Gene Expression Omnibus (GEO) database. The researchers used these tools, including SVM, receiver operating characteristic curve (ROC), and survival analyses, to predict the diagnostic value of hub genes as CRC biomarkers. The results showed that the area under ROC curve (AUC) values of all genes were more than 0.92, confirming that these genes are likely biomarkers for CRC. With the development of sequencing technology, many non-coding RNAs (ncRNAs) have been discovered. The ncRNAs include messenger RNAs (mRNAs), microRNA (miRNAs), and long non-coding RNAs (lncRNAs). MicroRNAs (miRNAs) are a class of endogenous ncRNAs with a length of approximately 22 nucleotides. They have a variety of important regulatory functions in cells and are associated with the development and metastasis of cancer. There is increasing evidence that miRNAs are potential biomarkers of CRC. Investigators have also investigated whether miR-31 could be used as a biomarker for the diagnosis of CRC lymph node metastasis (LNM) using bioinformatics analysis techniques, including the Kyoto Encyclopedia of Genes and Genomes (KEGG) enrichment analysis, correlation analysis, survival analysis, validation of expression levels, protein–protein interactive (PPI) network construction, and gene ontology (GO). It was found that miR-31 was significantly increased in the plasma and tissue of CRC patients with LNM.

Histopathology

Many studies have shown that the application of AI technology can help pathologists improve diagnosis efficiency by increasing the diagnosis rate and reducing the misdiagnosis rate. In a retrospective study, researchers obtained more than 100,000 H and E image patches from 86 CRC tissue slides, and they used these images to train a CNN based on transfer learning (TL). The results showed an accuracy of over 94%, confirming that CNN can separate histological images and predict the survival rate of CRC patients after treatment. Wang et al. (2021) proposed a CNN-based method to classify a large number of histopathological images. The AUC of this model was up to 0.988, with the ability to distinguish CRC from other benign tissues.

A monogram model combined with ML - pathomics, immunoscore, radiomics, and clinical factors effectively predicted the postoperative prognosis of patients with CRC lung metastases. These data indicate significant progress in AI-assisted pathological reading.

Radiomics

The combination of AI and radiomics can extract information from imaging data. It can be used for tumor segmentation, feature extraction, and model establishment, leading to tumor quantitative evaluation. In 2018 a study used a label assignment generative adversarial network (Lagan), and accurately segmented regions of interest (ROI) in the analysis and diagnosis of CRC. Other investigators developed a rectal cancer segmentation software based on a U-Net deep neural network. They used this software for MRI image simulation analysis of 201 preoperative patients. It segmented the rectum, mesorectum, and tumors respectively, and eventually obtained diverse counterfactual explanations (DICE) similarity coefficients to artificial segmentation (rectum: DSC = 0.930, mesorectum: DSC = 0.917, tumor: DSC = 0.727).

Conclusions

AI algorithms that combine multiple medical imaging big data will help to improve the early detection rate and diagnosis of CRC.

Prostate cancer

Diagnosis and grading of prostate cancer biopsies

In men prostate cancer is the most commonly diagnosed non-skin malignancy and the second leading cause of mortality from cancer. The diagnosis and management of prostate cancer involves the interpretation of data from multiple modalities to aid in decision making. Tools like prostate specific antigen (PSA) levels, MRI-guided biopsies, genomic biomarkers, and Gleason grading are used to diagnose, risk stratify, and then monitor patients during follow-up. Because of this intra- and inter-variability of human experts in prostate pathology Ström and colleagues (2020) developed an artificial intelligence (AI) system with clinically acceptable accuracy for prostate cancer detection, localisation, and Gleason grading (Figure 63). They digitised 6,682 slides from needle core biopsies from 976 randomly selected participants aged 50-69 in a Swedish prospective and population-based diagnostic study carried out between May 28, 2012, and Dec 30, 2014, as well as another 271 from 93 men from outside the study. The resulting images were used to train deep neural networks for assessment of prostate biopsies. The networks were evaluated by predicting the presence, extent, and Gleason grade of malignant tissue for an independent test dataset comprising 1,631 biopsies from 246 men and an external validation dataset of 330 biopsies from 73 men. They also evaluated grading performance on 87 biopsies individually graded by 23 experienced urological pathologists from the International Society of Urological Pathology. They assessed discriminatory performance by receiver operating characteristics and tumour extent predictions by correlating predicted cancer length against measurements by the reporting pathologist. They quantified the concordance between grades assigned by the AI system and the expert urological pathologists using Cohen's kappa.

The AI achieved an area under the receiver operating characteristics curve of 0·997 (95% CI 0·994-0·999) for distinguishing between benign (n=910) and malignant (n=721) biopsy cores on the independent test dataset and 0·986 (0·972-0·996) on the external validation dataset (benign n=108, malignant n=222). The correlation between cancer length predicted by the AI method and assigned by the reporting pathologist was 0·96 (95% CI 0·95-0·97) for the independent test dataset and 0·87 (0·84-0·90) for the external validation dataset. For assigning Gleason grades, the AI achieved a mean pairwise kappa of 0·62, which was within the range of the corresponding values for the expert pathologists (0·60-0·73).

The authors concluded that an AI system could be trained to detect and grade cancer in prostate needle biopsy samples at a ranking comparable to that of international experts in prostate pathology. Clinical application could reduce pathology workload by reducing the assessment of benign biopsies and by automating the task of measuring cancer length in positive biopsy cores. An AI system with expert-level grading performance might contribute a second opinion, aid in standardising grading, and provide pathology expertise in parts of the world where it does not exist.

Figure 63. The Gleason scoring system for prostate cancer

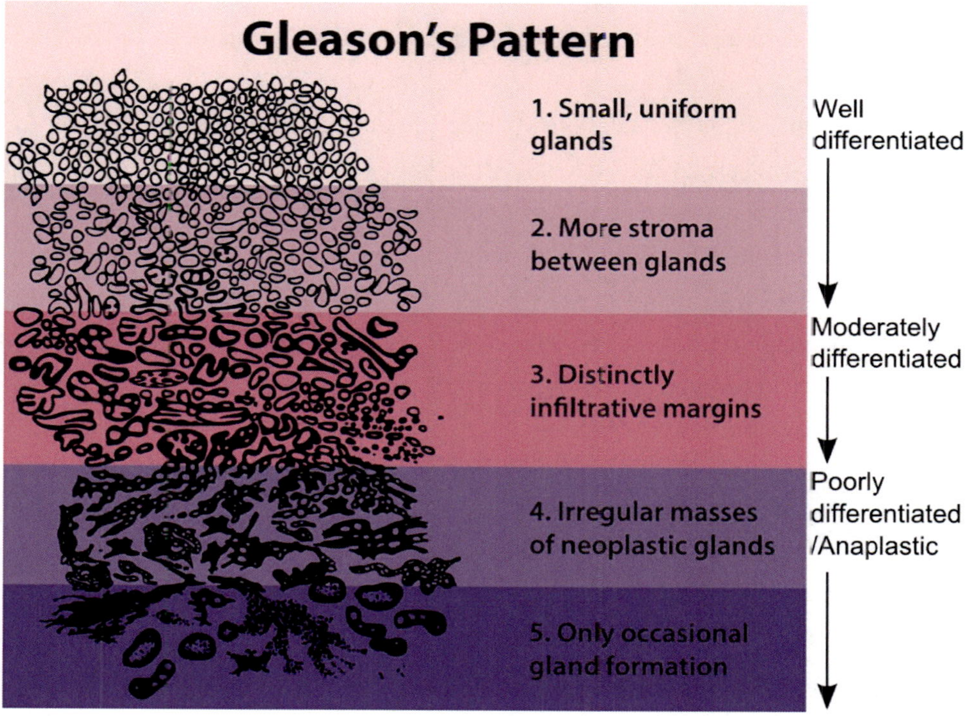

Risk factors

An early study by Naguib et al (1998) evaluated a combined approach of ANN and statistics known about various risk factors. The neural network in this study was trained on conventional factors including age, stage, bone scan findings, grade, PSA and treatment along with 2 experimental markers of immunostaining for bcl-2 and p53. By considering conventional risk factors alone, the prediction models achieved only 60% accuracy in identifying the patients with condition. However, this efficiency was improved to 80% when the experimental markers were included. Thus, there was a significant improvement in accuracy of the model with an increase in the amount of data fed to the algorithm. This study also underscored the importance of including experimental markers for testing into building the networks as each piece of data could impact the model accuracy profoundly.

In a study by Lawrentschuk et al. (2011), a polychotomous logistic regression (PR) model and an ANN was developed for predicting the biopsy results using 3,025 men undergoing biopsy with PSA <10 ng/dl. Clinical predictors of age, PSA, abnormal digital rectal examination, positive transrectal ultrasound (TRUS) and prostate volume were also considered during the development. It was suggested that an inclusion of additional predictors might improve the performance of the models. However, the ANN was unable to distinguish between the four biopsy outcomes that were utilized in their validation. The authors suggest that a more tempered enthusiasm should be used with ANN and that great care must be used in training them properly for effective application.

PSA

Numerous studies have evaluated the utility of PSA and other clinical characteristics in the setting of an ANN in detecting prostate cancer and/or its progression. For example, Djavan et al. (2002) developed an ANN to enhance the sensitivity and specificity of prostate cancer detection. The study consisted of 1,246 men with the primary aim of predicting the presence of prostate cancer or benign prostatic tissue in men with serum PSA levels from 2.5 to 4 ng/mL and from 4 to 10 ng/mL compared to conventional tools. At 95% sensitivity, the ANN model for patients with total PSA levels from 4 to 10 ng/mL produced specificity, positive predictive value, negative predictive value, and receiver operator characteristic (ROC) curve area under the curve values that were superior to any of the other comparative parameters.

A study by Stojadinovic et al. (2018) assessed various factors and determined that PSA density was the most decisive variable and showed the decision tree providing a net benefit compared to a logistic regression model. In this retrospective study, the model had a potential to reduce unnecessary biopsies without missing significant diagnoses.

Finne et al. (2000) developed an ANN using free PSA with the goal of eliminating unnecessary prognostic testing in false positive PSA results. The model was constructed using data on total PSA, the proportion of free PSA, digital rectal examination (DRE), and prostate volume from 656 men with total serum PSA concentrations of 4 to 10 ng/mL in Finland. Results showed that, at a 95% sensitivity level, 19% of the false-positive PSA results could be eliminated by using the proportion of free PSA versus 24% with the logistic regression model and 33% with the ANN model. These findings suggested that an ANN method has value if incorporated into prostate cancer screening to decrease the number of false-positive results.

Ge et al. (2015) developed a logistic regression and ANN model to aid in diagnosis of prostate cancer. To train their algorithms they utilized predictors including age, percent free PSA, prostate volume, and PSA density from 586 men with prostate cancer confirmed by biopsy. While they found no significant difference between the two models, they concluded that both models had high diagnostic validity and the potential to be included in practice to prevent unnecessary biopsies.

Stephan et al. (2002) developed an ANN utilizing percentage of free PSA (%fPSA) to identify men at increased risk of a positive prostate biopsy for cancer. The study enrolled 1,188 men with benign prostates or prostate cancer with input data that included total PSA, %fPSA, patient age, prostate volume, and digital rectal examination (DRE) status. The use of the ANN in men with 2–10 µg/L total PSA enhanced the specificity of %fPSA by 20–22%. Thus, the use of an % fPSA-based ANN was able to enhance detection accuracy over %fPSA alone and prevent unnecessary biopsies. Together, there are multiple studies which reflect the relevance of using artificial intelligence-based ANN tools which could be effectively integrated with some of the other tools commonly used in prostate cancer detection.

In a study by Remzi et al. (2003) an ANN was developed to predict the presence of prostate cancer and predict the outcome in repeat biopsies. This model was trained using variables such as age, PSA, f/t PSA ratio, digital rectal examination findings, PSA velocity, and the transrectal ultrasound-guided variables of prostate volume, transition zone volume, PSAD, and PSA-TZ from 820 men with PSA levels between 4 and 10 ng/mL. This ANN showed a strong pattern of prediction for prostate cancer in patients who had an initial negative biopsy. Overall, the ANN achieved a 68% specificity and 95% sensitivity. Thus, there are multiple studies which reflect the potential of AI ANNs to allow more accurate counselling of patients and overcome histopathologic variabilities.

Diagnosis when PSA levels are borderline

Identification of elevated PSA level is regarded as one of the most common clinical tools for the diagnosis of prostate cancer. However, an elevated PSA level is present in several other benign prostatic conditions that can lead to unnecessary procedures. Generally, a PSA level greater than 4 ng/mL is considered significant for the early detection of prostate cancer, but up to 20% of patients diagnosed with prostate cancer never reach that threshold. There has been a great need to diagnose prostate cancer in men with borderline PSA levels. Numerous studies have evaluated the utility of PSA and other clinical characteristics in the setting of an ANN in detecting prostate cancer and/or its progression. For example, Djavan et al. (2002) developed an ANN to enhance the sensitivity and specificity of prostate cancer detection. The study consisted of 1,246 men with the primary aim of predicting the presence of prostate cancer or benign prostatic tissue in men with serum total PSA levels from 2.5 to 4 ng/mL and from 4 to 10 ng/mL compared to conventional tools. At 95% sensitivity, the ANN model for patients with total PSA levels from 4 to 10 ng/mL produced specificity, positive predictive value, negative predictive value, and receiver operator characteristic (ROC) curve area under the curve values that were superior to any of the other comparative parameters.

Finne et al. (2000) developed an ANN using free PSA with the goal of eliminating unnecessary prognostic testing in false positive PSA results. The model was constructed using data on total PSA, the proportion of free PSA, digital rectal examination (DRE), and prostate volume from 656 men with total serum PSA concentrations of 4 to 10 ng/mL. Results showed that, at a 95% sensitivity level, 19% of the false-positive PSA results could be eliminated by using the proportion of free PSA versus 24% with the logistic regression model and 33% with the ANN model. These findings suggest that an ANN method has value in being incorporated into prostate cancer screening to decrease the number of false-positive results.

Ge et al. (2015) developed a logistic regression and ANN model to aid in diagnosis of prostate cancer. To train their algorithms they utilized predictors including age, percent free PSA, prostate volume, and PSA density from 586 men with prostate cancer confirmed by biopsy. While they found no significant difference between the two models, they concluded that both models have high diagnostic validity and have potential to be included in practice to prevent unnecessary biopsies.

Diagnosis, staging and treatment

Van Booven and colleagues (2021) used Pubmed, Embase, and Web of Science to identify and screen manuscripts pertaining to the use of machine learning and active surveillance in the diagnosis, staging, and treatment of prostate cancer. This review was conducted according to the Preferred Reporting Items for Systematic Review and Metaanalysis (PRISMA). The keywords used include: ((((((((((prostate cancer) OR prostatic cancer) OR guided prostate biops*) OR guided prostatic biops*) OR ultrasound guided prostate biops*) OR ultrasound guided prostatic biops*) OR prostate biops*) OR prostatic biops*) OR Gleason scor*)) AND (((((artificial intelligence) OR deep learning) OR machine learning) OR artificial neural network) OR neural network)) AND (((clinical trial*) OR active surveillance) OR active surveillance trial).

The authors concluded that by using AI algorithms and reducing the level of subjectivity, it is possible to use fewer resources while improving the overall efficiency and accuracy in trials.

Recurrence of disease

Neeraj et al. (2017) focused on disease recurrence prediction by creating 2 different convolutional neural networks (CNN) analyzing H&E images. The first CNN detected individual nuclei while the second CNN classified the patches around the nuclear centres. There was a voting process which yielded probabilities of recurrence from the patients. The model was trained on 80 case/control pairs and then validated on 30 recurrent and 30 non-recurrent controls. The end yield was 0.81 AUC for accuracy. Thus, this study provided a deep learning tool that could look at recurrence in conjunction with other risk factors in order to come up with a new scoring system that could be more accurate than those currently used.

Artificial Neural Network and Magnetic Resonance Imaging (MRI)

Diagnosis of prostate cancer by magnetic resonance imaging (MRI) has been investigated as a modality for prostate cancer detection and determination of aggressiveness. MR spectroscopic T2-weighted MR imaging, and apparent diffusion coefficient (ADC) have been valuable tools to assess prostate cancer, but their use still lacks consensus. Using these tools, users can easily detect malignant tumors, but determining their aggressiveness using MRI with good reliability is more difficult. Thus, automatic classification using machine learning has been proposed as a solution to provide more accurate and consistent results to aid clinicians' management.

In a similar context, Fehr et al. (2015) proposed a technique of utilizing machine learning-based automatic classification of prostate cancer aggressiveness by combining apparent diffusion coefficient (ADC) and T2-weighted MRI-based texture features. This technique was able to differentiate between the high Gleason score (GS) (>7) and low GS. Furthermore, this model could distinguish between high and low Gleason grades with 93% accuracy for cancers occurring in both peripheral (PZ) and transition (TZ) zones and 92% for cancers occurring in the PZ alone. These results were far superior to using only apparent diffusion coefficient (ADC) and suggested that this method could help provide reasonably accurate classification of Gleason patterns. In addition, in another study by Antonelli et al. (2019) the authors used quantitative MRI and clinical features from 164 men to construct machine learning classifiers. Following model validation, these classifiers were able to predict Gleason 4 in prostate tumors with greater accuracy than the three board-certified radiologists who participated in the study. It was suggested that these AI classifier tools could be useful to non-invasively detect the progression of tumours and aid in decisions regarding active surveillance programs. In a study by Toivonen et al. (2019) the authors developed machine learning tools to predict prostate cancer aggressiveness by using optimized high-quality MRI data sets. A classifier system was created based on multiple texture features of high-quality T2 weighted images, diffusion weighted imaging (DWI), and T2 relaxation maps from 100 patients for prediction of PCa Gleason score dichotomized as 3+3 (low risk) vs >3+3 (high risk). Results suggested that texture feature analysis of DWI, post-processed using monoexponential and kurtosis models, and T2w demonstrated a good classification performance for the Gleason score. Together, these multiple studies reflect the potential of AI ANNs to allow more effective integration with modern surveillance tools such as MRI to effectively help in prostate cancer surveillance. Thus, ANNs can play an instrumental role in analyzing and validating the biomarkers. For example, one study suggested that Ki-67 is an important marker of survival and disease progression. To confirm this, Green et al. (2016) created an ANN that was designed to validate Ki-67 gene expression while comparing it to another potential candidate - DLX2. Univariate analysis showed that both Ki-67 and DLX2 significantly predicted future metastases. However, only 6.8% of prostate cancer patients have high expression of Ki-67. Thus, this study showed that these 2 biomarkers could be used to identify candidates for targeted therapy only. In addition to gene expression, proteomics can also be useful when identifying potential biomarkers. For example, Kim et al. (2016) developed a novel approach by combining targeted proteomics with computational biology to discover new potential proteomic signatures for prostate cancer. The study started with 133 differentially expressed proteins that were evaluated with synthetic peptides in a 74-patient cohort. They then applied machine learning approaches to develop clinical predictive models using these candidates. Results showed that computationally guided proteomics can be used to discover novel non-invasive biomarkers. Overall, there are numerous studies which reflect the potential of AI ANNs to allow more effective identification and validation of biomarkers to aid in prostate cancer surveillance.

Chapter 15. How AI will improve outcomes in arthritis

The most common forms of arthritis are rheumatoid arthritis and osteoarthritis.

Rheumatoid arthritis

Rheumatoid arthritis (RA) is a long-term autoimmune disorder that primarily affects joints. It typically results in warm, swollen, and painful joints. Pain and stiffness often worsen following rest. Most commonly, the wrist and hands are involved, with the same joints typically involved on both sides of the body. The disease may also affect other parts of the body, including skin, eyes, lungs, heart, nerves, and blood. This may result in a low red blood cell count, inflammation around the lungs, and inflammation around the heart. Fever and low energy may also be present. The underlying mechanism involves the body's immune system attacking the joints. This results in inflammation and thickening of the joint capsule. It also affects the underlying bone and cartilage.

Figure 64. A hand severely affected by rheumatoid arthritis

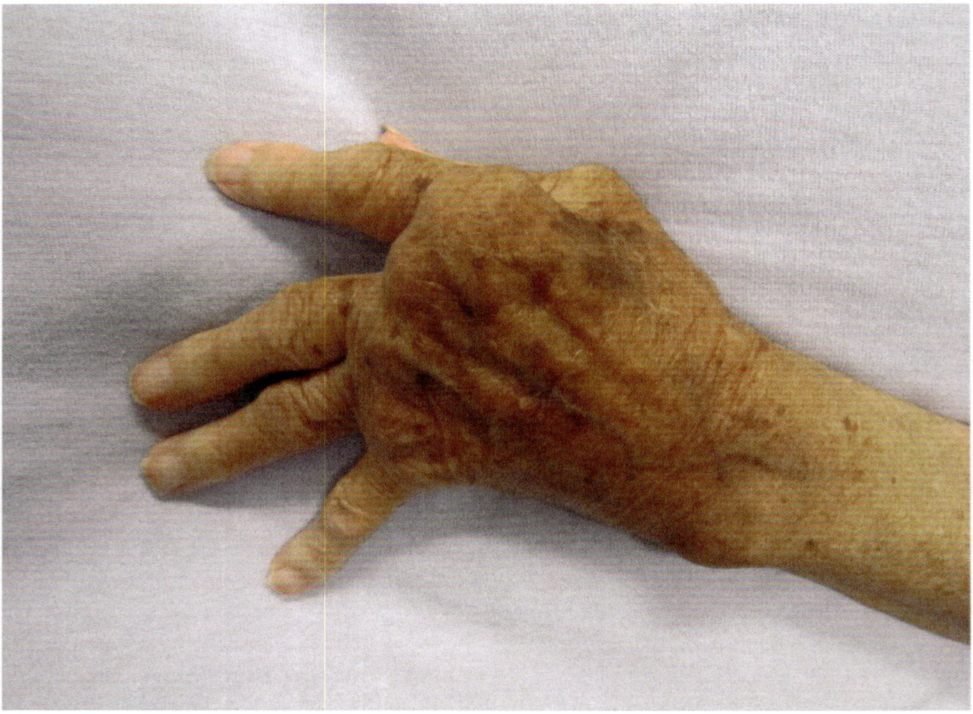

Figure 65. X-ray of the wrist of a 66 year old woman with rheumatoid arthritis, showing ankylosing fusion of the carpal bones. Previous X-ray showed unaffected carpal bones.

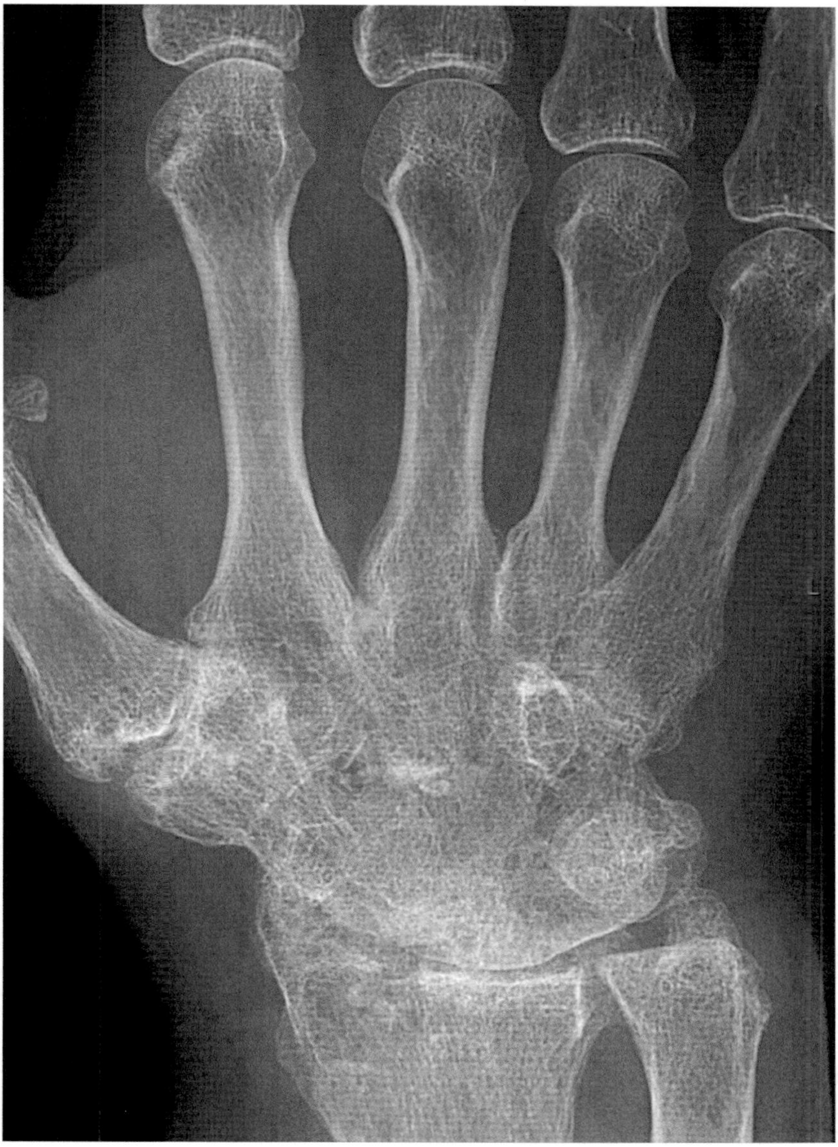

Bone erosion is a central feature of rheumatoid arthritis. Bone continuously undergoes remodeling by actions of bone-resorbing osteoclasts and bone-forming osteoblasts. One of the main triggers of bone erosion in the joints in rheumatoid arthritis is inflammation of the synovium, caused in part by the production of pro-inflammatory cytokines and receptor activator of nuclear factor kappa B ligand (RANKL), a cell surface protein present in Th17 cells and osteoblasts.

Figure 66. Bone erosions due to rheumatoid arthritis

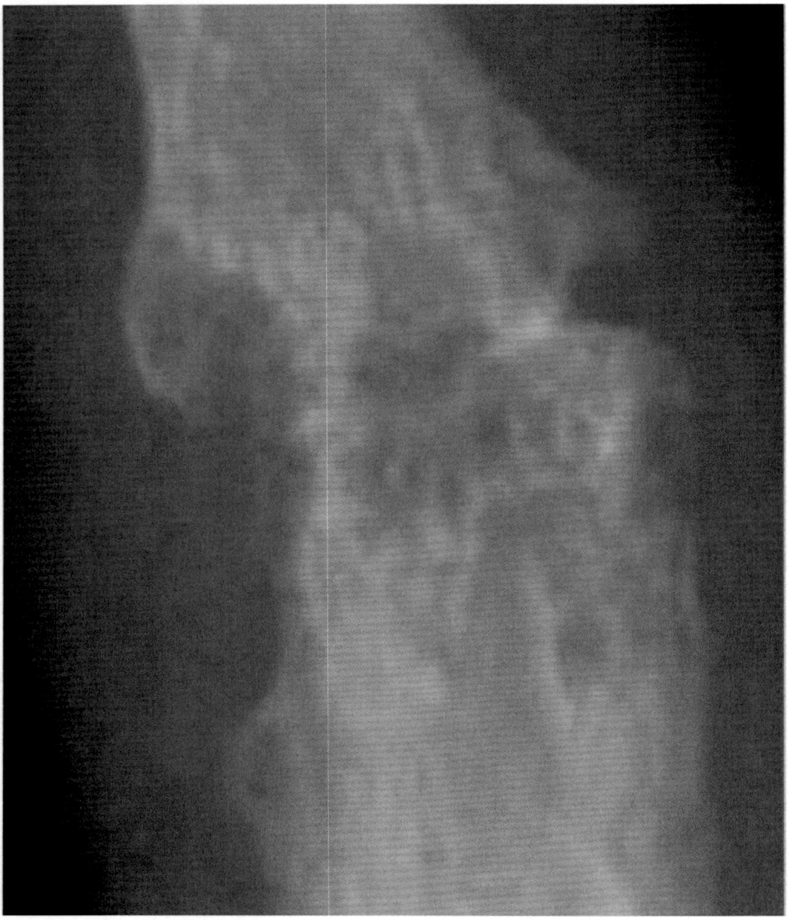

This image is by Haruko Ideguchi, Shigeru Ohno, Hideaki Hattori, Akiko Senuma and Yoshiaki Ishigatsubo - (2006). " Bone erosions in rheumatoid arthritis can be repaired through reduction in disease activity with conventional disease-modifying antirheumatic drugs" Arthritis Research & Therapy 8 (3): R76. DOI:10.1186/ar1943. ISSN 14786354. (CC-BY-2.0), CC BY 2.0, https://commons.wikimedia.org/w/index.php?curid=63609849; https://upload.wikimedia.org/wikipedia/commons/6/6c/X-ray_of_right_fourth_PIP_joint_with_bone_erosions_by_rheumatoid_arthritis.jpg. This file is licensed under the Creative Commons Attribution 2.0 Generic license. No changes were made to this image.

AI in rheumatoid arthritis

The application of AI in the fields of RA has the potential to enable healthcare professionals to detect RA at an earlier stage, thereby facilitating timely intervention and better disease management. AI algorithms, such as naive Bayes, convolutional neural network (CNN), logistic regression, and support vector machine (SVMs) or deep learning can analyse imaging data, such as X-rays, magnetic resonance imaging (MRI), and computer tomography (CT), to detect subtle changes in the joints that may indicate early RA. MRI can provide accurate data on early signs of inflammatory arthritis, particularly in the identification of bone marrow oedema and tenosynovitis. X-rays is also most commonly used and easily accessible non-invasive method for monitoring disease progression and can also detect bone structural changes at an early stage. One group developed a method for detecting finger joint involvement in patients with RA using hand X-ray images, and they achieved an accuracy of 91.8% by training an artificial neural network (ANN) for this task.

Many AI tools can help identify biomarkers that are indicative of RA and provide more accurate diagnoses. Investigators developed a random forest model that evaluated serum protein biomarkers and demonstrated good performance in discriminating between patients with RA and those with psoriatic arthritis. The model achieved an area under the curve (AUC) of 0.79 in the initial phase and 0.85 in the subsequent validation phase. The researchers created a robust matching learning feature selection pipeline, which identified new biomarkers for RA in over 2000 blood samples from RA patients.

AI assessment of risk of developing RA

One group designed regression models with serum proteome as input to identify patients who are likely to eventually develop RA among first-degree relatives of those with confirmed disease. Multiple studies have attempted to identify single-nucleotide polymorphisms (SNPs) associated with RA development risk and the epistatic relationships among them. One gene in which polymorphisms are associated with RA is PTPN22. Briggs et al. (2010) identified epistatic relations between PTPN22 and several SNPs that could augment the effect of PTPN22 on susceptibility to RA.

AI in the diagnosis of RA

Analysis of omics (for example, genomics, transcriptomics, proteomics, metabolomics, lipidomics, and glycomics) using ML approaches enables simultaneous assessment of the association of numerous biomolecules with RA. Incorporating omics data into medical decision-making has several benefits. They are easily acquired from body fluids and are objectively interpreted. Furthermore, their extensiveness provides a vast amount of information. Improved data analysis using AI can facilitate early detection of the disease and more efficient use of human resources.

Several studies developed panels of multiple coding or non-coding ribonucleic acids (RNAs) within the serum or plasma to establish an accurate RA diagnosis using ML approaches. In one study investigators assessed gene expression profiles of peripheral blood cells and identified 52 differentially expressed genes in patients with RA. Further protein - protein analysis identified nine hub genes with crucial roles in the development of RA, which are fundamental in immune regulation, namely CFL1, COTL1, ACTG1, PFN1, LCP1, LCK, HLA-E, FYN, and HLA-DRA. Logistic regression and random forest models showed an AUC ≥ 0.97 for the panel of the nine messenger RNAs (mRNAs) of these genes in distinguishing RA from healthy samples. Another investigation of gene expression profiling showed that a 12-gene transcriptional pattern in a peripheral blood cluster of $CD4^+$ T cells could predict the development of RA in patients with undifferentiated arthritis during a median follow-up of 28 months. While the autoantibody showed a higher sensitivity in the ACPA-positive patients, the newly developed expression signature had a higher sensitivity and specificity in seronegative patients. Notably, the expression of most of these genes was induced by interleukin (IL)-6-mediated STAT3 upregulation. The combination of the 12-gene risk metric with the Leiden prediction rule outperformed the Leiden prediction rule alone in seronegative patients (AUC = 0.78), highlighting the clinical significance of these biomarkers. Additionally, non-coding RNAs have garnered considerable research attention as diagnostic biomarkers in RA. Ormseth and colleagues used LASSO variable selection with logistic regression to develop a panel of microRNAs (miRNA) differentiating patients with RA from controls, which resulted in the selection of miR-22-3p, miR-24-3p, miR-96-5p, miR-134-5p, miR-140-3p, and miR-627-5p, all of which were upregulated in patients with RA. The miRNA panel showed an AUC of approximately 0.8 in discriminating patients with RA (seropositive or seronegative) from controls. However, the panel might be a non-specific signature for autoimmune diseases as it could not differentiate RA from systemic lupus erythematosus.

Multiple investigations have employed proteomic approaches to discover circulating diagnostic biomarkers using mass spectrometry. In such studies the sample sizes are often relatively small, whereas each sample includes a large number of input variables. This atypical data pattern makes decision tree-based algorithms suitable for analysis of the data as they can handle the disproportionate high dimensionality of the input data compared to the number of samples. In such settings, it has been shown that the boosted decision tree outperformed other ML approaches, including SVM and k-nearest neighbors (kNN). Using this method, several patterns of protein peaks were proposed to differentiate patients with RA from controls and patients with other autoimmune diseases with high sensitivity and specificity.

Several other diagnostic models have been developed using omics data derived from serum, particularly inflammatory and oxidative stress markers. Analysis of circulatory levels of 38 cytokines using an artificial neural network (ANN) resulted in a model with a sensitivity and specificity of 100% in differentiating patients with RA from controls and patients with osteoarthritis (OA). Therefore, investigators utilized a single decision tree to identify cytokines leading the program to its output. These cytokines included CD40L, transforming growth factor (TGF)-α, epidermal growth factor (EGF), interferon (IFN)-γ, eotaxin, macrophage inflammatory protein (MIP)-1β, tumor necrosis factor (TNF)-α, IL-1α, granulocyte colony-stimulating factor (G-CSF), fractalkine, growth-regulated oncogene (GRO), and vascular endothelial growth factor (VEGF) in descending order of importance for classification of RA, OA, and controls. Of the mentioned cytokines, eotaxin, G-CSF, IL-1alpha and TNF-α levels were not statistically different between the groups when analyzed using conventional statistics. This finding highlights the necessity of applying ML algorithms in addition to conventional statistical methods for the development of optimal diagnostic panels.

Machine learning approaches using metabolomics and glycomics have also shown promising results in the diagnosis of RA. One study assessed the diagnostic value of damaged proteins of the joints, including oxidized, nitrated, and glycated proteins and oxidation, nitration, and glycation free adducts released in the circulation by investigating plasma, serum, and synovial samples. Their algorithm, which featured levels of ten damaged amino acids in plasma, hydroxyproline, and anti-CCP antibody status, successfully differentiated early RA from controls and patients with other types of arthritis. Notably, the levels of damaged amino acids were higher in patients with advanced RA compared to early stage RA.

In addition to circulating biomarkers, advances have been made in the diagnosis and patient stratification by assessment of synovial tissue. One study using supervised ML approaches found a 16-gene profile expressed in synovial samples differentiated patients with RA from those with OA. This can be useful in seronegative and elderly patients with an inflammatory presentation of OA. Correspondingly, Yeo and colleagues (2016) found a panel of ten informative chemokine genes discriminating patients with established RA from uninflamed controls using ML methods. This study showed that synovial biomarkers can also assist in the early identification of patients developing RA. It found that mRNA levels of the chemokines CXCL4 and CXCL7 can accurately distinguish early RA from resolving arthritis, with higher levels in early RA compared to longer established RA or controls.

Within RA patients, ML algorithms can facilitate patient stratification. One study identified three patterns of synovial gene expression using a clustering algorithm, including a high inflammatory subtype with extensive infiltration of leukocytes, a low inflammatory subtype specified by enrichment in pathways mediated by TGF-β, glycoproteins, and neuronal genes, and a mixed subtype.

The human microbiome has recently drawn research attention. Dysbiosis can be associated with various diseases, including RA. Machine learning-based approaches analysing metagenomic data are optimal for exploiting the large biological datasets created by evolving microbiome research. One study used a logistic regression prediction algorithm to improve multiclass classification between patients with RA, type 2 diabetes mellitus, liver cirrhosis, and controls. While no biomarker was specific for type 2 diabetes mellitus or RA, the model had a favourable diagnostic performance with an AUC near 0.95, highlighting the value of microbiome biomarkers in disease diagnostics, especially disease screening, within a large-scale population. A meta-analysis found specific features in the gut microbiome distinguishing RA from healthy controls and other autoimmune diseases using random forest algorithms. Increased levels of *Clostridiaceae, Clostridium* and *Lachnospiraceae* and reduced abundance of *Erysipelotrichaceae* were the most distinctive features in RA compared to other autoimmune diseases.

Sensor data, which are rich datasets of disease diagnosis and monitoring, were acquired using technologies such as wearable devices, thermography sensors, and image sensors. In one study, ML algorithms, using features extracted from lymphocyte images generated by an electronic image sensor, were highly elevated for RA classification, with accuracy rates as high as 97.5%.

AI in the early intervention of RA

AI has shown the potential to improve early intervention of RA (Yoosuf et al. 2021). Gene expression analysis in baseline samples revealed notably higher expression of the gene EPPK1 in future responders. The study detected the suppression of genes and proteins following treatment, including suppressed expression of the T cell inhibitor gene CHI3L1 and its protein YKL-40. The gene expression results were replicated in an independent cohort. Additionally, machine learning models mainly based on transcriptomic data showed high predictive utility in classifying non-response to anti-TNF treatment in RA.

AI for the prediction of treatment response in RA

ML have been utilized to predict treatment responses to DMARDs, which are classified into conventional synthetic disease-modifying antirheumatic drugs (csDMARDs), biologic disease-modifying antirheumatic drugs (bDMARDs) and targeted synthetic DMARDs (tsDMARDs). Research conducted by Myasoedova et al. (2022) was one of the initial attempts to use machine learning techniques that combine clinical and genomic information to make personalized predictions about the response to methotrexate in individuals diagnosed with early RA. Along with baseline Disease Activity Score in 28 joints (DAS28) scores and intergenic single nucleotide polymorphisms (SNPs) such as rs12446816, rs13385025, rs113798271, and ATIC (rs2372536), this study demonstrated utility in predicting methotrexate response in RA patients.

AI in disease management of RA

Another application of AI in RA disease management is monitoring the disease, including scheduling follow-ups and notification for medications. In the past several decades, the field of mobile health (mHealth) has made significant advances, resulting in a multitude of smartphone apps designed for people with RA. One study utilized data from wearable activity trackers that used machine-generated models for predicting flare sensitivity, while a connected monitoring interface on a smartphone significantly lowered the number of physical visits. ML techniques have the ability to transform RA-related research and enhance disease management (Humbert -Droz et al., 2023). Disease activity score in 28 joints (DAS28) is one of the most utilized severity measures of RA. This index can be calculated based on various inflammatory markers, including ESR or CRP. An adaptive deep neural network was able to outperform non-DL methods in predicting DAS28-ESR from demographical and clinical data with an AUC of 0.73 (categorical prediction) and mean standard error of 0.9 (numerical prediction).

The clinical disease activity index (CDAI) is another scoring system for RA. It only uses clinical data and can be calculated more rapidly than DAS28. One group developed a model using neural networks with a remarkable AUC of 0.91 in predicting disease activity according to the CDAI.

Predicting risk of needing treatment step-up to tocilizumab in patients who do not respond to prior therapy is another example of the application of AI in monitoring disease course in RA. A logistic regression model showed that higher age and remission were the most important risk and protective factors for tocilizumab monotherapy, respectively (OR = 1.04 and 0.17, respectively) when excluding other treatments as variables.

Osteoarthritis

Osteoarthritis is the most common form of arthritis. It can affect both the larger and the smaller joints of the body. This includes the hands, wrists, feet, back, hip, and knee. The disease is essentially one acquired from daily wear and tear of the joint. Osteoarthritis begins in the cartilage, which erodes the cartilage, eventually causing the two opposing bones to grate into each other.

Figure 67.The formation of hard knobs at the middle finger joints (known as Bouchard's nodes) and at the distal joints of the fingers (known as Heberden's nodes) is a common feature of osteoarthritis in the hands.

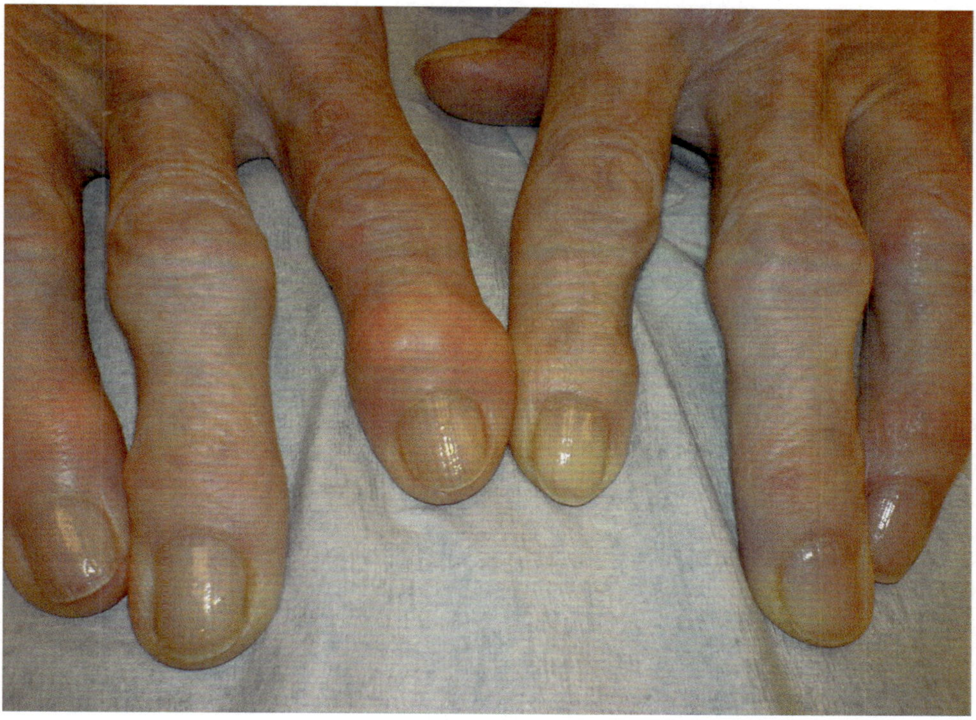

The condition starts with minor pain during physical activity, but soon the pain can become continuous and even occur while in a state of rest. The pain can be debilitating and prevent carrying out some activities. Osteoarthritis typically affects the weight-bearing joints, such as the back, knee and hip, as well as the hands. Unlike rheumatoid arthritis, osteoarthritis is most commonly a disease of the elderly. The strongest predictor of osteoarthritis is increased age, likely due to the declining ability of chondrocytes to maintain the structural integrity of cartilage. More than 30 percent of women have some degree of osteoarthritis by age 65. Other risk factors for osteoarthritis include prior joint trauma, obesity, and a sedentary lifestyle.

Figure 68. MRI of osteoarthritis in the knee, with characteristic narrowing of the joint space

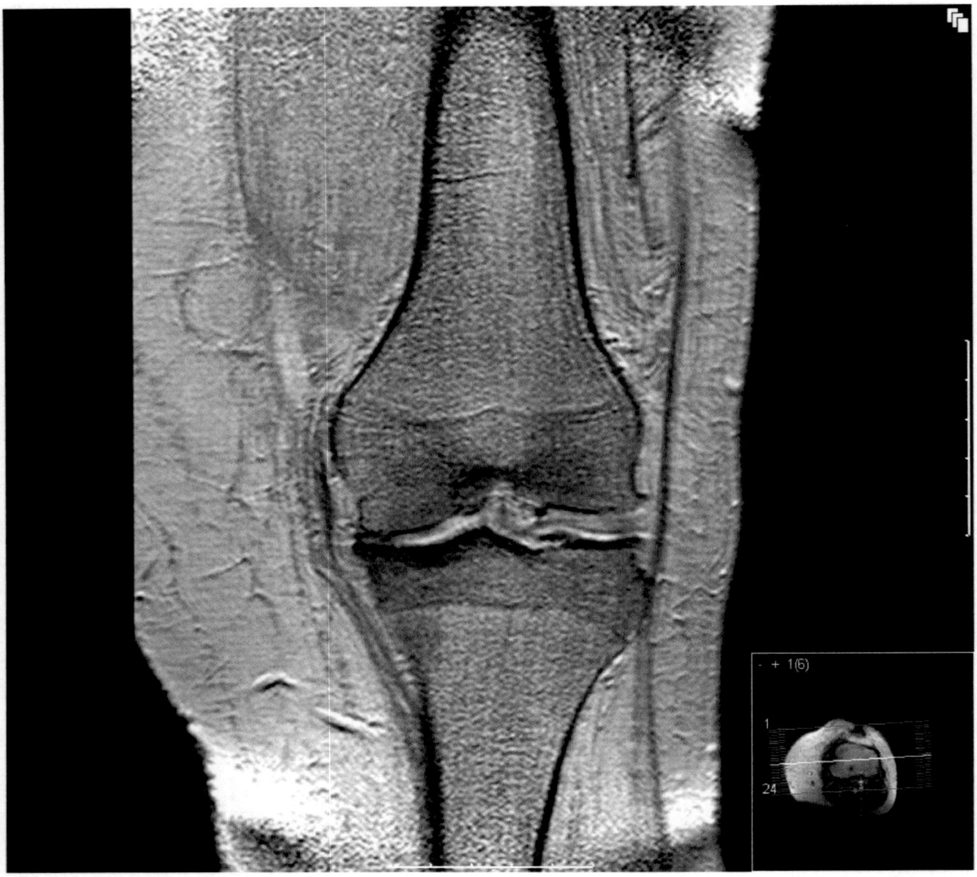

Flynn and colleagues (2023) identified 1931 (178%) more cases of OA than currently diagnosed in the electronic health record of the patients in the study. Individuals diagnosed as cases by their model had higher rates of self-reported knee pain, for longer durations and with increased severity compared to control individuals. They trained another deep-learning model to measure the knee joint space width, a quantitative phenotype linked to knee osteoarthritis severity. In performing genetic association analysis, they found that use of a quantitative measure improved the number of genome-wide significant loci they discovered by an order of magnitude compared with a binary model of cases and controls despite the two phenotypes being highly genetically correlated. In addition, they discovered associations between their quantitative measure of knee osteoarthritis and increased risk of adult fractures- a leading cause of injury-related death in older individuals-, illustrating the capability of image-based phenotyping to reveal epidemiological associations not captured in the electronic health record. For diseases with radiographic diagnosis, the results demonstrated the potential for using deep learning to phenotype at biobank scale, improving power for both genetic and epidemiological association analysis.

Joseph and colleagues (2022) stated that deep learning applications for OA research, including analysis of both radiographs for automatic detection of OA severity, and MR images for detection of cartilage/meniscus lesions and cartilage segmentation for automatic T2 quantification have been developed.

A study by Calivà and colleagues (2022) showed that the application of deep learning to accelerate MRI acquisition and reconstruction was useful; nevertheless, fundamental questions remained regarding the most appropriate metrics for evaluating the quality of reconstructed images. Image segmentation errors from artificial intelligence models lie within intra-reader variability. Deployment in clinical practice still required some form of quality assurance, such as visual inspection of segmentation outputs. They concluded that the role of AI in osteoarthritis is not to provide a final diagnosis but rather to serve as an additional input for decision-making.

Chapter 16. How AI will improve outcomes in musculo-skeletal diseases

Musculoskeletal disorders (MSDs) are injuries or pain in the human musculoskeletal system, including the joints, ligaments, muscles, nerves, tendons, and structures that support limbs, neck and back. Examples of MSDs include carpal tunnel syndrome, epicondylitis, tendinitis, back pain, tension neck syndrome, and hand-arm vibration syndrome.

AI-based techniques applied in musculoskeletal ultrasound (US) imaging focus on automated segmentation, image enhancement, detection and classification. AI-based ultrasound imaging can thus improve accuracy, time efficiency and offer a framework for standardization between different examinations.

Applications in musculoskeletal radiology

One of the characteristics of the radiology field is its incorporation of technological advances into clinical practice. Throughout the history of radiology, there have been several paradigm shifts. Computed tomography (CT) started a revolution in the diagnosis of brain conditions. Another fundamental advance was the advent of magnetic resonance imaging (MRI). AI will likely be the next paradigm shift.

Aspects that artificial intelligence (AI) could bring to radiology include designing imaging protocols and individualized protocols for each patient, reducing image acquisition and processing time, automatic image correction for images with noise or poor image quality, automatic identification of features within images, and automated diagnostic input.

AI can improve efficiency by optimizing workflows in image interpretation and can reduce the imaging workload, which is especially important in modern scanning and MRI techniques that require dozens of sequences for analysis. AI could also improve clinical decision making, increasing the accuracy in interpreting clinical images.

The application of AI in ultrasonography could improve healthcare equity in developing countries and rural areas due to its benefits in detection, diagnosis and image segmentation.

To analyze how a DL system works in image processing, heat map analyses can be useful. The technique identifies the part of the image that requires the largest processing load and can help to better understand whether the algorithm is using incorrect data. For example, to assess an algorithm's ability to detect fractures, a heat map can indicate whether a portion of the image far from the fracture is being analyzed, thereby indicating that the algorithm is processing incorrect data.

AI has been used to detect anterior cruciate ligament ruptures, with no differences in sensitivity or specificity compared with analyses by expert radiologists (Liu et al., 2019). AI has shown good results in diagnosing meniscal tears (Roblot et al., 2019). DL has also been employed to assess acute and chronic cartilaginous lesions (Liu et al., 2018.

Figure 69. Right knee showing the position of the anterior cruciate ligament

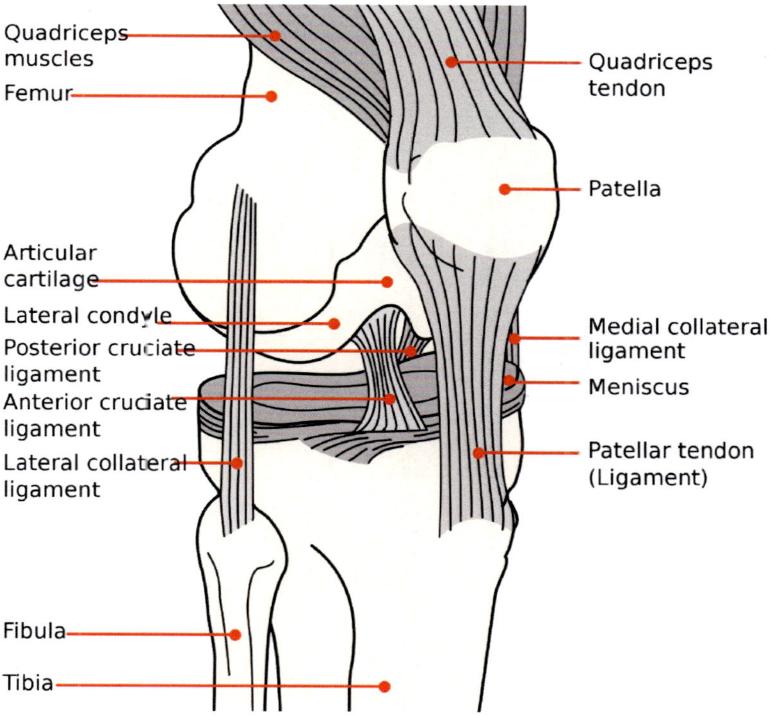

This image is by Mysid - vectorized and colorized in Inkscape, based on Image:Knee diagram.png., Public Domain, https://commons.wikimedia.org/w/index.php?curid=4004042; Knee diagram - Anterior cruciate ligament - Wikipedia. This work is in the public domain in the United States because it is a work prepared by an officer or employee of the United States Government as part of that person's official duties under the terms of Title 17, Chapter 1, Section 105 of the US Code. No changes were made to this image.

The anterior cruciate ligament is composed of strong, fibrous material and assists in controlling excessive motion. This is done by limiting mobility of the knee joint. The anterior cruciate ligament is one of the four main ligaments of the knee, providing 85% of the restraining force to anterior tibial displacement at 30 and 90° of knee flexion. The ACL is the most frequently injured ligament of the four located in the knee.

Figure 70. Bucket-handle tear of the lateral meniscus (red). Medial meniscus intact (green). MRI, coronal T2 *-weighted GRE sequence.

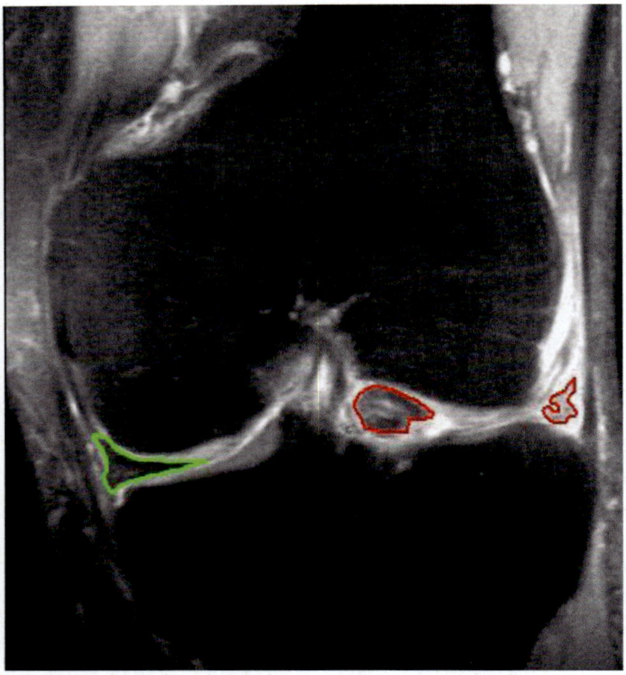

This image is by MBq - Selbsterstellt, public-domain. --MBq (Disk) 14:54, 7. Nov 2005 (CET), Public Domain, https://commons.wikimedia.org/w/index.php?curid=23991857; MBq korbhenkelriss - Meniscus tear - Wikipedia. This work has been released into the public domain by its author, MBq, at the German Wikipedia project. No changes were made to this image.

AI can be used to improve clinical workflows and prioritize the tasks to be performed by clinicians. For example, AI can be used to analyze a large number of images awaiting review, prioritizing the study of those images that are most likely to show lesions/injuries which can have important implications, such as the detection of intracranial haemorrhage in brain scan images.

AI can also be used to accelerate image acquisition. AI systems have been employed to obtain rapid MRI scans (within 5 minutes compared to 15 min for scans without AI). These can be interpreted in a similar manner to conventional MRI scans and are considered of higher quality by clinicians who review the images.

AI has been used as an assistant for automated image segmentation, which enables the extraction of useful biomarkers to facilitate the diagnosis. AI algorithms can differentiate the part of the image that corresponds to the mass to be studied/removed and the part that constitutes healthy tissue, allowing this time-consuming task to be performed quickly and automatically.

Application in skeletal trauma

Extremity trauma is one of the main reasons for emergency department visits and requires high healthcare expenditures. Managing trauma patients almost always involves diagnostic imaging, which can range from radiographs and ultrasound to MRI. Errors in interpreting trauma imaging results can be associated with in increased morbidity and mortality. It has been estimated that the error rate is as high as 30%, even with imaging specialists. Due to the increased use of imaging, there is increasing pressure on physicians to interpret these images.

Figure 71. Fractures of the radius and ulna before surgery (left hand images) and after surgery with metal plates used to unite the fractures (right hand images).

This image is by Sjbrown at English Wikipedia - Transferred from en.wikipedia to Commons., Public Domain, https://commons.wikimedia.org/w/index.php?curid=2001775; Broken fixed arm - Bone fracture - Wikipedia. This work has been released into the public domain by its author, Sjbrown at English Wikipedia. No changes were made to this image.

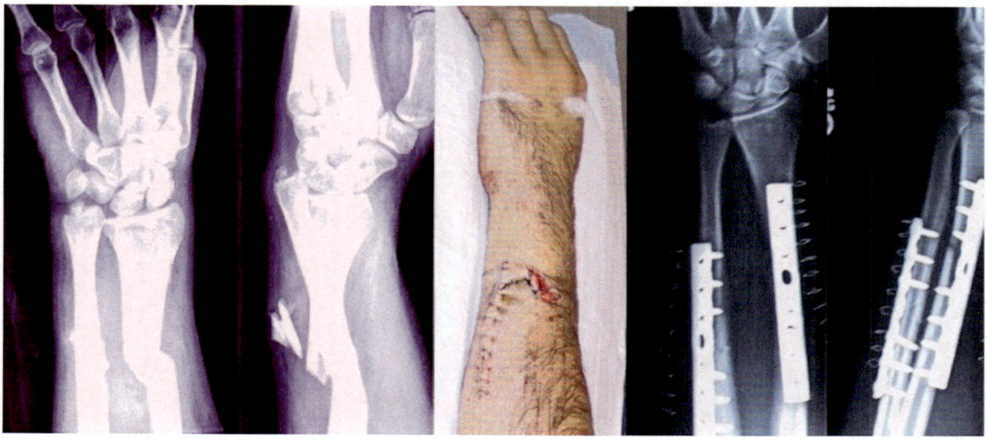

CNNs have been used to detect fractures in radiographs at various anatomical locations, including the extremities, pelvis and spine. Most CNN systems are developed for specific locations, although there are ongoing efforts to integrate several such algorithms. The published algorithms for identifying fractures have shown a performance that has not exceeded the capabilities of a musculoskeletal specialist. The use of these AI tools should therefore be limited to specific clinical tasks. Physicians who are not musculoskeletal radiology specialists would benefit the most from these AI tools.

AI has also been used to classify fractures. There are algorithms that have shown a hip fracture classification accuracy of 93.7%, a femur fracture classification accuracy of 86%, a proximal humerus fracture classification accuracy of 65–86% and good performance in classifying fractures around the knees and ankles.

AI has been used to detect fragility fractures, such as osteoporotic fractures, in plain radiographs with an accuracy of 86%. CNNs have also been used to detect osteoporotic fractures using MRI with an accuracy of up to 88%.

Figure 72. Multiple osteoporotic wedge fractures demonstrated on a lateral thoraco-lumbar spine X-ray

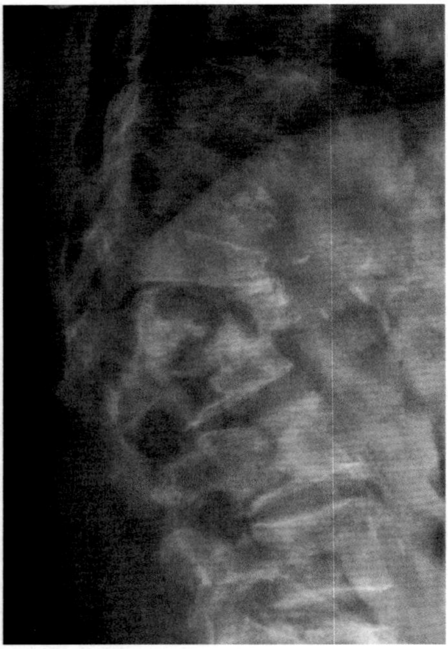

DL has been used to detect occult fractures. For example, a model has been developed that can detect scaphoid fractures that go undetected by human specialists. However, the system capable of detecting previously undetectable fractures missed radiographically obvious fractures. Algorithms combining clinical and radiological data have also been designed. Algorithms have been developed that combine the results of image test analyses with clinical data on rib fractures, which, compared with expert radiologists, could improve the sensitivity and reduce the diagnostic time by a couple of minutes, while maintaining similar accuracy.

Figure 73. X-ray showing a suspected compressive subcapital fracture as a radiodense line

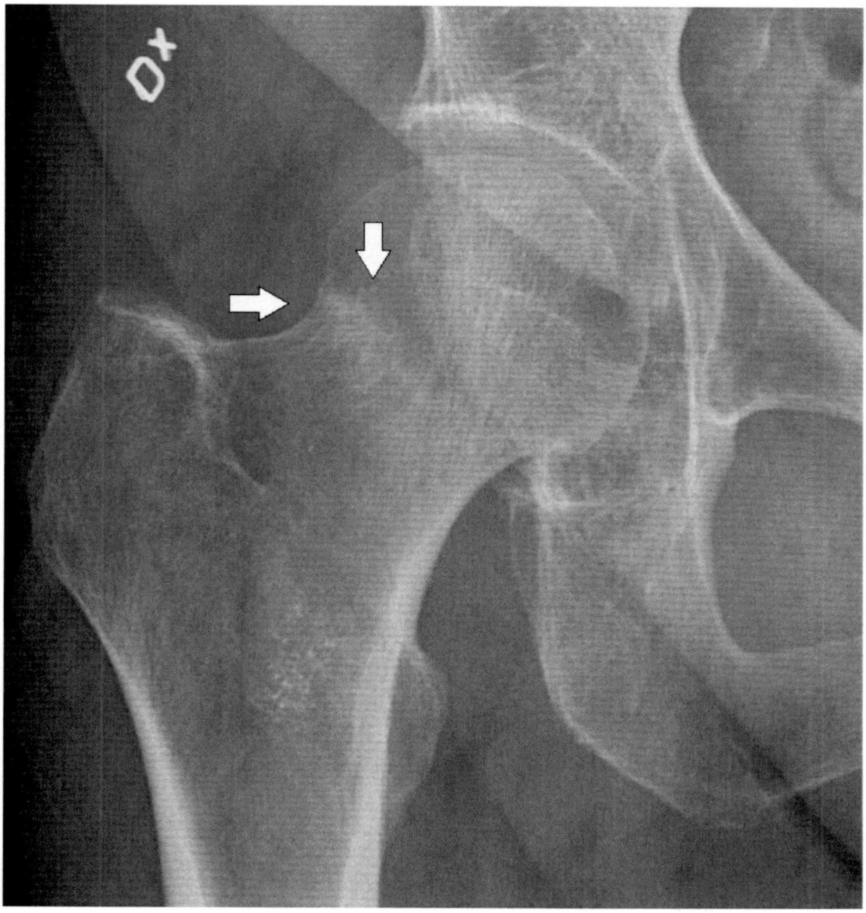

Applications in elective orthopedic surgery

In orthopedic surgery the success of an intervention does not only imply anatomical restoration for the injury or improvements in parameters such as mobility and strength. As important, if not more so, is the subjective result perceived by the patient. Efforts have therefore been made in recent years to collect patient-reported outcome data. AI could help integrate these subjective data with other measures to perform an overall assessment and predict intervention outcomes.

The advantage of AI techniques such as DL is that they can process large amounts of input data (patient age, comorbidities, and sports activity) and generate a single outcome variable with predictive capacity (for example, cost of hospital stay). AI has been used to help decide whether to perform surgery and to preoperatively estimate the risk of mortality and postoperative complications, thereby furnishing surgeons and patients with more accurate data for making better decisions and providing better informed consent.

One study employed artificial neural networks to analyze data from 111,147 patients who underwent total shoulder prosthesis and reverse shoulder prosthesis to predict length of stay, discharge status and inpatient costs, showing good accuracy and reliability.

Figure 74. X-ray of a shoulder prosthesis

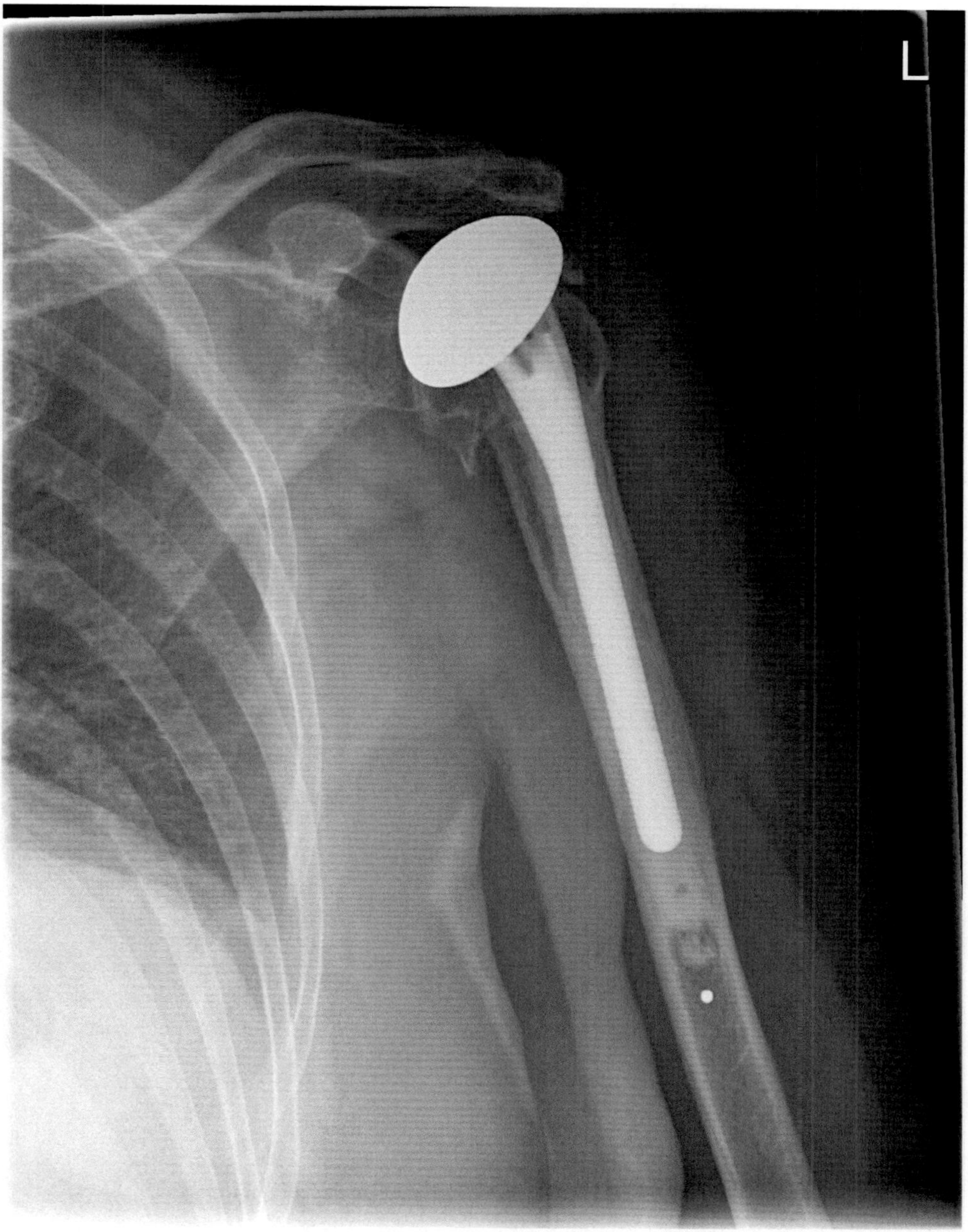
L

Applications in sports medicine

In sports medicine AI can measure the risk of injury to athletes by analyzing the factors involving the athletes and their environment. Injuries can occur as a consequence of these factors. For example, to assess the risk of injury in soccer, the characteristics of the ball, playing field and its environment should be included, as well as the athlete's factors include age, sex and previous injuries.

Another interesting aspect is the development of new technologies that allow high-quality data to be extracted from training and sporting events. There is a large number of wearable devices capable of providing an immense amount of biomedical data. AI can use these data and integrate them with other sources of information to generate algorithms for planning training and matching loads.

Chapter 17. How AI will improve outcomes in vascular diseases

Vascular disease is a group of diseases of the vessels of the circulatory system which includes the arteries and veins, and the lymphatic vessels. Vascular disease is a subgroup of cardiovascular disease. Disorders in this vast network of blood and lymph vessels can cause a range of health problems that can sometimes be severe and fatal. Those of the arterial system are associated with blood supply to tissues and its obstruction due to blockages or narrowing. In the venous system disorders are often caused by a slow return of blood due to insufficiency of valves or to a blood clot.

Venous diseases

Most disorders of the veins involve obstruction such as a thrombus or insufficiency of the valves, or both of these.

Phlebitis

Phlebitis is inflammation of a vein. It is usually accompanied by a blood clot when it is known as thrombophlebitis. When the affected vein is a superficial vein in the leg, it is known as superficial thrombophlebitis, and unlike deep vein thrombosis there is little risk of the clot breaking off as an embolus.

Venous insufficiency

Venous insufficiency is the most common disorder of the venous system, and is usually manifested as varicose veins. Postphlebitic syndrome is venous insufficiency that develops following deep vein thrombosis.

Figure 75. Varicose veins in a 49 year old man

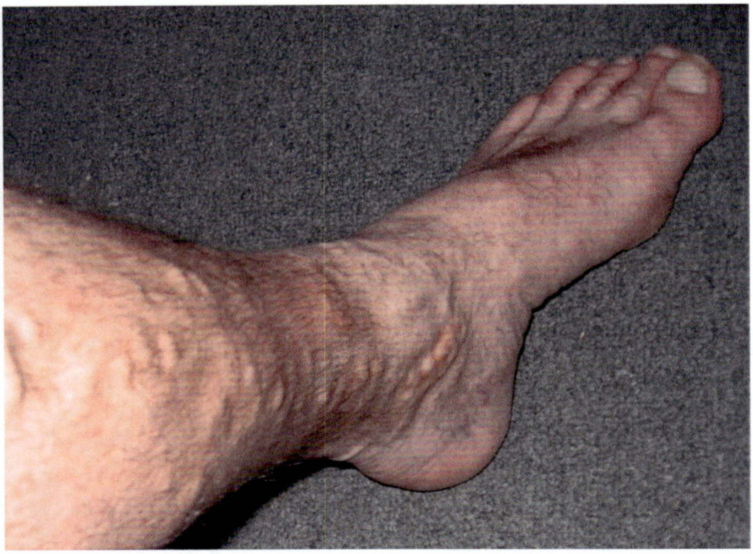

Venous thrombosis

Venous thrombosis is the formation of a thrombus in a vein. This most commonly affects a deep vein and is known as deep vein thrombosis (DVT). DVT usually occurs in the veins of the legs, although it can also occur in the veins of the arms. Immobility, active cancer, obesity, traumatic damage and congenital disorders that make clots more likely are all risk factors for deep vein thrombosis. It can cause the affected limb to swell, and cause pain and an overlying skin rash. A part of a clot can break off as an embolus and lodge in a pulmonary artery in the lungs - a pulmonary embolism. Treatment generally involves anticoagulation to prevents clots or to reduce the size of the clot.

Figure 76. A deep vein thrombosis of the right leg. Note the swelling and redness (blue arrow).

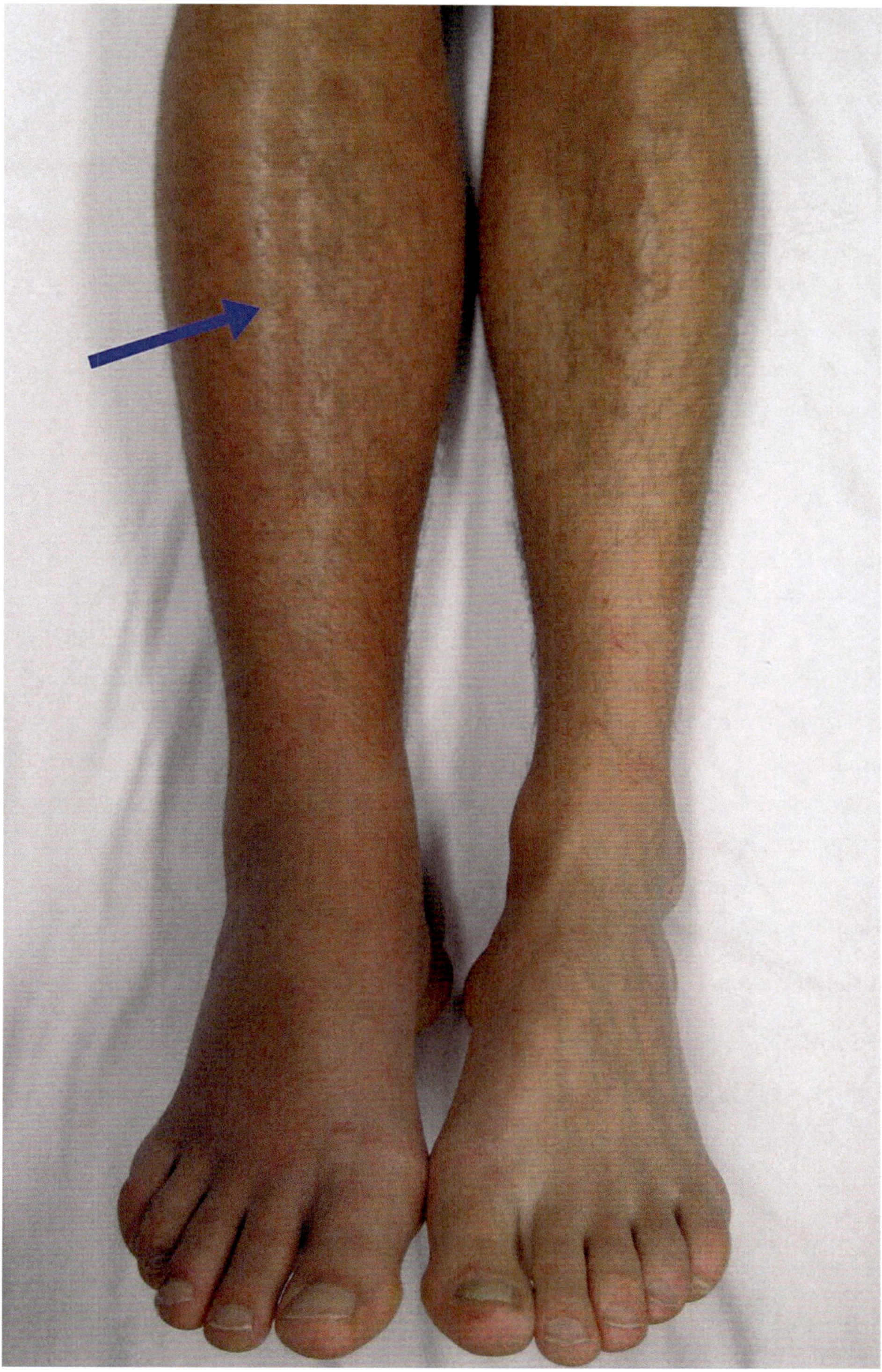

A clot can also form in a superficial vein (superficial venous thrombosis) which is normally not clinically significant, but the thrombus can migrate into the deep venous system where it can also give rise to a pulmonary embolism.

Portal hypertension

The portal vein, also known as the hepatic portal vein, carries blood drained from most of the gastrointestinal tract to the liver. Portal hypertension is mainly caused by cirrhosis of the liver. Other causes can include an obstructing clot in a hepatic vein (Budd-Chiari syndrome) or compression from tumors or tuberculosis lesions. When the pressure increases in the portal vein, a collateral circulation develops, causing abnormal veins such as esophageal varices.

Application of AI to deep vein thrombosis, pulmonary embolism and portal hypertension

Wang et al (2021) performed the first meta-analysis to assess the role of AI in the diagnosis and prediction of venous thromboembolism, which included deep vein thrombosis, pulmonary embolism and portal hypertension. Their results showed that AI had good ability to diagnose and predict venous thrombosis with high sensitivity, specificity and area under the SROC curve values. AI models performed well regardless of the different thrombus types and the different AI methods used. With the development and application of AI in the field of venous thrombosis research, more in-depth and accurate analyzes can be performed in the future, which should allow for a highly applicable and convenient AI model to be developed for widespread use in clinical practice.

Arterial diseases

Carotid artery stenosis – any narrowing of the carotid arteries.

Figure 77. Carotid arteries: the right and left carotid arteries arise from the arch of he aorta.

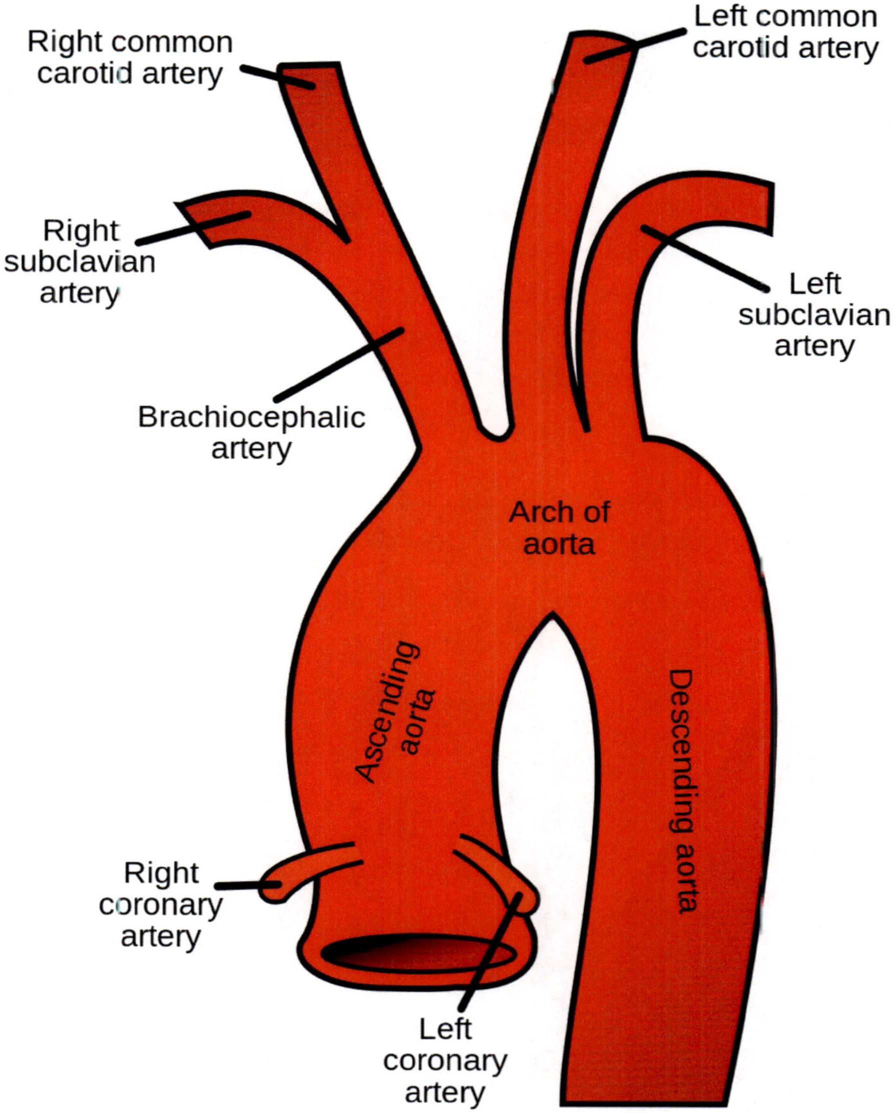

Right common carotid artery
Left common carotid artery
Right subclavian artery
Left subclavian artery
Brachiocephalic artery
Arch of aorta
Ascending aorta
Descending aorta
Right coronary artery
Left coronary artery

AI application for carotid artery stenosis

Kigka and colleagues (2021) developed a machine learning model for the diagnosis and identification of individuals of asymptomatic carotid artery stenosis. The overall model was trained on demographics, clinical data, risk factors and medical treatment data and was able to classify individuals into high risk and low risk individuals. They implemented a statistical analysis to check the data quality and the distribution into the two classes. Different feature selection techniques, in combination with classification schemes were applied for the development of the machine learning model. The overall methodology was trained and tested using 881 cases (443 subjects in low risk class and 438 in high risk class). The highest accuracy 0.82 and an area under curve 0.9 were achieved using the relief feature selection technique and the random forest classification scheme.

Peripheral artery disease

This occurs when atheromatous plaques build up in the arteries that supply blood to the arms and legs, causing the arteries to narrow or become blocked.

Figure 78. Gangrene of three toes resulting from peripheral artery disease due to diabetes mellitus.

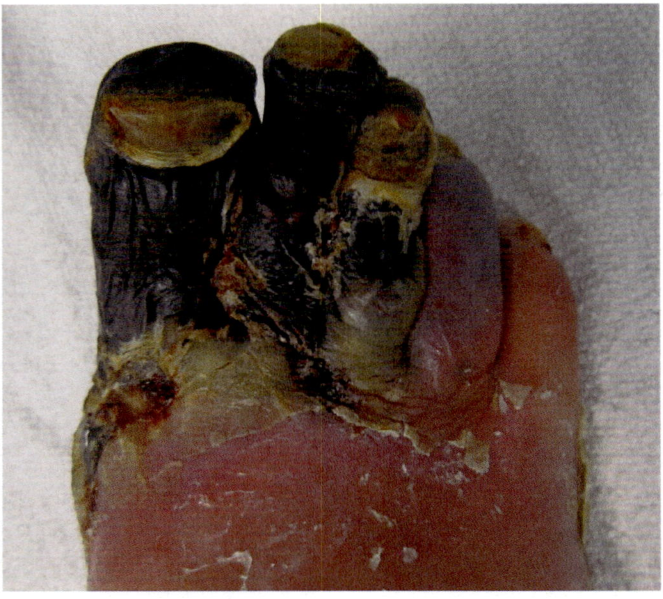

This image is by James Heilman, MD - Own work, CC BY-SA 3.0, https://commons.wikimedia.org/w/index.php?curid=14572015; https://en.wikipedia.org/wiki/Peripheral_artery_disease#/media/File:GangreneFoot.JPG. This file is licensed under the Creative Commons Attribution-Share Alike 3.0 Unported license. No changes were made to this image.

Figure 79. Dorsal foot ulceration (2.5 cm X 2.4cm) that had been chronically open for nearly 2 years in a 71-year-old diabetic male smoker with severe peripheral arterial disease

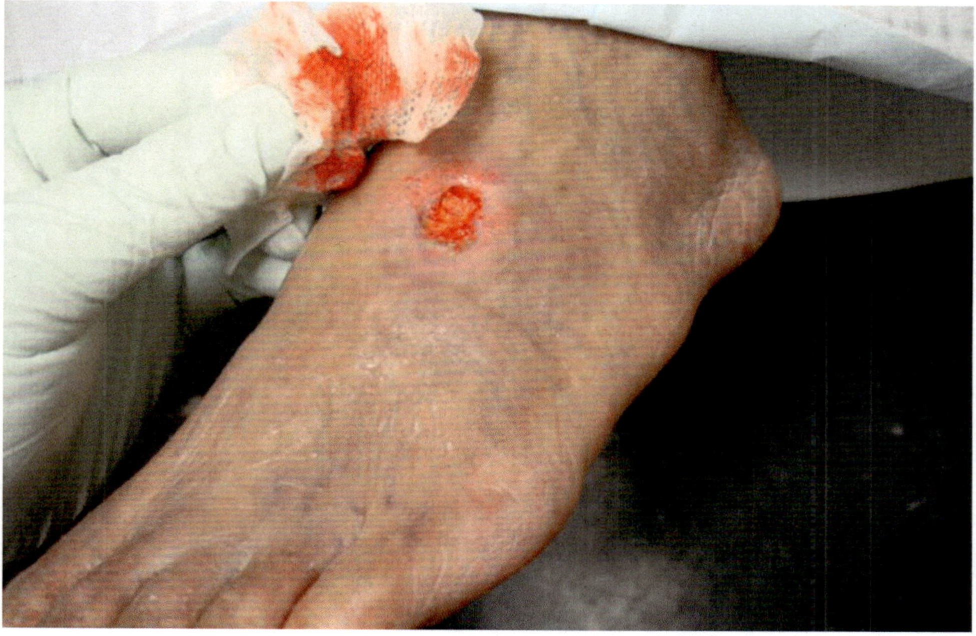

This image is by Jonathan Moore - Creating the Ideal Microcosm for Rapid Incorporation of Bioengineered Alternative Tissues Using An Advanced Hydrogel Impregnated Gauze Dressing: A Case Series. The Foot and Ankle Online Journal 1 (9): 2., CC BY 3.0, https://commons.wikimedia.org/w/index.php?curid=6886430; https://en.wikipedia.org/wiki/Peripheral_artery_disease#/media/File:Arterial_ulcer_peripheral_vascular_disease.jpg. This file is licensed under the Creative Commons Attribution 3.0 Unported license. No changes were made to this image.

Applications of artificial intelligence to peripheral arterial disease (PAD)

Lareyre and colleagues (2023) summarized current knowledge on applications of AI in patients with PAD. Three main types of AI were investigated including natural language processing (NLP), computer vision and machine learning (ML). They found that NLP and ML brought new tools to improve the screening, the diagnosis and classification of the severity of PAD. ML was also used to develop predictive models to better assess the prognosis of patients and develop real-time prediction models to support clinical decision-making. Studies related to computer vision mainly aimed at creating automatic detection and characterization of arterial lesions based on Doppler ultrasound examination or computed tomography angiography. Such tools could help to improve screening programs, enhance diagnosis, facilitate presurgical planning, and improve clinical workflow. They concluded that AI offers several applications to support and likely improve the management of patients with PAD.

Aortic aneurism

Figure 80. Diagram of aortic aneurysm. Panel A shows a normal aorta. Panel B shows a thoracic aortic aneurysm (which is located behind the heart). Panel C shows an abdominal aortic aneurysm located below the arteries that supply blood to the kidneys.

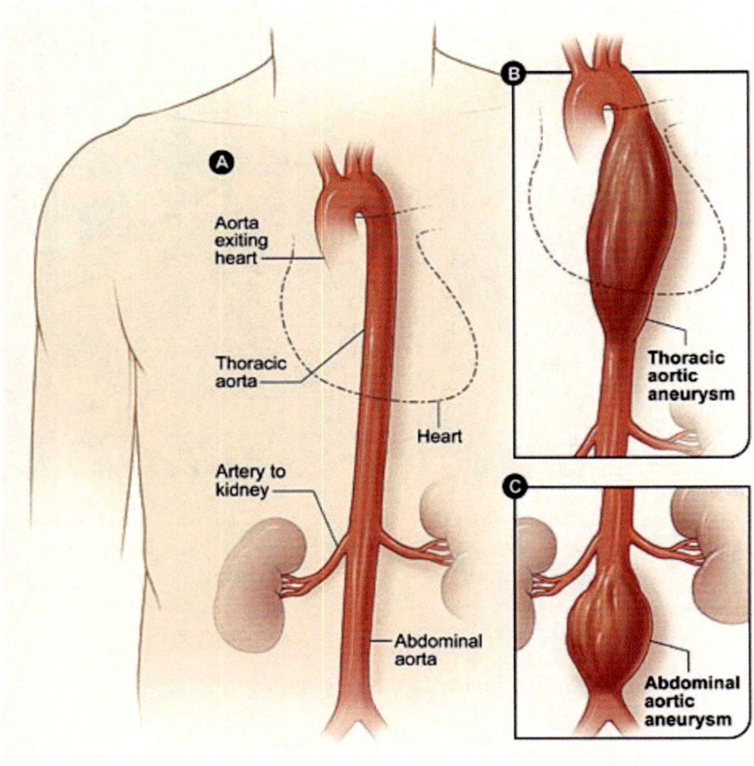

This image is by en:National Institutes of Health - http://www.nhlbi.nih.gov/health/health-topics/topics/arm/types.html, Public Domain, https://commons.wikimedia.org/w/index.php?curid=12180868; Aortic aneurysm - Aortic aneurysm - Wikipedia. This image is a work of the National Institutes of Health, part of the United States Department of Health and Human Services, taken or made as part of an employee's official duties. As a work of the U.S. federal government, the image is in the public domain. No changes were made to this image.

Application of AI to the management of aortic aneurysms

Raffort and colleagues (2020) reviewed the literature on the application of AI to abdominal aortic aneurisms (AAA). AI was used in patients with AAA to improve image segmentation and for quantitative analysis and characterization of AAA morphology, geometry, and fluid dynamics. AI allowed computation of large data sets to identify patterns that may be predictive of AAA growth and rupture. Several predictive and prognostic programs were also developed to assess patients' postoperative outcomes, including mortality and complications after endovascular aneurysm repair. They concluded that AI represents a useful tool in the interpretation and analysis of AAA imaging by enabling automatic quantitative measurements and morphologic characterization. It could be used to help surgeons in preoperative planning. AI-driven data management may lead to the development of computational programs for the prediction of AAA evolution and risk of rupture as well as postoperative outcomes. AI could also be used to better evaluate the indications and types of surgical treatment and to plan postoperative follow-up. AI represents an attractive tool for decision-making and may facilitate development of personalized therapeutic approaches for patients with AAA.

Chapter 18. How AI will improve outcomes in surgery

AI is expanding its footprint in clinical systems ranging from databases to intraoperative video analysis. The unique nature of surgical practice puts surgeons well-positioned to help usher in the next phase of AI, one focused on generating evidence-based, real-time clinical decision support designed to optimize patient care and surgeon workflow (Hashimoto et al., 2018).

Surgical anastomoses after colo-rectal resections

In surgical patients natural language processing (NLP) has been used to automatically comb through electronic medical records (EMRs) to identify words and phrases in operative reports and progress notes that predicted anastomotic leak after colorectal resections. Many of its predictions reflected simple clinical knowledge that a surgeon would have (e.g. operation type and difficulty), but the algorithm was also able to adjust predictive weights of phrases describing patients (e.g. irritated, tired) relative to the postoperative day to achieve predictions of leak with a sensitivity of 100% and specificity of 72%.

Figure 81. A hand-sewn bowel anastomosis, in this case of the sigmoid colon

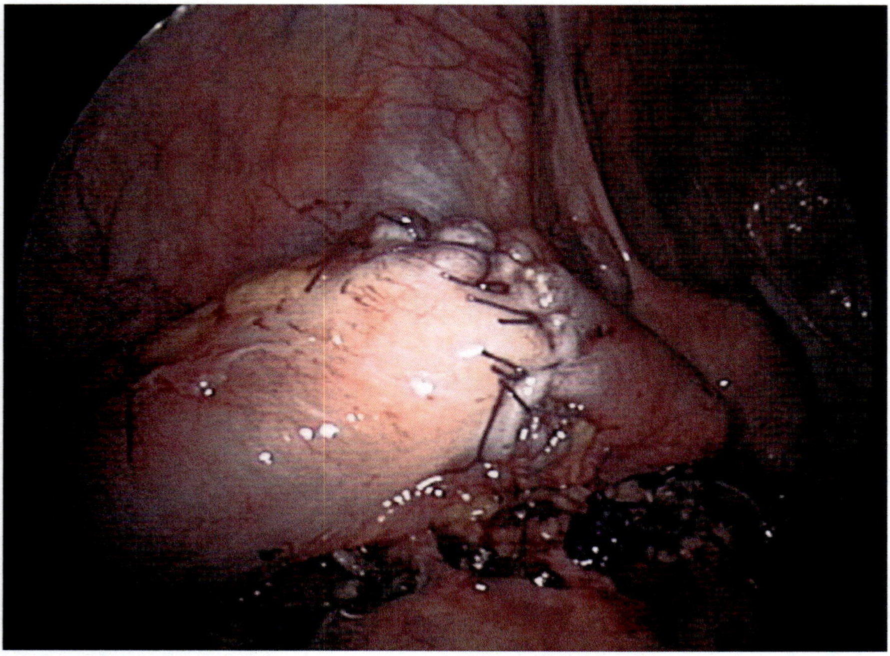

The ability of algorithms to self-correct can increase the utility of their predictions as datasets grow to become more representative of a patient population. NLP and ML analyses of postoperative colorectal patients demonstrated that prediction of anastomotic leaks improved to 92% accuracy when different data types were analyzed in concert instead of individually (accuracy of vital signs – 65%; lab values – 74%; text data – 83%).

Laparoscopy

Real-time analysis of laparoscopic video has yielded 92.8% accuracy in automated identification of the steps of a sleeve gastrectomy and noted missing or unexpected steps. With one minute of high-definition surgical video estimated to contain 25 times the amount of data found in a high-resolution computed tomography image, video could contain a wealth of actionable data. Thus, while predictive video analysis is in its infancy, such work provides proof-of-concept that AI can be leveraged to process massive amounts of surgical data to identify or predict adverse events in real-time for intraoperative clinical decision support.

Figure 82. Surgeons performing laparoscopic stomach surgery. The surgery was performed to remove the gall bladder and to alleviate acid reflux disease.

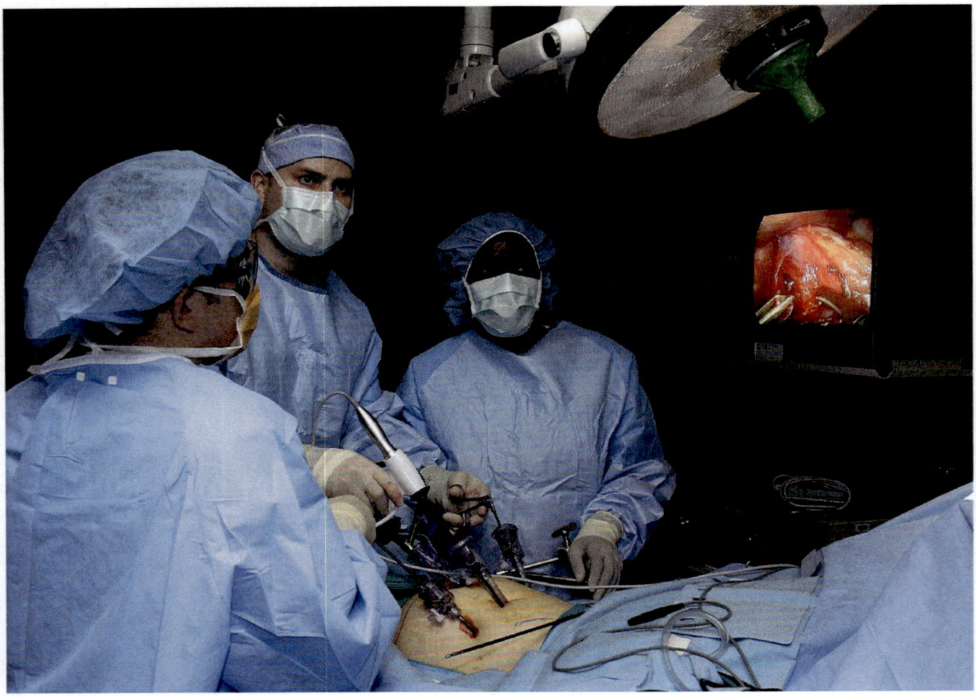

Metastatic lymph nodes

The first widespread uses of AI are likely be in the form of computer-augmentation of human performance. Clinician-machine interaction has already been demonstrated to augment decision-making. Pathologists have utilized AI to decrease their error rate in recognizing cancer-positive lymph nodes from 3.4% to 0.5%.

Figure 83. Histopathology of a lymph node with metastatic invasive ductal carcinoma from the breast, H&E stain, with the presence of extranodal (or "extracapsular") extension (arrows), seen as tumor outside the fibrous capsule of the lymph node.

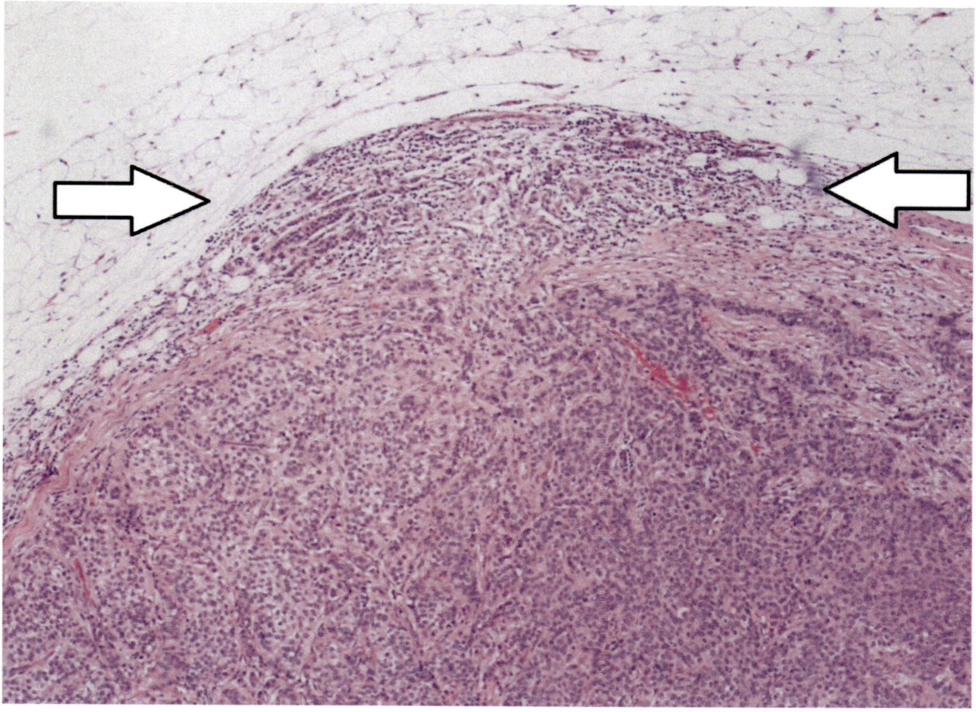

Breast surgery

By improving identification of high risk patients, AI can assist surgeons and radiologists in reducing the rate of lumpectomy by 30% in patients whose breast needle biopsies are considered high risk lesions but ultimately found to be benign after surgical excision.

Bariatric surgery

In the future, a surgeon will likely see AI analysis of population and patient-specific data augmenting each phase of care. Preoperatively, a patient undergoing evaluation for bariatric surgery may be tracked for weight, glucose, meals, and activity through mobile applications and fitness trackers, with the data feeding into their EMR. Automated analysis of all preoperative mobile and clinical data could provide a more patient-specific risk score for operative planning and yield valuable predictors for postoperative care. The surgeon could then augment their decision-making intraoperatively based on real-time analysis of intraoperative progress that integrates EMR data with operative video, vital signs, instrument/hand tracking, and electrosurgical energy usage. Intraoperative monitoring of such different types of data could lead to real-time prediction and avoidance of adverse events. Integration of pre-, intra-, and post-operative data could help to monitor recovery and predict complications. After discharge, post-operative data from personal devices could continue to be integrated with data from their hospitalization to maximize weight loss and resolution of obesity-related comorbidities. Such an example could be applied to any type of surgical care with the potential for truly patient-specific, patient-centred care.

If appropriately developed and implemented, AI has the potential to revolutionize the way surgery is taught and practiced with the promise of a future optimized for the highest quality patient care. AI is expanding its footprint in clinical systems ranging from databases to intraoperative video analysis. The unique nature of surgical practice leaves surgeons well-positioned to help usher in the next phase of AI, one focused on generating evidence-based, real-time clinical decision support designed to optimize patient care and surgeon workflow.

Chapter 19. How AI will improve outcomes in congenital diseases

Congenital heart disease (and see Chapter 6 on cardiology)

Congenital heart disease (CHD) is a complex condition affecting various age groups, with up to 4 to 5/1,000 live births affected by its diverse structural abnormalities. Artificial intelligence (AI) has gained prominence as a transformative technology that can revolutionize the diagnosis, prognosis, and treatment of CHD. The capacity of AI to analyze extensive datasets, recognize patterns, and generate insights has immense implications for CHD management. It excels in predicting CHD occurrence and progression, enabling early interventions and preventive measures. The technology aids in risk stratification by factoring in patient specific variables, facilitating personalized monitoring, and targeting interventions. AI optimizes diagnosis, treatment planning, and outcomes, ushering in a new era of CHD management.

A review of this subject by Mohsin and colleagues (2023) comprehensively examined the role of AI in predicting CHD, understanding risk factors, and facilitating personalized treatment planning. They also explored how AI algorithms analyse diverse datasets to predict and understand CHD risk factors. Additionally, they investigated how AI contributes to risk stratification by considering patient-specific factors associated with CHD complications. Additionally, they delved into the application of AI in crafting personalized treatment strategies for CHD patients. By assessing individual patient traits, therapeutic responses, and treatment outcomes, they found that AI aids in formulating tailored and evidence-based plans.

Prediction of CHD

The potential applications of AI encompass a range of critical functions in the early detection and prognosis of CHD. These tasks include image acquisition, optimization, automated measurements, outlier detection, diagnostic classification, and outcome prediction. AI addresses the limitations of traditional 2D fetal imaging techniques, which often fall short of providing conclusive information due to fetal movement, heart size, and the expertise of the sonographer.

The integration of AI and machine learning (ML) has significantly improved the visualization of cardiac defects. By processing data and identifying patterns, AI algorithms can enhance the accuracy of fetal heart pictures and assist in evaluating cardiac form and function. This is particularly relevant given the challenges posed by factors like rapid fetal heartbeat, small heart size, and limited access to the fetus. Machine learning algorithms have shown promise in diagnosing both critical and non-critical CHDs. Various AI models have gained traction, yielding promising breakthroughs. One notable achievement is the combination of human-performed ultrasound (US) and machine analysis, leading to a remarkable 95% detection rate of CHDs in a test sample. This indicates the potential of automated prenatal screening to significantly reduce newborn mortality by identifying CHDs early. AI-enabled algorithms can estimate prognosis for conditions like the tetralogy of Fallot, enhancing the accuracy of mortality risk assessments and making the process more efficient. Fallot's tetralogy consists of four congenital abnormalities (Figure 84):

- pulmonary stenosis, which is narrowing of the exit from the right ventricle;
- a ventricular septal defect, which is a hole allowing blood to flow between the two ventricles;
- right ventricular hypertrophy, which is thickening of the right ventricular muscle; and
- an overriding aorta, which is where the aorta expands to allow blood from both ventricles to enter.

Figure 84. A diagram showing a healthy heart and one suffering from the tetralogy of Fallot.

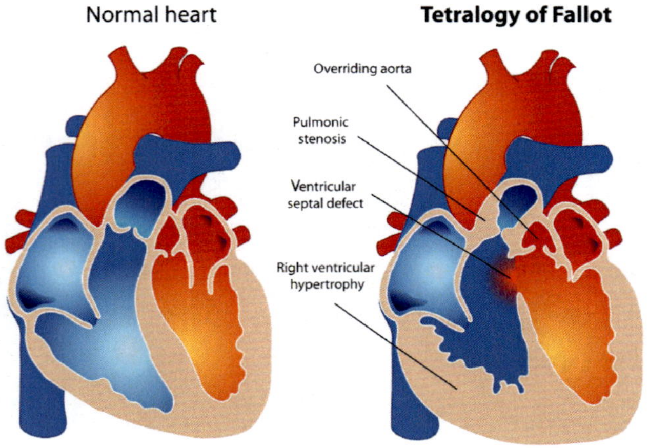

This image is by Mariana Ruiz LadyofHats - the image i made myself using adobe ilustrator using this images including a diagram found on the book "Pädiatrie" from Karl Heinz Niessen., Public Domain, https://commons.wikimedia.org/w/index.php?curid=860748; Tetralogy of Fallot - Tetralogy of Fallot - Wikipedia. This work has been released into the public domain by its author, LadyofHats. No changes were made to this image.

Clubbing of the fingernails is a common abnormality in Fallot's tetralogy, as well as in other diseases. In the case of Fallot's it results from the hypoxia associated with the condition.

Figure 85. Severe clubbing of the fingernails

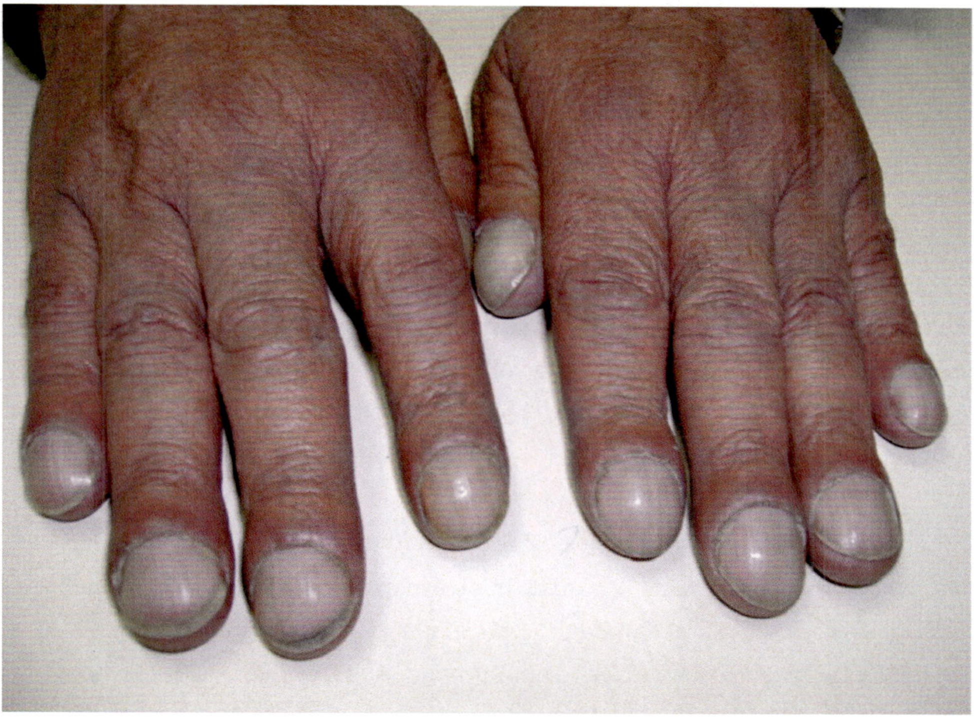

This image is by Desherinka - Own work, CC BY-SA 4.0, https://commons.wikimedia.org/w/index.php?curid=7605105; Dedos con acropaquia - Nail clubbing - Wikipedia. This file is licensed under the Creative Commons Attribution-Share Alike 4.0 International, 3.0 Unported, 2.5 Generic, 2.0 Generic and 1.0 Generic license. No changes were made to this image.

AI-powered software can offer a second view to sonographers during fetal echocardiography, providing valuable guidance in the absence of experienced colleagues. This technology can be integrated into ultrasound machines, allowing real-time assistance during examinations.

Prediction of outcomes and support for clinical decisions

In cardiology, ML-based prediction models are gaining traction for forecasting outcomes and supporting clinical decisions. For instance, these models have been employed to predict mortality following heart transplantation in adults with congenital heart disease, aiding physicians in delivering personalized treatment strategies.

Risk stratification of CHDs

The potential benefits of AI extend to various domains of healthcare, including adult CHD. Developing and using risk scores based on AI predictions can enhance patient care by guiding appropriate follow-up frequencies, treatment escalations, and referrals for procedures or transplantation. The impact of AI on auscultatory results can improve diagnosis accuracy, while ensemble learning models can aid in diagnosing foetal congenital heart defects through imaging. In the field of paediatric cardiology, AI-based algorithms play a vital role in clinical assessment, diagnosis, procedure planning, and intervention management. Machine learning models have the ability to predict various outcomes, such as hospital length of stay, ventilator support time, and mortality after congenital heart surgery. Interpretable machine learning approaches enable accurate predictions of post-surgery complications and patient-specific factors contributing to these predictions. By combining interpretability and model performance, AI empowers clinicians to make more informed decisions. For neonates who undergo complex procedures, AI-driven risk prediction models aid in forecasting one-year death or cardiac transplantation risks, as well as extended hospital stay risks. Several AI models, including Multilayer Perceptron, Random Forest, Extra Trees, Stochastic Gradient Boosting, Ada Boost Classification, and Bag Decision Trees are employed for risk prediction, leveraging factors such as diagnostic groups, patient attributes, and medical history to achieve high levels of accuracy.

Personalized treatment for CHDs

AI is transforming the field of CHD by enabling precision medicine through the analysis of large datasets from these patients. This approach holds the potential to revolutionize diagnosis, treatment planning, and interventions for individual patients. The ability of AI to amalgamate diverse layers of medical data, including clinical records, imaging data, environmental factors, and social influences, offers personalized analytics that can improve patient outcomes. Precision AI in precision medicine for CHD is revolutionizing diagnosis and treatment by leveraging vast datasets to provide personalized care. This wealth of data serves as the foundation for developing predictive models that can guide individualized treatment plans. For instance, serum metabolite panels and DNA methylation are being explored as tools for CHD screening, showcasing the potential of AI in identifying unique biomarkers for early detection.

Digital twin technology takes personalization a step further by creating virtual patient models that mirror real-time clinical data. This technology integrates data from mobile health monitoring, clinical reports, and medical imaging to enhance clinical insights and offer tailored interventions. The potential of AI is evident in studies that utilize deep learning algorithms to diagnose, predict prognosis, and direct therapy for adult patients with CHD. With impressive accuracy rates, these algorithms analyze vast medical records to provide insights into diagnosis, disease complexity, and disease progression. One study investigated how deep learning-based algorithms can be used to diagnose, predict prognosis, and direct therapy in adult patients with congenital cardiac disorders. Over the course of 18 years, the deep learning-based system was applied to over 44,000 medical records from over 10,000 individuals. The analysis was utilized to describe the diagnosis, disease complexity, and New York Heart Association (NYHA) class of adult congenital heart disease. It demonstrated accuracy of 91.1%, 97.0%, and 90.6%, respectively, in the test sample. AI techniques like reinforcement learning, supervised learning, and unsupervised learning are used to analyze extensive datasets, uncover patterns, and generate predictive models. These models enhance diagnostic accuracy, early disease detection, and specialized cardiac care access, offering valuable insights for neonatal and pediatric CHD populations. AI algorithms analyze medical imaging data, such as cardiac MRIs and echocardiograms, to precisely identify anatomical changes and abnormalities. Techniques like picture segmentation and feature extraction contribute to personalized treatment regimens based on individual anatomical traits. Natural language processing (NLP) methods extract valuable information from unstructured data sources like electronic health records and clinical notes. This information aids in creating individualized treatment plans and provides a comprehensive understanding of patients' conditions, facilitating better clinical decisions. AI algorithms utilize patient-specific variables to develop risk prediction models. These models calculate probabilities of complications, disease progression, and treatment outcomes, guiding individualized treatment plans based on unique risk profiles. AI-powered decision support systems offer clinicians recommendations for treatments based on patient-specific data and available research. These systems optimize resource allocation, minimize errors, and enhance patient outcomes by providing evidence-based suggestions. Reinforcement learning techniques tailor treatment plans through trial and error, modelling the patient's state and treatment choices. This adaptive approach responds to patient feedback and preferences. Collaborative filtering techniques consider patient preferences by analyzing data from similar patients, enabling the customization of treatment regimens based on individual preferences and histories. AI-driven decision support systems offer several advantages for CHD treatment. The ability of AI to analyze extensive patient data enhances the accuracy and precision of diagnosis and treatment recommendations. AI algorithms consider various factors to provide personalized treatment strategies that consider anatomical variations, comorbidities, and patient preferences. Decision support systems rely on evidence-based medicine and the latest clinical recommendations, ensuring patients receive the most current and effective treatments. AI systems provide alerts and reminders for potential risks, reducing the likelihood of medical errors.

Hirschsprung disease

Hirschsprung disease (HSCR) is characterized by a lack of ganglion cells in the distal bowel, which may extend proximally for varying lengths. A transition zone (TZ) is almost always seen proximal to the colon’s aganglionic segment (AZ) and distal to the histologically identifiable ganglionic section.

Copy number variant (CNV) analysis on Hirschsprung disease (HSCR) identified a novel candidate gene, NRG3, with an increased burden of intronic CNVs (both deletions and duplications) in patients with Hirschsprung disease. CNV analysis also revealed the differential genetic architecture in relation to CNVs, such that syndromic HSCR was associated with longer CNVs whereas isolated HSCR were found to have an increased burden of shorter CNVs.

Figure 86. A: Plain abdominal radiograph showing a PARTZ at rectosigmoid, arrow. B: Plain abdominal radiograph showing a PARTZ at midsigmoid, arrow. C: Plain abdominal radiograph showing a PARTZ at descending colon, arrow. D: Contrast enema showing a CETZ at rectosigmoid, arrow. E: Contrast enema showing a CETZ at midsigmoid, arrow. F: Contrast enema showing a CETZ at descending colon arrow.

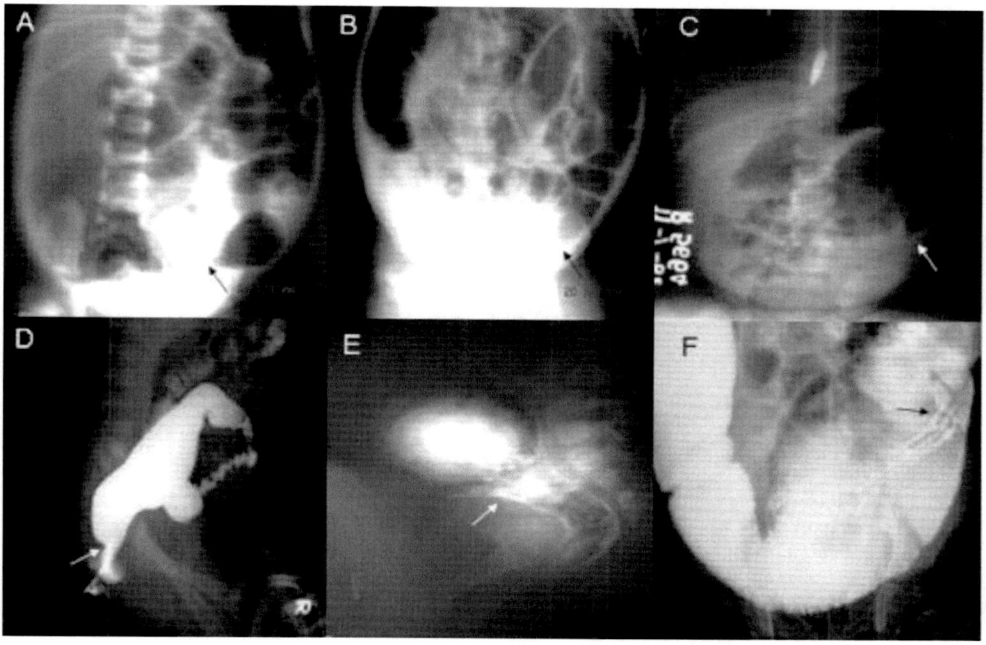

Biliary atresia (BA)

Biliary atresia is a childhood disease in which one or more bile ducts are abnormally narrow, blocked, or absent. It can be congenital or acquired. It has a multifactorial etiology. It is characterized by progressive fibro-inflammatory obstruction of the bile duct. The exact cause of BA is still unknown, but it is thought to be caused by both genetic and environmental factors. One study found BA-private CNVs from SNP array data of BA patients and controls using PennCNV, Birdseye and iPattern. By exploring the interconnectivity of CNVs, SNPs and genetic networks in BA patients, they observed a significant enrichment in the immune-inflammatory pathway for genes associated with these BA-associated CNVs.

Chapter 20. How AI will improve outcomes in infectious diseases

Infectious diseases are caused by microorganisms such as bacteria, viruses, fungi, and parasites. These pathogens are transmitted, directly or indirectly, and can lead to epidemics or even pandemics. The resulting infection may lead to mild-to-severe symptoms such as life-threatening fever or diarrhea. Infectious diseases may be asymptomatic in some individuals but may lead to disastrous effects in others. Despite the advances in medicine, infectious diseases are a leading cause of death worldwide, especially in low-income countries (Agrebi and Larbi, 2020).

Diagnosis

Tuberculosis

Existing systems such as the artificial immune recognition system (AIRS) for the diagnosis of various diseases have been used by investigators to develop early diagnostic tests for several infectious diseases. AIRS uses k-nearest neighbour (kNN) as a classifier. Investigators have improved the accuracy of such a classification aid by using SVM instead of kNN as classifier. SVM is a much more robust classifier and was applied to a cohort of people with tuberculosis. With an accuracy of 100%, sensitivity of 100%, specificity of 100%, Youden's Index of 1, area under the curve (AUC) of 1, and root mean squared error (RMSE) of 0, the new AIRS method was able to successfully classify tuberculosis patients.

Figure 87. An anteroposterior X-ray of a patient diagnosed with advanced bilateral pulmonary tuberculosis. This AP X-ray of the chest reveals the presence of bilateral pulmonary infiltrate (white arrows), and cavity formation (black arrows) present in the apical region of the right lung.

This image is by Unknown author - This media comes from the Centers for Disease Control and Prevention's Public Health Image Library (PHIL), with identification number #2543. Public Domain, https://commons.wikimedia.org/w/index.php?curid=978580; Tuberculosis-x-ray-1 - Tuberculosis - Wikipedia. This image is a work of the Centers for Disease Control and Prevention, part of the United States Department of Health and Human Services, taken or made as part of an employee's official duties. As a work of the U.S. federal government, the image is in the public domain. No changes were made to this image.

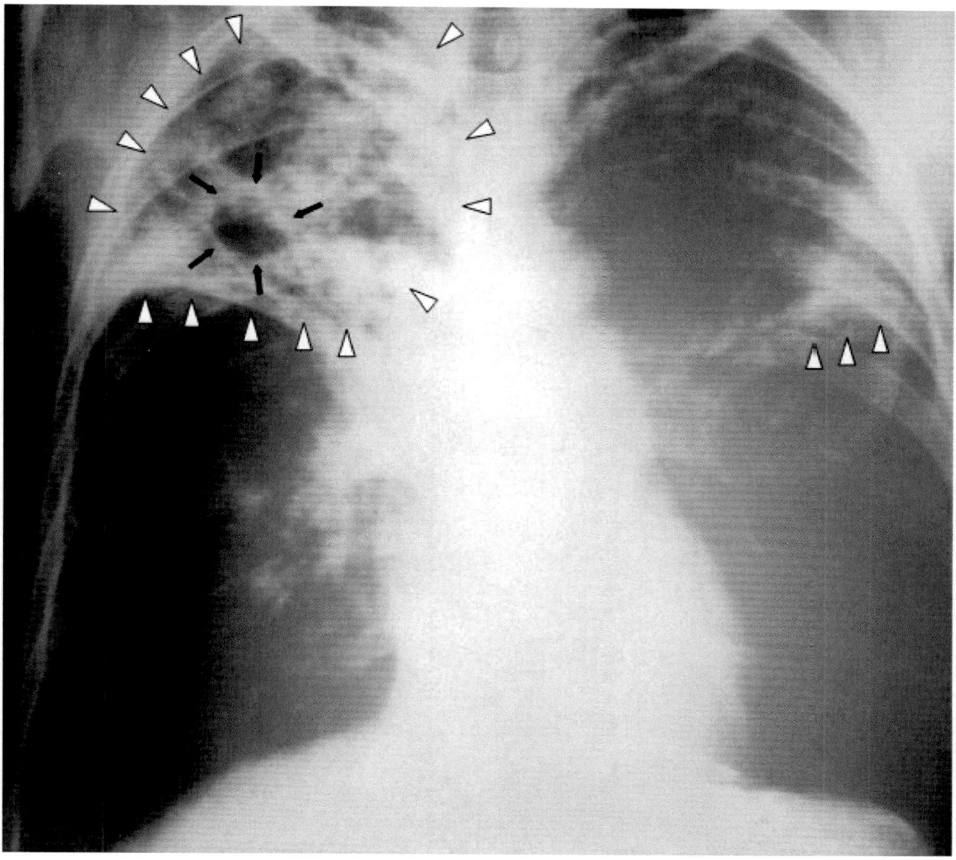

Malaria

Machine learning algorithms were developed to detect red blood cells (RBCs) infected with malaria from digital in-line holographic microscopy (DIHM) data, a fairly cheap technology. Segmented holograms from individual RBCs were tagged with several parameters and 10 of these were statistically different between healthy and infected RBCs. Several machine learning algorithms were applied to improve the malaria diagnostic capacity and the model trained by the SVM showed the best accuracy in separating healthy from infected RBCs for training (n = 280, 96.78%) and testing sets (n = 120, 97.50%). This DIHM-based AI methodology is simple and does not require complex blood sample processing.

Figure 88. Electron micrograph of a *Plasmodium falciparum*-infected red blood cell (center), illustrating adhesion protein "knobs"

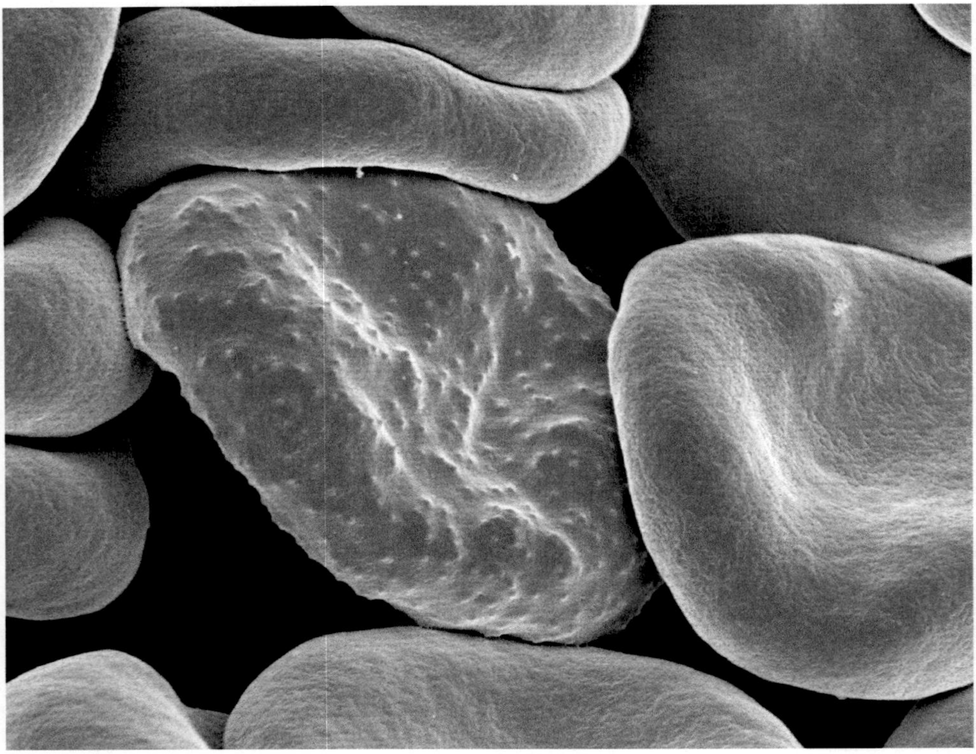

This image is by Rick Fairhurst and Jordan Zuspann, National Institute of Allergy and Infectious Diseases, National Institutes of Health - https://www.flickr.com/photos/nihgov/25534997493/in/photolist-EUrx8t-CvR53a-B3Ad52-ydGygr-wZzPff-C5BN5H, Public Domain, https://commons.wikimedia.org/w/index.php?curid=49182050; Red blood cells infected with malaria - Malaria - Wikipedia. This work is in the public domain in the United States because it is a work prepared by an officer or employee of the United States Government as part of that person's official duties under the terms of Title 17, Chapter 1, Section 105 of the US Code. No changes were made to this image.

Infections after surgery

The University of Iowa Hospitals & Clinics have used machine learning to reduce surgical site infections by 74% over the past 3 years. Using DASH analytics systems, the hospitals are using the high-definition care platform (HDCP), which integrates with the hospital's electronic health records to assess the risk for individual patients. Focusing on surgery-derived infections, the system uses the WHO surgical safety checklist. The checklist comprises three phases of the surgery: (1) before the induction of anesthesia, (2) before the first incision of the skin, and (3) before the patient leaves the operating room. Once these data and those from the existing electronic health records are collected, the DASH system inputs it all into a prediction model and identified potential risks. This enabled the hospitals to provide costly treatments only to patients who needed them.

Clostridium difficile infection

In another hospital, a new algorithm predicted the risk of contracting *Clostridium difficile*, a serious nosocomial infection. Every year in the United States, > 400,000 people contract a *C. difficile* infection following hospitalization and about 30,000 of them die because of the infection. Using a dataset from > 300,000 patients admitted and the knowledge that *C. difficile* spreads through physical contacts, every possible interaction between patients was taken into account when developing the algorithm. Another tool reduced by 87% the time for identification of nosocomial infection in hospitals, suggesting that wider utilization of such application could significantly reduce the morbidity and mortality of hospital-acquired infections.

Figure 89. A pathological specimen showing pseudomembranous colitis due to C. difficile infection

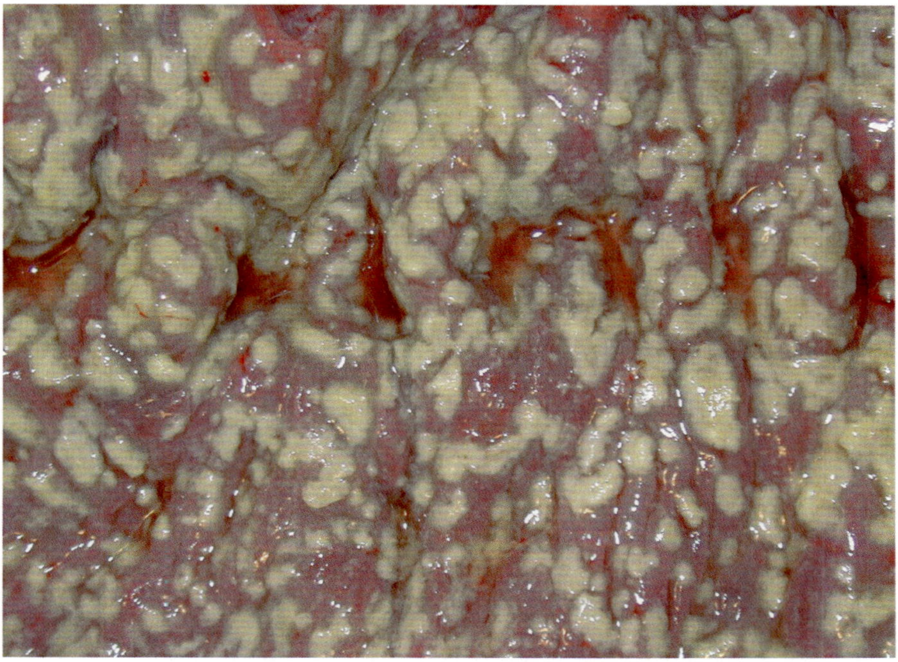

https://en.wikipedia.org/wiki/Clostridioides_difficile_infection#/media/File:Pseudomembranous_colitis.JPG. The copyright holder of this file allows anyone to use it for any purpose, provided that the copyright holder is properly attributed. No changes were made to this image.

Epidemiology and transmission

Ebola

Using machine learning, a single-layer artificial neural network (ANN), logistic regression (LR), decision tree (DT), and SVM classifiers scientists generated an ensemble of predictors that could be applied to different combinations of Ebola-related data.

Hemorrhagic fever, dengue fever, and tuberculosis

The autoregressive integrated moving average (ARIMA) for predicting infectious diseases has been used in domains such as infections that occur in cyclic or repeating patterns. Time series models such as ARIMA have been used to predict future outbreaks since they filter out high frequency noise in the data to detect local trends based on linear dependence in observations in the series. ARIMA models have been widely used for epidemic time series forecasting including hemorrhagic fever, dengue fever, and tuberculosis. Using seasonal ARIMA (SARIMA) and neural network auto-regression (SARIMA-NNAR), the incidence and seasonality of tuberculosis incidence and seasonality was analysed in South Africa. This machine learning approach indicated the need to tackle coinfection issues, especially HIV, and also indicated that festival peak periods are risk factors driving transmission. Derivatives of ARIMA, such as an optimized ARIMA-generalized regression neural network (GRNN) model, were used for forecasting and control of tuberculosis in a far from ideal environment of high population movement and coinfection history (HIV) in China. This showed a superior performance compared to previous models to predict the future incidence of tuberculosis. This suggested that several strategies should be run in parallel and adapted to the local environment and context.

Rift Valley fever

Other methods than ARIMA can indicate the potential risk associated with an infection outbreak. In a study on Rift Valley Fever (RFV) outbreaks in Africa and the Arabian Peninsula, maximum entropy machine learning methods identified the key determinants associated with infectious risk. RVF is a vector-borne viral zoonosis and the ML output identified intermittent wetland, wild Bovidae density, and sheep density as the main associations for RVF outbreaks. (Bovidae are cloven-hoofed, ruminant mammals that includes cattle, bison, buffalo, antelopes, sheep and goats).

H5N1 (bird flu, which can infect humans)

A comparative analysis of H5N1 outbreak in Egypt identified random forest as a more robust method for prediction of H5N1 than ARIMA. This was exemplified by a study showing how modelling (using three-step floating catchment area [3SFCA]) can help optimize health-care utilization by reallocating health-care resources to sites where the ratio of demand/supply is increasing dramatically.

Dengue

Following inoculation of the dengue virus by mosquitoes, dengue hemorrhagic fever occurs in 5% of cases. Applying SVM with the radial basis function (RBF) kernel, scientists have been able to forecast those people with a potential high morbidity rate. The parameter that was able to reach a high level of accuracy was not linked to climate but to the infection rate of the mosquitoes that transmit dengue virus. It most cases of infectious diseases the success transmission blockade is usually linked to outreach.

Figure 90. *Aedes aegypti* mosquito (which can transmit, dengue, yellow fever and malaria) feeding on human blood.

This image is by James Gathany - This media comes from the Centers for Disease Control and Prevention's Public Health Image Library (PHIL), with identification number #9258.Note: Public Domain, https://commons.wikimedia.org/w/index.php?curid=4269685; Aedes aegypti CDC-Gathany - Aedes aegypti - Wikipedia. This image is a work of the Centers for Disease Control and Prevention, part of the United States Department of Health and Human Services, taken or made as part of an employee's official duties. As a work of the U.S. federal government, the image is in the public domain. No changes were made to this image.

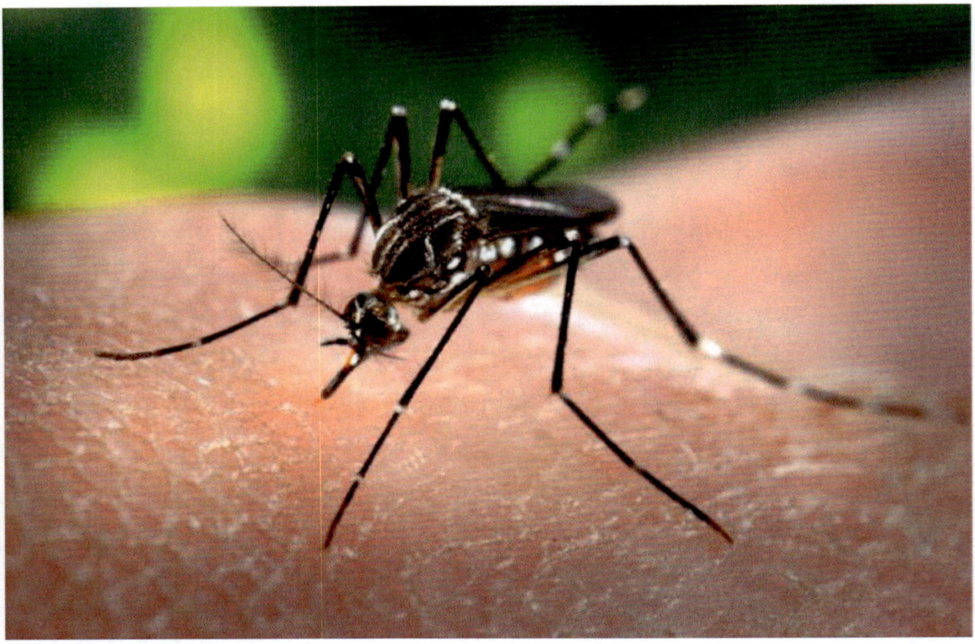

Treatments and antimicrobial drug resistance

The artemisinin-based combination therapies introduced for malaria 20 years ago is now being challenged by the emergence of *Plasmodium falciparum* malaria parasites with decreased susceptibility to artemisinin-based combination therapies. Mathematical modelling using intra-host parasite stage-specific pharmacokinetic-pharmacodynamic relationships predicted that artemesinin resistance was a result of ring stages of the parasite becoming refractory to the anti-malaria drugs.

Figure 91. Blood smear from a *P. falciparum* culture: several red blood cells have ring stages of the parasite inside them.

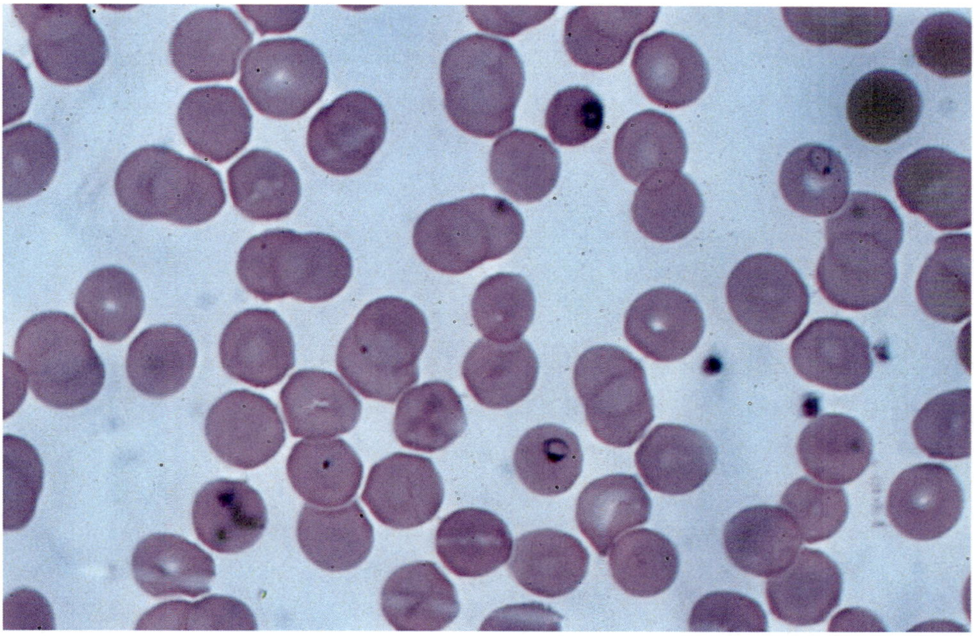

The comprehensive antibiotic resistance database (CARD) contains high-quality reference data on the molecular basis of antimicrobial resistance (http://arpcard.mcmaster.ca). CARD is ontologically structured, model centric, and spans the breadth of antimicrobial resistance drug classes and mechanisms. The database is an interconnected and hierarchical structure allowing optimized data sharing and organization. Recent studies have also shown the use of machine learning in effectively identifying the potential antimicrobial capacity of candidate compounds. In a more systematic way, other investigators used a series of machine learning approaches to predict responsiveness to tuberculosis infection in mice. This included Laplacian-corrected naïve Bayesian classifier models and SVM models using Discovery Studio 4.1. Bayesian model with SVM, recursive partitioning forest (RP forest), and RP single tree models were compared. For each tree, a bootstrap sample of the original data was taken, and this sample was used to grow the tree. (A bootstrap sample is a data set of the same total size as the original one, but a subset of the data records can be included multiple times). Their data clearly suggested that Bayesian models constructed with data generated by different laboratories in various mouse models can have predictive value and can be used in conjunction with other datasets for the selection of the most effective antimicrobial compound. The same mathematical approaches can be performed either on a very specific target for potential drugs or for a more systematic analysis such as performed for the known inhibitors of fructose bisphosphate aldolase, an enzyme central to the glycolysis pathway in *M. tuberculosis*, and an essential player in the bacteria's metabolism. Naïve Bayes, random forest, and C4.5 J48 algorithms were used to improve models by avoiding over fitting and generating faster and cost-effective models. Overall, this suggested that machine learning provides good accuracy, thus confirming other studies validating in silico methods used for screening large datasets to identify potential new drug candidates. Other investigators proposed a decision support system to suggest an antibiotic therapy adapted to the patient based on factors such as the body temperature, infection sites, symptoms/signs, complications, antibacterial spectrum, contraindications and drug-drug interactions. The ontology of this model contained 1,267,004 classes, 7,608,725 axioms, and 1,266,993 members of "SubClassOf" that pertained to infectious diseases, bacteria, syndromes, anti-bacterial drugs and other relevant components. The system included 507 infectious diseases and their therapy methods in combination with 332 different infection sites, 936 relevant symptoms of the digestive, reproductive, neurological and other systems, 371 types of complications, 838,407 types of bacteria, 341 types of antibiotics, 1,504 pairs of reaction rates (antibacterial spectrum) between antibiotics and bacteria, 431 pairs of drug interaction relationships and 86 pairs of antibiotic-specific population contraindicated relationships. It was shown that applying a random forest approach could identify the best set of predictors from laboratory variables measured at onset.

Antibodies are very effective in protecting against viral infection. Studies have shown that the use of machine learning was important for identifying the best candidate vaccines to stimulate antibody production. Antibody features can predict qualitative and quantitative functional outcomes which provide a novel and objective approach to assess immune correlates to antibody features. In the case of the HIV, a way to follow the evolution of the infection is to obtain the blood level of HIV RNA. This is efficient for adjusting therapy but rarely affordable in poor resources settings. As the evolution of HIV infectivity depends highly on antiretroviral therapy, it becomes important to ensure the therapy is taken appropriately and that viral loads are not affected because of loose adherence to treatments. The use of machine learning was very efficient and was able to improve classification of virological failure in a cohort of > 1,000 patients in the United States. The combination of machine learning with standard HIV follow-up ($CD4^+$ T cell count) and antiretroviral therapy regimen significantly improved classification (ROC ≈ 0.8) compared to electronic monitoring system alone. The contribution of machine learning in this context reduced the necessity to perform viral load tests (by 1/3) with a sensitivity for virological failure detection at > 95%.

While these studies show the enormous potential of AI, there are still many aspects that need adjusting in order to fully utilize the capacity of AI to help eradicate pathogens, reduce the burden of seasonal viruses, and better understand the interactions between pathogens and humans.

Making improvements

In order to improve the utilization of AI in the context of infectious diseases, Agrebi and Larbi (2020) believed that identification of the earliest signs of transmission was crucial and used the combination of extreme value theory and robust statistical methods-based analysis for this. The first two steps of correlation/event analysis framework were aimed at filtering most of the data and only letting a small fraction pass to the last step. The goal was to scrutinize the unfiltered data in order to detect suspicious observations. Here again, the main issue lay in the learning of the dynamic Bayesian network (BN). For this purpose, the first step was to store the dataset in a convenient way, often in a specific database to enable fast extraction. The second issue lay in the scores used by learning algorithms to determine the conditional independences required to define the graphical structure of the BN. The focus should be on the rare events and to apply statistical methods suited for this context. This paradigm shift is important because, in their opinion, it is one of the keys to better detect outliers in medical databases. An important aspect of uncertainty discovery is the focus on rare events, which characterize precisely what the analysis is looking for. For this purpose, it was necessary to integrate into algorithms the most recent statistical techniques for the study of large multimodal datasets.

Extreme values and rare events are of utmost importance for extreme risk evaluation In the context of problematic infectious diseases, the low-frequency risk makes extreme value theory and rare event analysis the models of choice for representing appropriately infectious risk-related uncertainties. The study and application of the extreme value theory allows the detection of weak signals in large structured and unstructured data. It should be known that when dimension reduction methods are used, the weak signal at the extreme may be lost. Extreme value theory is a branch of statistics that seeks to assess, from a given ordered sample the probability of events that are more extreme than any previously observed. It is thus a high-dimensional statistical approach. There were several attempts to use extreme value theory in machine algorithms and deep learning. By combining high-dimensional statistics and AI, there should be enough synergy to convince stakeholders and decision-makers to test their potential for predicting and modelling rare events such as pandemics, with a level of certainty.

Chapter 21. How AI will improve outcomes in sepsis

Many studies have been published on a variety of clinical applications of artificial intelligence for sepsis. Sepsis is a life-threatening condition in which early detection and intervention are key to reducing mortality. As per the sepsis-3-criteria, sepsis is currently defined as an acute increase in Sequential Organ Failure Assessment (SOFA) score of ≥2 points, indicating life threatening organ dysfunction, due to suspected infection. This is associated with an in-hospital mortality of about 10%. In the early stages of the disease, sepsis is relatively easy to treat with source control and broad spectrum antibiotics. However, diagnosing sepsis in this stage of the disease remains a challenge. In the later stages of the disease, sepsis becomes much easier to diagnose, but hard to treat successfully. With current diagnostic and prognostic tools, it is difficult for physicians to identify patients with sepsis early and to predict their prognoses to decide upon the best treatment strategy for the individual patient. One of the many reasons behind this, is that sepsis is a very heterogeneous syndrome. Patients may develop sepsis based on different pathophysiological mechanisms and may present with different clinical phenotypes. About one in five patients that present to the emergency department with suspected sepsis does not show any signs of organ dysfunction, while they will develop this within 48 h of admission. Furthermore, bedside screening tools to detect these patients, like the quick Sequential Organ Failure Assessment (qSOFA), lack sensitivity. To improve patient outcomes, it is of the essence to improve time to diagnosis and accuracy of the prognosis for patients with sepsis. Some patients who are initially not even categorized as having sepsis might benefit greatly from early administration of antibiotics. AI prediction models, which have been shown to be useful for diagnosing and prognostication in other fields of medicine, could potentially add much value to these areas for patients with sepsis.

Diagnosis of sepsis

In a literature review Schinkel and colleagues (2019) identified twenty-two articles on the diagnosis or prognosis of sepsis using AI that reported AUROC as the outcome measure.

Fifteen articles on the diagnosis of sepsis with AI models were included. The best performing model reached an AUROC of 0.97. Of the included articles, eleven reported on diagnosing sepsis. In one study the investigators created an algorithm that predicted sepsis onset 48 hours in advance with an AUROC of 0.83, using just vital signs. In another study the investigators created a model to predict the onset of sepsis during hospital admission. This Risk of Sepsis score (RoS) reached an AUROC of 0.93 in the first hour of admission and increased to 0.97 after 24 h. Investigators in another study created an algorithm (InSight) to predict sepsis onset in an intensive care unit (ICU) population. The model used vital signs and age and reached an AUROC of 0.880. Others validated the InSight algorithm on a different ICU dataset and detected sepsis 4 hours before onset with an AUROC of 0.9238. Also, 4 h before onset, the algorithm predicted septic shock with an AUROC of 0.96. In another study investigators created a model to predict sepsis with an AUROC of 0.92937. Kaji and colleagues predicted same-day and next-day sepsis. Same-day sepsis onset prediction models achieved an AUROC of 0.952, while this was 0.876 for prediction of next-day sepsis.

Four articles reported on predictions regarding the pathogens that caused sepsis. One study used an AI model to predict positive blood cultures. The AUROC was 0.98 when 72 hours of data was used for the prediction, while other researchers predicted bacteraemia with an AUROC of 0.73 at the time blood cultures were drawn. In another study the best model to predict whether a pathogen was susceptible to certain antibiotics reached an AUROC of 0.80, for predicting susceptibility to ceftriaxone.

Prognosis of sepsis

There were seven articles on prognosis, predicting mortality over time with an AUROC of up to 0.895. In one study investigators created an algorithm to predict in-hospital mortality in patients with sepsis. The model reached an AUROC of 0.863. Two other studies reported on a model to predict in-hospital mortality with an AUROC of 0.8633 and a model predicting in-hospital mortality with an AUROC of 0.84529, respectively.

Assistance with treatment

There were three articles on assistance of treatment of sepsis, where the use of AI was associated with the lowest mortality rates. Schinkel and colleagues identified three articles regarding assistance of treatment of sepsis using AI. In one study the investigators created an "artificial intelligent clinician" using reinforcement learning. The aim was to create an algorithm that assisted clinicians by suggesting the best treatment at the right time. The model was built based on data from two large ICU databases, Medical Information Mart for Intensive Care (MIMIC)-III and eICU Research Institute Database, that are available online. The "AI clinician" suggested doses of intravenous fluids and vasopressors. On average, the AI recommended higher doses of vasopressors and lower doses of fluids when compared to clinicians. The AI suggested doses correlated with the lowest risk of mortality.

Concerns about these studies

Of these articles, all were judged to be at high risk of bias or had major concerns regarding applicability. This was mostly because predictor variables in these models, such as blood pressure, were also part of the definition of sepsis, which led to overestimation of the performance.

Conclusions

AI models have great potential for improving early identification of patients who may benefit from administration of antibiotics. Some AI prediction models seem to outperform current diagnostic tools by a fair margin, but there are many problems with these models, such as the fact that predictor variables like blood pressure, are also part of the current definition of sepsis. Furthermore, generalizability of these models was very poor. Until these problems have been resolved, a large gap remains between the creation of an AI algorithm for sepsis and its successful implementation in clinical practice.

Chapter 22. How AI will improve outcomes in psychiatric disease

In 2016 about 1 billion people globally were affected by mental health and addiction disorders, constituting about 6% of the world population at the time, with a relatively proportional representation between men and women (Lee et al., 2021). This amounted to about 162.5 disability-adjusted life years (DALY) lost. In recent years and due to COVID-19 mental health illnesses have increased, with a marked increase in loneliness, suicide, and substance abuse.

Types of AI used in mental health

As of 2020, there was no Food and Drug Administration (FDA) approval for AI in the field of psychiatry. This may be due to the large and complex dataset which is required to train any AI model in psychiatric decision making or analysis. The biggest two domains of AI that are currently widely available for multiple applications are Machine learning (ML) and Natural Language Processing (NLP).

Machine Learning

ML begins by looking at the data and finding its own hypothesis based on the patterns it detects. It then creates algorithms to be able to predict new information, based on the created algorithm and the pattern it was able to generate from the original dataset. This model of AI is data driven; it requires a huge amount of structured data, an obstacle in the field of psychiatry which relies mostly on complex DSM-5 definitions for diseases, with a lot of its patient encounters being based on interview and story telling on the part of the patient. (DSM-5 is The Diagnostic and Statistical Manual of Mental Disorders, Fifth Edition).

Because of this, some researchers adopted a different method for creating ML models to be used in psychiatry based on trained models in different fields, a process termed transfer learning.

Transfer learning

This was used by researchers to develop a modified algorithm to detect alcoholism vs. non-alcoholism, and on another occasion the same method was used to detect the signs of post-traumatic stress disorder.

Natural Language Processing (NLP)

One of the obstacles for AI is finding or creating an organized dataset to train and develop a useful algorithm. NLP can be used to create such a dataset. NLP is a technique that involves semantic, lexical, speech recognition, and optical character recognition in order to turn unstructured data into structured data. This is crucial because many of the diagnoses and DSM-5 mental health disorders are diagnosed by speech and doctor/patient interview, utilising the clinician's skill for behavioural pattern recognition and translating it into medically relevant information to be documented and used for diagnoses. NLP can be used to extract, order and structure data on patients from their everyday interactions and not just during a clinical visit.

Diagnosis

AI, through the use of NLP and ML, can be used to diagnose individuals with mental health disorders. It can be used to differentiate closely similar disorders based on their initial presentation to inform timely treatment before disease progression. For example, it may be able to differentiate unipolar from bipolar depression from imaging and medical scans or differentiating between different forms of dementia. AI has the potential to also identify novel diseases that were overlooked due to the heterogeneity of presentation of a single disorder; this means that while many people get diagnosed with depression, that depression may take on different forms and be enacted in different behaviours. AI may parse through the variability of human expression and potentially identify different types of depression.

Prognosis

AI can be used to create accurate predictions for disease progression once diagnosed. AI algorithms do not have to follow current assumptions on diseases and can formulate their own hypotheses and tests to validate new algorithms to predict disease progression and quality of life. Some studies have used neuroimaging, electronic health records, genetic, and speech data to predict how depression would present in patients, their risk for suicide or substance abuse, or functional outcomes.

Treatment

In psychiatry, multiple drugs are trialled with patients until the effective combination or regimen is reached to treat their ailment. AI can be used to predict treatment response based on observed data collected from the various sources that it would have at its disposal.

Benefits

AI in mental health offers several benefits including

- Improving the accuracy of diagnosis: AI-based systems can analyse data from various sources, such as brain imaging and genetic tests, to identify biomarkers of mental health conditions and improve the accuracy of diagnosis.
- Personalized treatment: AI-based systems can analyse data from EHRs, brain imaging, and genetic tests to identify the most effective treatment for specific individuals.
- Improving access to mental health care: AI-based systems can be used to deliver mental health interventions, such as cognitive behavioural therapy, in virtual environments, which can improve access to mental health care in areas where access is limited.

Affective disorders

Much work has been done using artificial intelligence on affective disorders (Ray et al., 2021). Electroencephalograms (EEGs) have been used extensively to study mental illness such as depression as it is a non-invasive, portable and inexpensive method and also because it has high temporal resolution information. Studies involving EEG- based deep learning methods such as one or two dimensional convolutional neural networks have been used to discriminate depressed patients from healthy controls with accuracy of more than 90%. The three D convolutional neural network has also been used to extract short-term dynamic visual representation of depression from video segments, and studies have shown that these network systems can accurately predict depression from video segments.

.

Artificial intelligence supports virtually embodied psychotherapeutic devices are rapidly developing, such as apps like Tess and other chatbots such as Sara, Woebot, and Wysa These work over short message, service text messaging. They have an interactive screen presence. The Woebot engages with patients in the form of a virtual psychological review, helps patients to identify their emotions and thought patterns and to learn skills such as resilience or methods to reduce anxiety. Studies have shown that the use of the Woebot application can successfully reduce depressive symptoms.

Tess is another application which uses natural language processing to flag expressions that indicate emotional distress, and it has been shown to reduce depression and anxiety among users. WhatsApp, or other internet platforms, are also being explored for addressing anxiety and depression.

Psychotic disorders

Machine learning algorithms have successfully discriminated healthy patients from patients with psychotic disorders with the accuracy more than 70%.

It has also been used in studies to assay disordered language production and to differentiate speech samples of patient with psychotic disorders from healthy controls. Algorithms can localize where speech incoherence occurred, predict levels of incoherence and was found to be sensitive to very subtle deviations in lengthy clinical interviews.

Schizophrenia

Avatars have been successfully used in the treatment of schizophrenia to improve medication adherence. Virtual reality-assisted therapy for schizophrenia usually encourages patients to engage with the voices they hear through the use of an AI avatar. Studies have found that this therapy could help in developing therapeutic targets. Virtual reality therapy has helped in improvement of symptoms like visual and auditory hallucinations, depressive symptoms and in overall quality of life particularly in difficult cases of schizophrenia such as treatment-resistant schizophrenia.

Childhood and adolescent disorders

Machine learning techniques have successfully been used to differentiate adult attention deficit hyperactivity disorder (ADHD) from healthy controls and in classification of ADHD subtypes based on power spectra of EEG measurements (Tenev et al., 2014).

Robot-mediated interventions

Robots are being used for children with autism spectrum disorder. One such robot is KASPAR. Six roles for KASPAR have been identified: provoker, reinforcer, trainer, mediator, prompter and diagnostic information provider. The strengths of KASPAR are related to personalization possibilities, its playfulness, the action-reaction principle, its neutral expression, consistent and repetitive application of actions, possibilities to vary behaviour in a controlled manner and having an extra hand. However, certain challenges like limited reaction possibilities such as the likelihood of children being afraid of KASPAR; difficulties with generalization or transfer and the potential dependence on KASPAR, have also been identified.

RoboTherapy is another example of socially assistive robotics designed to help children with autism spectrum disorder to develop social skills. Robot Nao helps in enhancing facial recognition and appropriate gaze response. Such interventions mainly aim at improving social skills like such as imitation, taking turns, staying engaged, and empathy, with the target that children can then apply these learned skills to their relationships with human peers. Initial studies have been very promising. Children with Autism Spectrum Disorder (ASD) have been seen to perform better with their robot partners than with human therapists; they responded with social behaviours toward robots, and their spontaneous language improved during therapy sessions.

Geriatric psychiatry

Companion robots commonly called 'companion bots' are increasingly being used to help patients with dementia. Artificially intelligent animal-like robots such as Paro or e-Bear engage individuals as at-home health care assistants, respond to speech and movement with dynamic 'dialog', or assist in helping elderly or depressed patients by providing companionship and interaction. Studies have found that such robots are fruitful in reducing stress, agitation and loneliness and improve mood and social connections.

Addiction psycniatry

Studies have shown that a conversational agent can improve engagement in digitalized mental health care. Research on psychoeducation delivery has found that text-based conversational agents can lead to higher program adherence compared to verbal presentation. Additionally, such conversational agents cause significant reduction in substance abuse and cravings.

Drug repurposing is a strategy that can help identify potential new therapies for complex diseases. An integrated drug repurposing strategy which combined computational-based drug prediction, patient electronic health records (EHRs)-based clinical corroboration and mechanisms of action analysis was used in a study which could identify five repurposed candidate drugs for treating patients with opioid use disorders.

Sleep disorders

An information support robot (ISR) has been used to influence the daily activities of older people. With changing times, the proportion of older people living alone has increased. Living alone in old age increases the risk of cognitive dysfunction, low mood, and a disturbed sleep/wake cycle. Robots can support older people in maintaining their independence and daily activities. Older people with balanced daily activities have been seen to have lesser disturbance of sleep/wake cycle. Information-supported robots have been used to remind people of the time to wake up, go to bed, and to eat. One study showed that after use of ISR, subjects showed faster wake-up times, decreased sleep duration, and improvement in amount of activity during the day.

Anxiety spectrum disorder

Artificial intelligent models have been used to investigate predictors of fear and perceived ill health using machine learning. Results showed that the model could accurately predict fear of Covid virus using factors like worrying about shortage of food supplies and perceived health using factors like physical exercise, attachment anxiety.

Chapter 23. How AI will improve the evaluation of symptom complexes

Eriksen et al (2023) assessed the performance of the newly released AI chatbot Chat Generative Pre-trained Transformer-4 (GPT-4) in diagnosing complex medical case challenges and compared the success rate to that of medical journal readers. GPT-4 correctly diagnosed 57% of cases, outperforming 99.98% of simulated human readers generated from online answers. The authors highlighted the potential for AI to be a powerful supportive tool for diagnosis; however, further improvements, validation, and addressing ethical considerations are needed before clinical implementation.

The continuous development of AI, including the large language model (LLM) known as the Generative Pretrained Transformer (GPT), has enabled research in new areas, such as the generation of discharge summaries and patient clinical letters. Recently, a paper exploring the potentials of GPT-4 showed that it was able to answer questions in the U.S. Medical Licensing Examination correctly. However, how well it performs on real-life clinical cases is less well understood. For example, it remains unclear to what extent GPT-4 can aid in clinical cases that contain long, complicated, and varied patient descriptions and how it performs on these complex real-world cases compared with humans.

Eriksen et al. assessed the performance of GPT-4 in real-life medical cases by comparing its performance with that of medical journal readers. Their study utilized available complex clinical case challenges with comprehensive full-text information published online between January 2017 and January 2023. Each case presented a medical history and a poll with six options for the most likely diagnosis. To solve the case challenges, the authors provided GPT-4 with a prompt and a clinical case. The prompt instructed GPT-4 to solve the case by answering a multiple-choice question followed by the full unedited text from the clinical case report. Laboratory information contained in tables was converted to plain text and included in the case. The version of GPT-4 available could not accept images as input, so the unedited image description given in the clinical cases was added to the case text. The March 2023 edition of GPT-4 was provided with each case five times in order to assess reproducibility across repeated runs. This was also performed using the current (September 2023) edition of GPT-4 to test the behaviour of GPT-4 over time.

Because the applied cases were published online from 2017 to 2023 and GPT-4's training data included online material until September 2021. Additionally a temporal analysis was performed to assess performance before and after potentially available training data. For medical journal readers, they collected the number and distribution of votes for each case. Using these observations, they simulated 10,000 sets of answers to all cases, resulting in a pseudopopulation of 10,000 generic human participants. The answers were simulated as independent Bernoulli-distributed variables (correct/incorrect answer).

The authors identified 38 clinical case challenges and a total of 248,614 answers from online medical journal readers. The most common diagnoses among the case challenges were in the field of infectious disease, with 15 cases (39.5%), followed by 5 cases (13.1%) in endocrinology and 4 cases (10.5%) in rheumatology. Patients represented in the clinical cases ranged in age from newborn to 89 years old; 37% were female. The number of correct diagnoses among the 38 cases occurring by chance would be expected to be 6.3 (16.7%) due to the six poll options. The March 2023 edition of GPT-4 correctly diagnosed a mean of 21.8 cases (57%) with good reproducibility (55.3%, 57.9%, 57.9%, 57.9%, and 57.9%), whereas the medical journal readers on average correctly diagnosed 13.7 cases (36%). GPT-4 correctly diagnosed 15.8 cases (52.7%) of those published up to September 2021 and 6 cases (75.0%) of those published after September 2021. Based on the simulation, it was found that GPT-4 performed better than 99.98% of the pseudopopulation.

Limitations

An important study limitation was the use of a poorly characterized population of human journal readers with unknown levels of medical skills. Moreover, the authors could not assess whether the responses provided for the clinical cases reflected their maximum effort. Consequently, the results may represent a best-case scenario in favour of GPT-4. The assumption of independent answers on the 38 cases in the pseudopopulation was somewhat unrealistic, because some readers might have performed consistently differently from others and the frequency at which participants responded correctly to the cases might have depended on their level of medical skills. However, even in the extreme case of maximally correlated correct answers among the medical journal readers, GPT-4 still performed better than 72% of human readers.

Conclusions

In this pilot assessment, the diagnostic accuracy of GPT-4 in complex challenging cases was compared to that of journal readers who answered the same questions on the Internet. GPT-4 performed surprisingly well in solving the complex case challenges and was better than the medical journal readers. GPT-4 had high reproducibility, and temporal analysis suggested that the accuracy observed was not due to these cases appearing in the model's training data. However, performance did appear to change between different versions of GPT-4, with the newest version performing slightly worse. Although it demonstrated promising results in this study, GPT-4 missed almost every second diagnosis. However, a recently published letter reported research that tested the performance of GPT-4 on a closely related data set, demonstrating diagnostic abilities even without multiple-choice options.

Currently, GPT-4 is not specifically designed for medical tasks. However, it is expected that progress on AI models will continue to accelerate, leading to faster diagnoses and better outcomes, which could improve outcomes and efficiency in many areas of health care. Whereas efforts are in progress to develop such models, these results, together with recent findings by other researchers, indicate that the current GPT-4 model may hold clinical promise today. Clinical trials are needed to ensure that this technology is safe and effective for clinical use. Additionally, whereas GPT-4 in this study worked only with written records, future AI tools that are more specialized are expected to include other data sources, including medical imaging and structured numerical measurements, in their predictions. Importantly, future models should include training data from developing countries to ensure a broad, global benefit of this technology and reduce the potential for health care disparities. AI based on LLMs might be relevant not only for in-patient hospital settings but also for first-line screening that is performed either in general practice or by patients themselves. The ethical implications surrounding the lack of transparency by commercial models such as GPT-4 also need to be addressed, as well as regulatory issues on data protection and privacy. Finally, clinical studies evaluating accuracy, safety, and validity should precede future implementation. Once these issues have been addressed and AI improves, society is expected to increasingly rely on AI as a tool to support the decision-making process with human oversight, rather than as a replacement for physicians.

Chapter 24. How AI will improve outcomes in pathology testing

Pathology has already witnessed the successful application of AI algorithms in tissue analysis, markedly enhancing diagnostic accuracy and speed. Automated image analysis tools enable pathologists to scrutinise tissues microscopically, identifying subtle histopathological attributes often overlooked by the human eye (Kommura et al., 2018). AI is also accelerating the move towards digital pathology, converting traditional glass slides into digital scans for remote diagnostics and collaborative work - both of which are vital in the digital age of telemedicine.

Digital pathology images used in AI are mostly scanned from slides stained with H&E. Pathology specimens undergo multiple processes, including formalin fixation, paraffin embedding, tissue sectioning, and staining. Each step of the process and the different devices and software used with the digital imaging scanners can affect aspects of the quality of the digital images, such as colour, brightness, contrast, and scale. Normalization is one technique used to reduce such variations. When multiple image acquisition devices are used, scale normalization is of concern, since images acquired from different devices can have different pixel sizes, even at the same magnification level.

Detecting the region-of-interest (ROI) has been performed by combining several computer vision operations, such as colour space conversion, image blurring, sharpening, edge detection, morphological transformation, pixel value quantization, clustering, and thresholding. Colour space conversion is often performed before pixel clustering or quantization, to separate chromatic information and intensity information. Another type of colour space conversion targets direct separation of colour channels for hematoxylin (H), eosin (E) and diaminobenzidine from stained tissue images to effectively obtain nuclei area. Thresholding, based on a certain fixed value, leads to low-quality results when there are variations in luminance in the input images. Adaptive thresholding methods can generate better thresholding results. Recently, pixel-wise or patch-wise classifiers based on CNN have been used widely in ROI detection, where a deep CNN is trained to classify the type of target pixel or patch cantered on the larger input image patch in a sliding window manner. Semantic segmentation CNN is another recent trend for this task; this can detect multiple ROIs in a given image without a sliding window operation, resulting in much faster speed.

In the development of a CNN-based automated image analysis, data-limited situations are common, because it is costly and time-consuming to build a large amount of annotated, high-quality data. Transfer learning and data augmentation should be incorporated to get a better result. In transfer learning, convolutional layer parameters of a CNN, pre-trained with a well-known dataset like ImageNet, are imported into the target CNN as layer initialization, while later layers like fully connected layers or deconvolutional layers are initialized randomly. Additional training steps can update all the layer parameters, including the imported ones, or only the parameters of the layers that were randomly initialized. With sufficient data, building a model without transfer learning is reported to give better performance.

A common strategy of image data augmentation is, for a given image, applying various transformations that do not alter the essential characteristics; such transformations include rotation (90°, 180°, and 270°), flipping (horizontal/vertical), resizing, random amounts of translation, blurring, sharpening, adding jitters in colour and/or luminance, and contrasting histogram equalization. Another type of augmentation relates to the patch generation strategy. Applying large medical images directly to the CNN is impractical. From a large pathological image, with a size between 1024 × 1024 (camera) and > 104 × 104 (scanner) pixels, smaller patches with sizes between 32 × 32 and 512 × 512 pixels are retrieved for use in training and inference of CNNs. Instead of using the pre-generated set of image patches through the whole training process, resampling patches during each training epoch can introduce more variance in training data to reduce the chance of overfitting.

After the patch-level CNN is trained, another ML model is often developed for the whole image level decision. In this case, a patch-level decision is made for every single patch in the training images to generate heatmap-like output, from which several features are extracted via conventional image analysis methods. Then, collected feature values for the training images are fed into the target image level ML model.

An example workflow for two-stage pathology artificial intelligence.

Training phase

From the collected pathology images, a proper amount of annotation data is constructed. Firstly, image patch sets of balanced size are used in the training of a patch-level convolutional neural network (CNN). Secondly, after the patch-level CNN is trained sufficiently, heatmaps are generated for another set of pathology images using the CNN, from which features are extracted for the decision forest like image-level machine learning (ML) model training.

Inference phase

Patch-level CNN runs on every single patch in the input pathology to generate a heatmap (first stage). Features are then extracted as in the training phase and fed into the image-level ML model to determine the image-level result (second stage).

Examples of AI used in pathology tests

Breast cancer

CNN-based breast cancer diagnosis was attempted with fine needle aspiration (FNA) cytology images, optical coherence tomography (OCT) images, and H&E stained tissue images, each with varying numbers of data points and model structures. A total of 175 cytology images captured by a microscopic camera at 40 × magnification was manually split into 918 ROIs, 256 × 256 pixels in size, where each ROI had multiple cells. A CNN was trained to determine the malignancy of a given ROI, and the cytological image was classified as malignant when > 30% of the ROIs in the image were malignant. The reported accuracy was 89.7%, which was inferior to the 99.4% accuracy of a random forest classifier with 14 hand-crafted features. In order to attempt an automated intraoperative margin assessment, 4,921 frame images from the frozen section OCT were used, from which patches 64 × 64 pixels in size were extracted, resized to 32 × 32 pixels, and used for training and evaluation. Patch-level CNN performance was measured, giving an accuracy of 95.0% and AUC of 0.984 in the best setting. In another study, 2,387 H&E stained breast biopsies were scanned at a magnification of 20 ×. Multiple CNNs were used in this study: the first CNN classified each image pixel as fat, stroma, or epithelium; the second CNN predicted whether each stromal pixel was associated with a cancer, and the third CNN determined the whole-slide-level malignancy. The reported slide level AUC was 0.962. A notable result was that, while the CNNs were trained with stromal tissues in benign slides and invasive cancer slides only, the predicted cancer association probability of the stroma near the ductal carcinoma in situ (DCIS) lesion was related to the severity of the DCIS. CNN-based lymph node metastasis detection was also explored with a different model and dataset. Conditional random field was adopted on top of convolutional layers in order to regulate the metastasis prediction. From the whole slide images (WSIs) in the CAMELYON16 dataset, benign and tumour image patches of 768 × 768 pixels in size were sampled to train and validate the model, giving patch-level accuracy of 93.8% after incorporating data augmentation methods. In another study, 271 WSIs scanned at a magnification of 20 × were used in developing a CNN-based model for detecting micro- or macro-metastasis-free slides. Region-level annotations on training images were utilized. Slide-level metastasis detection was performed after metastasis probability map generation by patch-level CNN, incorporating probability thresholding (> 0.3) and connected component analysis to remove small lesions (< 0.02 mm diameter), resulting in a detection AUC of 0.90.

Figure 92. Mitosis appearances in breast cancer: snapshots from several whole slide images (WSI) of several breast resections diagnosed previously as an infiltrative ductal carcinoma using a light microscopy were used. These snapshots showed different appearances of mitotic figures encircled by green circles. Panels A–C show cells in early metaphase. Panels D–G show different forms of mitotic division in late metaphase. Panel H–L shows different forms of anaphase. Panels M–P show cells in telophase.

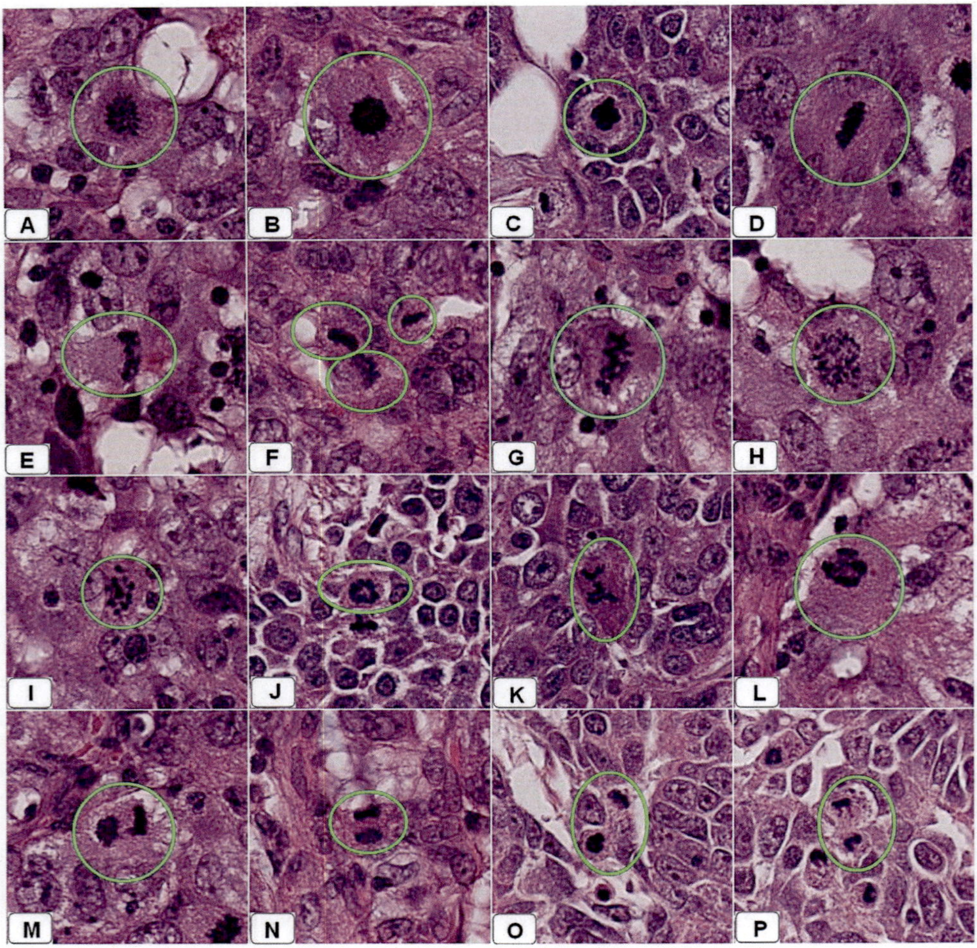

Mitosis detection was assessed with a CNN that decides whether the centre of the given image is mitotic or not, trained and evaluated with 50 images from five biopsy slides containing about 300 mitoses in total, and adopting data augmentation techniques including patch rotation and flipping. In the evaluation, a mitosis probability map was created for the given image, and pixels with locally maximal probabilities were considered as mitotic, resulting in detection F1-score 0.782.

Lung cancer

Automatic lung cancer subtype determination was explored with FNA cytology images and H&E stained WSIs. A total of 298 images from 76 cases acquired using a microscopic camera at 40 × magnification level was utilized in developing a CNN receiving 256 × 256 pixel images as input; the dataset comprised 82 adenocarcinomas, 125 squamous cell carcinomas, and 91 small cell carcinomas.

Figure 93. H&E stained samples from lung biopsies: (Top-left) Normal bronchiole surrounded by alveoli, (top-right) adenocarcinoma with papillary (finger-like) growth, (bottom-left) alveoli filled with mucin suggesting adenocarcinoma nearby, (bottom-right) squamous-cell carcinoma, with alveoli full of keratin.

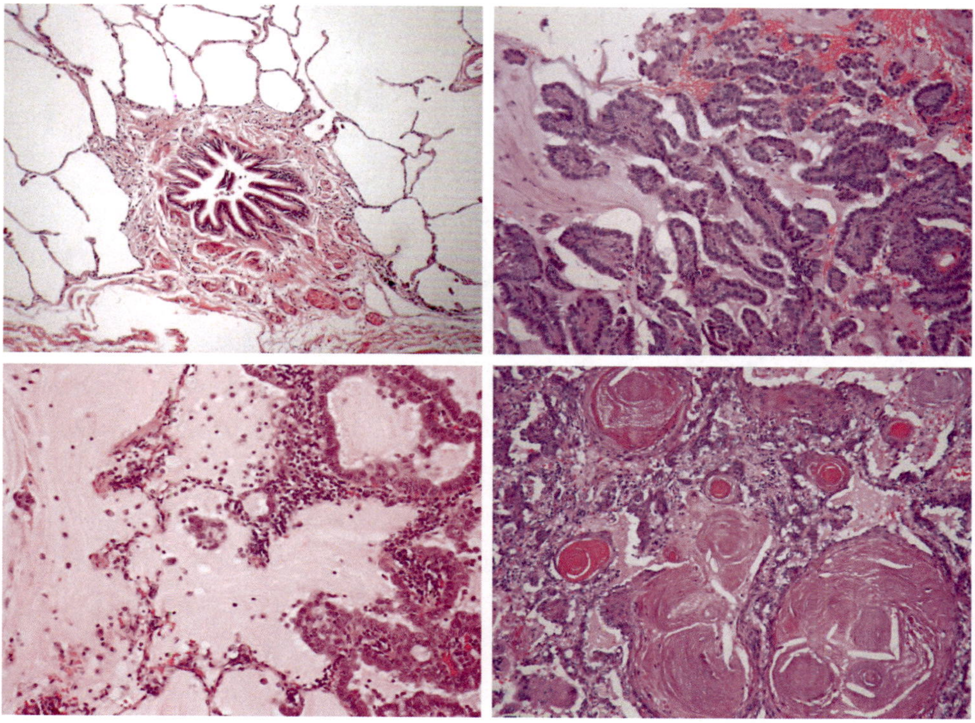

Data augmentation techniques like rotation, flipping, and Gaussian filtering were adopted to enhance the classification accuracy from 62.1% to 71.1%. A total of 1,635 WSIs from The Cancer Genome Atlas (TCGA) dataset were used in the detection of lung cancer type with CNN. Each input patch (512 × 512 pixels) was classified as adenocarcinoma, squamous cell carcinoma or benign, and then the averaged probability of non-benign patches was used in the slide-level decision, resulting in slide level classification with an AUC of 0.97, which is much superior to the previous SVM-based approach. Moreover, by using the multi-task transfer learning approach, mutations of six genes including KRAS, EGFR, and STK11 were independently able to be determined on the input WSI of lung adenocarcinoma patches. The mutation detection had an AUC of 0.86 for STK11 and an AUC of 0.83 for EGFR.

Prostate cancer

Prostate cancer diagnosis has been one of the most active fields in adopting DL because of its large dependence on tissue morphology. Prostatic tissues from various sources have been used for making therapeutic decisions. In one study, 225 prostate needle biopsy slides were scanned at 40 × magnification, and malignant regions were annotated in developing a cancer detector. A CNN-based patch-level cancer detection was performed for every overlapping patch in a slide to generate a probability map, and a cumulative probability histogram was created and analysed in slide-level malignancy determination (AUC 0.99). In another study, 12,160 needle biopsy images were utilized in developing a CNN-based slide-level malignancy detector. To train a patch-classifying CNN with no patch/region level manual annotation, multiple instance learning was used. With a large number of WSIs (> 8,000), the result was useful (AUC 0.98). A total of 886 tissue microarray (TMA) samples were used in a trial of automated Gleason scoring, where 508 TMA images for training were manually segmented into combinations of benign, Gleason pattern 3, 4, and 5; 133 TMA images were used for tuning and 245 images were used for validation. The TMA level score was determined by the two most dominant patterns measured from the per-pattern probability maps generated by a trained patch-level CNN classifier. In grading the validation set, Cohen's kappa between two pathologists was 0.71, while those between the model and each of the two pathologists were 0.75 and 0.71. Three hundred and forty cases from The Cancer

Genome Atlas (TCGA), teaching hospital and medical laboratory were utilized in training an automated Gleason scoring system, where CNN and k-NN classifier were ensembled. A total of 912 slide images were annotated with the region level to be used in training CNN to generate a pattern map for a given slide image; 1,159 slides were used to train the k-NN classifier that determines the Gleason group for the given pattern map statistics. The reported grading accuracy measured on 331 slides was 0.70, while the average accuracy of 29 general pathologists was 0.61, which is superior to the previous TCGA-based result that showed 75% accuracy in discriminating Gleason score 3 + 4 and 4 + 3.

Figure 94. A surgeon performing robot-assisted surgery: this is common practice now for performing a prostatectomy.

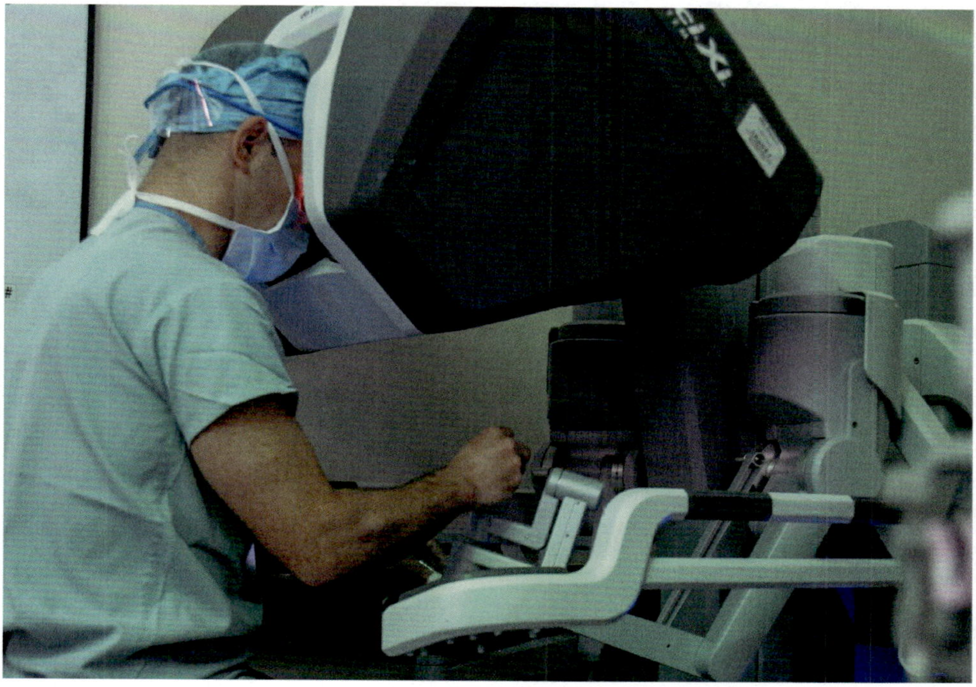

This image is by Navy Medicine - https://www.flickr.com/photos/navymedicine/50264453162/, Public Domain, https://commons.wikimedia.org/w/index.php?curid=139256953; https://en.wikipedia.org/wiki/Prostate_cancer#/media/File:Surgeon_performing_robot-assisted_surgery.jpg This file is a work of a sailor or employee of the U.S. Navy, taken or made as part of that person's official duties. As a work of the U.S. federal government, it is in the public domain in the United States. No changes were made to this image.

Brain cancer

The most common primary brain tumors are gliomas (50.4%), meningiomas (20.8%), pituitary adenomas (15%), and nerve sheath tumors (10%).

Figure 95. Two views of a low-grade brain glioma in a 28-year-old male visualized by MRI

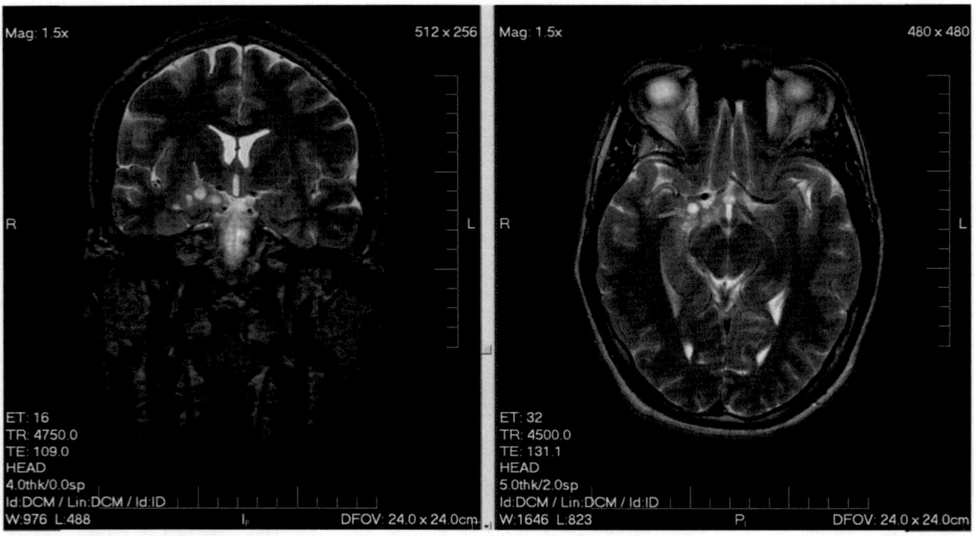

This image is by Blondis at English Wikipedia(Original text: Blondis (talk)) - Own work (Original text: self-made), Public Domain, https://commons.wikimedia.org/w/index.php?curid=3535195; https://en.wikipedia.org/wiki/Glioma#/media/File:MRI_glioma_28_yr_old_male.JPG. This work has been released into the public domain by its author, Blondis at English Wikipedia. No changes were made to this image.

An automated determination of brain cancer severity was tried with TCGA brain cancer data. A cascade of CNNs was used: an initial CNN was trained with 22 WSIs for discriminating between glioblastoma (GBM) and low-grade glioma (LGG), and a secondary CNN trained with an additional 22 WSIs for discriminating between LGG grades 2 and 3. Each H&E-stained RGB colour image was transformed into an H-stained channel and an E-stained channel, and only the H-stained channel was used for further analysis. The first CNN showed GBM/LGG discrimination accuracy of 96%, but the LGG grade discrimination was not so successful (71%). Survival analysis using CNN was also tried. Again, 1,061 WSIs from TCGA dataset were used. For each training epoch, 256 × 256 pixel patches were sampled from manually identified 1,024 × 1,024 pixel ROIs. At diagnosis, ROI-wise risk was determined as the median risk of nine patches sampled from the ROI, and the sample-level risk was determined as the second highest risk among ROI risks. The measured c-index of this kind of survival analysis was 0.75, which was elevated to 0.80 by modifying the CNN to receive mutation information at its fully connected layer.

Ovarian cancer

Ovarian cancer subtype classification based on CNN was explored. 7,392 images were generated by splitting and cropping the original images acquired by the microscopic camera at 40 × magnification level. Rotation and image quality enhancement were used in the data augmentation phase, which enhanced the classification accuracy from 72.8% to 78.2%.

Cervical cancer

Cervical cancer diagnosis on cytological images was also investigated. Without cell-wise segmentation, nuclei-centred cell patches were sampled from the original cytology image, followed by augmentation operations like rotation and translation. Convolutional layer parameters that were trained by using ImageNet data were transferred to actual CNN. Herlev and H&E manual liquid-based cytology (HEMLBC) datasets were used in evaluation, giving 98.3% and 98.6% accuracy, respectively, in five-fold cross-validation.

Figure 96. Invasive cervical squamous cell carcinoma on H&E histopathology and Ki-67 immunohistochemistry.

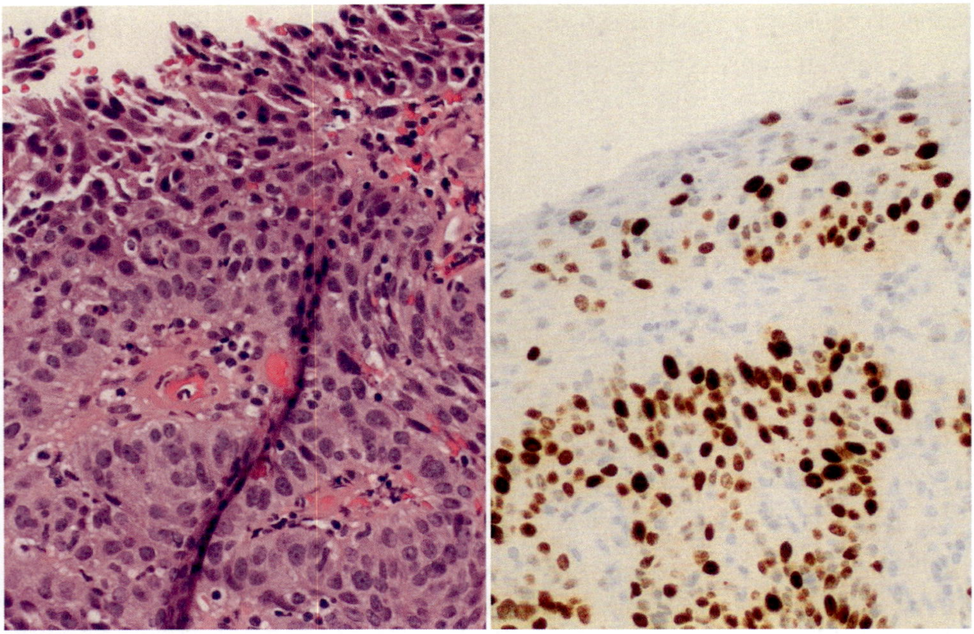

Gastric cancer

A total of 469 tissue microarray (TMA) cores from gastric cancer patients were used in a CNN-based survival analysis. $CD8^+$ and Ki-67 immunostained images were acquired and fed into separate patch-wise risk-predicting CNNs for each stain. From the differential analysis between the low-risk group and the high-risk group, it was claimed that the density of $CD8^+$ cells was largely related to the risk level.

Figure 97. Gastric cancer: endoscopic image of linitis plastica, a type of stomach cancer where the entire stomach is invaded, leading to a leather bottle-like appearance with blood coming out of it.

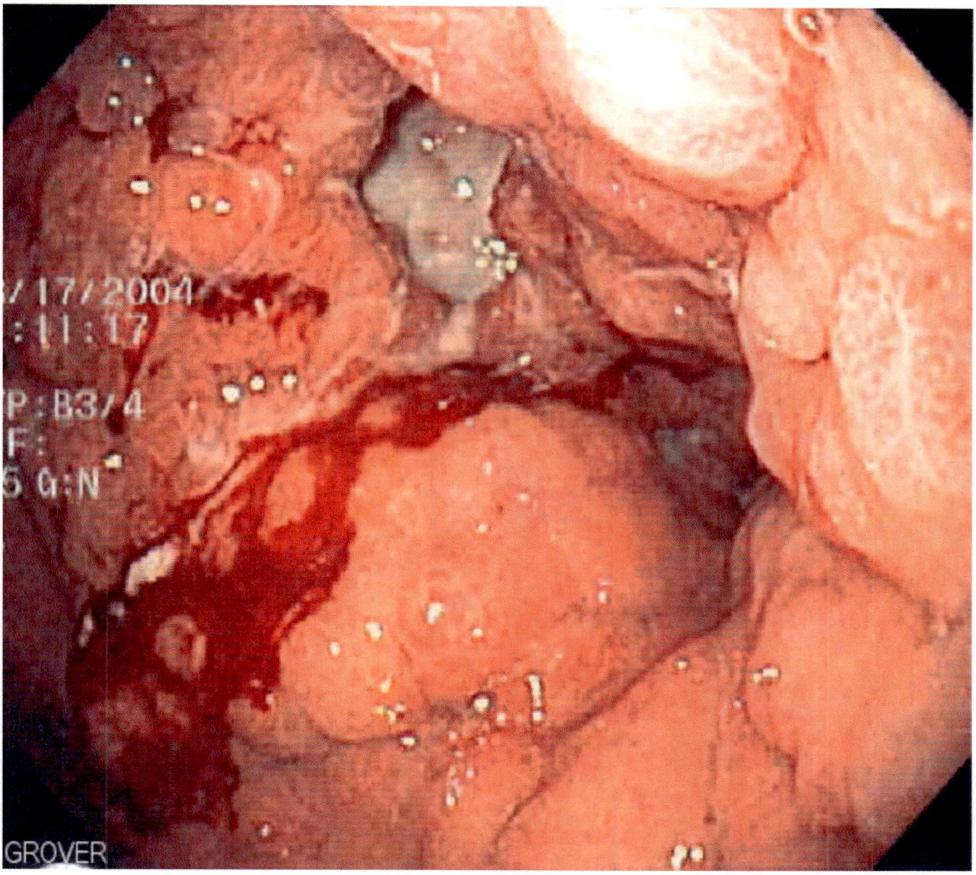

Sickle cell disease

Red blood cell (RBC) classification is critical for the diagnosis of sickle cell disease. A CNN-based automatic RBC classification was tried, where 7,206 cell patches were generated from 434 microscopic images and used for training and testing of the classifier. Rotation and flipping were used to augment training data. Five-fold cross-validation showed an average accuracy of 89.3% in five-class coarse classification, and 87.5% in eight-class refined classification.

Figure 98. Panel A shows normal red blood cells flowing freely in a blood vessel. The inset image shows a cross-section of a normal red blood cell with normal haemoglobin. Panel B shows abnormal, sickled red blood cells blocking blood flow in a blood vessel. The inset image shows a cross-section of a sickle cell with abnormal (sickle) haemoglobin forming abnormal strands.

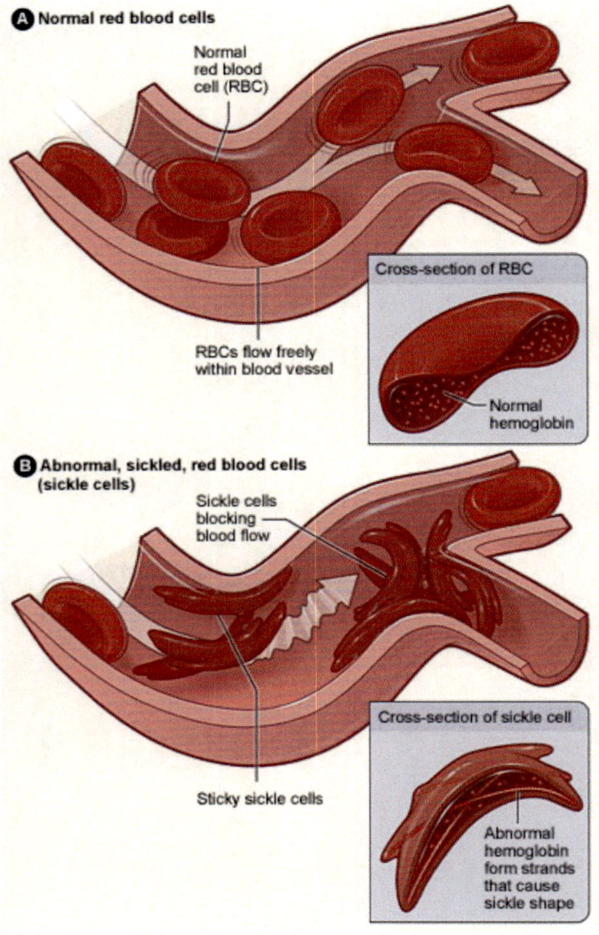

This image is by The National Heart, Lung, and Blood Institute (NHLBI) - http://www.nhlbi.nih.gov/health/health-topics/topics/sca/, Public Domain, https://commons.wikimedia.org/w/index.php?curid=19198765; https://en.wikipedia.org/wiki/Sickle_cell_disease#/media/File:Sickle_cell_01.jpg. This work is in the public domain in the United States because it is a work prepared by an officer or employee of the United States Government as part of that person's official duties under the terms of Title 17, Chapter 1, Section 105 of the US Code. No changes were made to this image.

How AI will improve outcomes in congenital diseases requiring surgery

Genetic mutations are critical factors leading to congenital surgical diseases and can be identified through genomic analysis. Early and accurate identification of genetic mutations underlying these conditions is vital for clinical diagnosis and effective treatment. In recent years, artificial intelligence (AI) has been widely applied for analysing genomic data in various clinical settings, including congenital surgical diseases. Current state-of-the-art AI-based approaches used in genomic analysis are described below and highlight some successful applications that deepen the understanding of the etiology of several congenital surgical diseases. AI methods have been designed for the detection of different variant types and the prioritization of deleterious variants located in different genomic regions, in order to uncover susceptibility genomic mutations that contribute to congenital surgical disorders.

Congenital surgical diseases refer to medical conditions present at birth that require surgical intervention as the first-line treatment. Myriad factors, including genetic mutations, chromosomal abnormalities, and environmental factors such as toxins or virus infection can contribute to these conditions.

Many of these congenital surgical diseases have been shown to have a strong genetic basis. For example, approximately 10%–30% of patients with congenital heart disease (CHD), the most common congenital anomaly that affects around 1% of newborns, may have an identified genetic cause. Chromosomal anomalies (such as trisomy 21 and 22q11.2 deletion) and mutations in genes such as GATA4, NOTCH1, NKX2-5 and TBX1 dysregulate cardiac morphogenesis and differentiation and have been identified in individuals with CHD. In addition, common regulatory variants and rare mutations also predispose to an increased risk of less common surgical disorders, such as Hirschsprung disease and biliary atresia.

Next generation sequencing (NGS) has revolutionized precision medicine, shifting the paradigm of genetic diagnosis toward big data analytics. It is now possible to elucidate the genetic etiology of congenital diseases by analyzing massive omics data generated from DNA, RNA and epigenetic sequencing. Although genomic analysis has been confirmed to be a potent approach for identifying disease-causal variants, the detection and prioritization of these variants predisposed to diseases from a mass amount of data is still a barrier for researchers to tackle. AI fills in this research gap by offering compelling solutions to big data genomic analysis in three major aspects: (i) detection of high-confidence genomic mutations from various genomic data; (ii) predicting the functional impact of these variants on protein structure or functions or regulatory elements; and (iii) prioritizing disease-causing variants in patients.

Conclusions

AI makes it possible to integrate and model vast amounts of genomic data quickly and accurately, facilitating the identification, annotation and prioritization of genetic mutations that contribute to disease development. AI has been confirmed to be a powerful tool that revolutionizes disease-specific genomic analysis by providing speedy and precise insights into the complex relationship between genetics and disease development. Ultimately, these findings that traditional methods might have missed will lead to earlier diagnosis and better prognoses for patients with complex congenital disorders.

Chapter 25. How AI will improve outcomes in genomics research

The complex nature of genomics renders it an ideal candidate for AI intervention. DL techniques decipher genomic data, aiding in identifying genetic variants linked to disease susceptibility, and opening avenues for tailored treatment strategies based on individual genetic profiles.

The major classes of problems that have been addressed by AI in clinical genomics are described below (Dias and Torkamani, 2019).

Variant calling

The clinical interpretation of genomes is sensitive to the identification of individual genetic variants among the millions populating each genome, necessitating extreme accuracy. Standard variant-calling tools are prone to systematic errors that are associated with the subtleties of sample preparation, sequencing technology, sequence context, and the sometimes unpredictable influence of biology such as somatic mosaicism. A mixture of statistical techniques including hand-crafted features such as strand-bias or population-level dependencies are used to address these issues, resulting in high accuracy but biased errors. AI algorithms can learn these biases from a single genome with a known gold standard of reference variant calls and produce superior variant calls. DeepVariant, a CNN-based variant caller trained directly on read alignments without any specialized knowledge about genomics or sequencing platforms, has been shown to outperform standard tools on some variant-calling tasks. The improved accuracy is thought to be due to the ability of CNNs to identify complex dependencies in sequencing data. In addition, results suggested that deep learning is poised to revolutionize base calling (and as a result, variant identification) for nanopore-based sequencing technologies, which have historically struggled to compete with established sequencing technology because of the error-prone nature of prior base-calling algorithms.

To detect high-quality genomic variants sensitively and specifically, numerous tools have been developed using different AI models (for example, Bayesian, Random Forest, and CNN). The majority of these tools have been established to identify single-nucleotide variations (SNVs), small insertions and deletions (indels), and copy number variants (CNVs), as these types of variation are the dominant sources of a genomic mutation linked to disease. Similarly, rare and novel CNVs can also be discovered from traditional SNP (single-nucleotide polymorphisms) array data using AI models trained on data with known copy number information.

As the major variant types, SNVs and indels could be detected by numerous variant calling tools, among which the Genome Analysis Toolkit (GATK), DeepVariants, and FreeBayes are the most frequently used. GATK is the most widely used programming framework for analyzing DNA sequencing data and for the discovery of SNVs and indels. It applies various machine learning methods like logistic regression, HMM, and Naïve Bayes classification to reduce base errors and capture high-quality variants. For example, in the variant quality score recalibration (VQSR) process to filter low-quality variants, GATK was trained on multiple variant annotations (such as genotype qualities, depth of coverage, mapping qualities, and local sequence context) of high-confident known variants like HapMap genotypes and Omni 2.5 genotypes for 1,000 Genomes samples. The trained model was then used to assign a well-calibrated variant quality score to each variant in a callset and refined the callset to a desired high level of truth sensitivity.

Unlike GATK, another deep learning-based variant caller called DeepVariants accurately identifies genetic variants using a single deep CNN model trained with known genotypes instead of a combination of multiple statistical models. Using the Inception architecture, the CNN model calculated the genotype likelihoods for each site using a pileup image of the reference genome and sequenced reads around each candidate variant. FreeBayes, a Bayesian variant-calling tool, uses a haplotype-based method to read short haplotypes directly from sequencing data. It offers many advantages for variants detection compared to approaches that manipulate a single site simultaneously. To maintain semantic consistency between the candidate variants, the haplotype-based method assesses all categories of alleles in the same sequencing context simultaneously, improving detection utilities and accuracy.

Prioritizing variants that may lead to alternative splicing

Alternative splicing is regulated by an extensive protein-RNA interaction network involving cis-elements within the pre-mRNA and trans-acting factors that bind to these cis-elements. It is a crucial regulator of gene expression, with around 15% of disease-causing mutations predicted to alter mRNA splicing. Disruption of splicing (for example, exon skipping and intron retention) would result in aberrant proteins that do not function correctly. Numerous tools have been developed to predict the effects of splice variants, emphasizing whether variants in the splice regions can potentially lead to the loss or gain of the splice donor or splice acceptor.

SpliceAI uses an ultra-deep CNN model to computationally predict the effects of genetic variants on splicing based on the sequence of the pre-mRNA transcript. SpliceAI trained on the dataset from GENCODE (an integrated annotation of gene features) and the RNA-seq data Genotype-Tissue Expression (GTEx). Training on the GTEx RNA-seq dataset enhanced the sensitivity of splicing-altering variation detection, particularly for detecting deep intronic splicing variants. Similar to SpliceAI, MMSplice (modular modeling of splicing) is a neural network-based model for predicting the effects of variants on exon skipping, splice site choice, splicing efficiency, and pathogenicity. It consists of six modules scoring sequences from different genomic regions, wherein the donor and acceptor modules are trained using GENCODE annotation features, while the exon modules (exon 5' and exon 3' modules) and intron modules (intron 5' and intron 3' modules) are trained using massively parallel reporter assays (MPRAs). These six modules were combined with a linear model to score the variant effects on exon skipping, alternative donor/acceptor site, and splicing efficiency separately. Furthermore, it was integrated with a logistic regression model to predict variant pathogenicity. For each input variant, MMSplice would output several scores, including (1) a main score that exhibits the effect of the variant on the inclusion level, (2) a pathogenicity score that shows the potential pathogenic effect, (3) an efficiency score that demonstrates the variant effect on splicing efficiency of the exon and (4) several scores for the effects of the acceptor/donor/exon/intron according to the reference allele and alternative allele.

In the context of genomic analyses, tools like SpliceAI and MMSplice are typically employed not in isolation but as part of a more extensive set of methods to prioritize pathogenic variants with deleterious effects. One study explored a cryptic splice variant in the ATP-binding cassette transporter gene sub-family A (ABCB4). ABCB4 was predicted to cause a splice acceptor loss by SpliceAI (score = 0.39) through an IBD-based (identity-by-descent) phenome-wide association study (PheWAS) analysis and fine-mapping. It was further validated to disrupt the splicing of the

ABCB4 pre-mRNA in vitro, leading to the skip transcription of exon 23, thus resulting in liver disease. Given the complex genetic architecture of the congenital disease, most of the time, researchers may not only employ tools for the prediction of coding variants but also adopt other tools for the prediction of splicing variants or regulatory variants. One study that concentrated on the detection of mosaic mutation implicated in CHD captured deleterious missense variant by REVEL (with a score > 0.5) and damaging splicing variants by SpliceAI (with a delta score > 0.5). Therefore, researchers would annotate the splice variants together with other variants using some ensemble tools or databases. As an example, CADD-Splice (same as CADD v1.6) integrated with several superior ML-based methods (including SpliceAI and MMSplice) to score the potential splicing effect led by the genetic variations.

dbNSFP (database for nonsynonymous SNPs' functional predictions) is a comprehensive database designed to annotate the functional impact of all SNPs in the human genome. It compiled dozens of prediction scores from various tools, consisting of (i) functional prediction (from SIFT, Polyphen, CADD), (ii) conservation scores (from phyloP, phastCons, GERP++), and (iii) many other variant annotations like allele frequency, gene information, protein information, splicing effect, regulatory elements, and the gene-associated phenotype of the mouse and zebrafish.

Prioritizing potentially damaging regulatory variants

Historically, pathogenic variants of diseases are detected in the protein-coding regions, although it only takes up around 2% of the human genome. Nonetheless, disease-causing variations in the coding areas could only elucidate about 20%–50% of the disease etiology, indicating that rare noncoding variations may contribute substantially to disease risk. Unlike coding variants that may affect protein structure, function and folding, noncoding variants disrupting functional regulatory elements (such as enhancers, insulators, and promoters) have the potential to dysregulate gene expression and thus contribute to genetic diseases. Deleteriousness prediction tools primarily trained with coding datasets, like CADD and REVEL, are insufficient to predict the pathogenicity of noncoding variation. Hence, other variation annotation tools specialized in predicting the regulatory effect of noncoding variants are needed.

DeepSEA is a deep learning model specialized in predicting the functional effects of noncoding mutations. It uses a multi-layer CNN architecture to decode the regulatory sequence from massive epigenomic profiles and predict the chromatin effects of the genomic mutations. DeepSEA takes a 1,000 base pairs (bp) DNA sequence centered on each variant as input and creates a couple of sequences harboring either the reference or alternative allele at the variant position. Then it calculates the chromatin effect size across each epigenomic feature for each reference and alternative allele, in which the absolute differences between wild-type and mutation could be obtained. Additionally, DeepSEA also takes evolutionary conservation into account and computes the conservation score for each variant using PhastCons, PhyloP and GERP++. By incorporating the variant-phenotype information on human pathogenic variants from the Human Gene Mutation Database (HGMD), DeepSEA has the capacity to forecast the deleterious regulatory impacts that regulatory variations may have, thereby aiding in the prioritization of functional variations.

DeepSEA is a general deep learning model to predict the regulatory effects of noncoding variants for all kinds of diseases. HeartENN, on the other hand, is a heart-specific neural network built on top of DeepSEA to predict the epigenomic outcomes of variants in relation to heart diseases (such as congenital heart disease) with a double number of convolution layers architecture. HeartENN is established with two neural network-based epigenomic effects models, one for predicting heart-specific human chromatin features (histone marks, transcription factors and DNase I accessibility) and the other for mice. To assess the utility of the HeartENN model, developers applied it to the WGS data from 749 CHD trios and 1,611 unaffected trios. They found that variants prioritized by HeartENN damaging score (scores ≥0.1) exhibited significant enrichment of the known human CHD genes in CHD cases. Cooperating with a strategy focused on human fetal cardiac enhancers, they confirmed that genes enriched for noncoding DNVs in human fetal cardiac enhancers also have an excess burden on the noncoding DNVs with HeartENN scores ≥0.1, suggesting the capability of the HeartENN in the prioritization of potentially disruptive regulatory noncoding DNVs implicated in CHD.

Multiscale Analysis of Regulatory Variants on the Epigenomic Landscape (MARVEL) is developed with a ML algorithm GLM-LARS (generalized linear model-based least angle regression) to prioritize phenotype-associated noncoding variants using WGS data and cell-type specific epigenomic profiles. It integrates gene annotation information, publicly available epigenetic data (e.g., enhancers, promoters, transcription factor motifs) from relevant tissues and the covariates of sample phenotypes to identify potential regulatory regions affected by the noncoding variants. The developers applied MARVEL to the WGS data of 431 short-segment Hirschsprung disease (S-HSCR) cases and 487 ethnically matched controls. Together with ChIP-seq and ATAC-seq data of the human pluripotent stem cell (hPSC)-derived enteric neural crest (NC) -like cells, they uncovered multiple novel genes implicated in S-HSCR by affecting neural crest migration and development.

Genome annotation and variant classification

After variant calling, the interpretation of human genome data relies on the identification of relevant genetic variants through prior knowledge and inference of the impact of genetic variants on functional genomic elements. AI algorithms can improve the use of prior knowledge by informing phenotype-to-genotype mapping. Both genome annotation and variant classification are discussed because many AI algorithms that are used to predict the presence of a functional element from primary DNA sequence data are also used to predict the impact of a genetic variation on those functional elements.

Classification of coding variants

Many methods have been developed for the classification of nonsynonymous variants. Some of these methods have been integrated into deep-learning-based meta-predictors (models that process and merge the predictions produced by several other predictors) that outperform both their individual predictive components and the combination of those predictive components when integrated using regression or other machine-learning approaches. As an example, the combined annotation-dependent depletion approach (CADD) combines a variety of predictive features in a machine-learning algorithm to predict the deleteriousness of genetic variants. A deep-learning-based extension of CADD, named DANN, demonstrated improved performance using the same set of input features as CADD but combined in a deep neural network. This technical extension of CADD suggests that deep learning may be a superior approach for integrating known features that are predictive of deleteriousness. However, the classification accuracies of these tools are not sufficient to drive clinical reporting, although they can be useful for guiding the interpretation of clinical genomic data by prioritizing potential candidate variants for further consideration.

More interesting are AI-based methods that make predictions directly from DNA or protein sequence data with minimal hand-crafting of features. One approach, PrimateAI, which used CNNs trained on variants of known pathogenicity with data augmentation using cross-species information, was shown to outperform prior methods when trained directly on sequence alignments. The network was able to determine important protein domains, conserved amino acid positions, and sequence dependencies directly from the training data consisting of about 120,000 human samples. PrimateAI substantially exceeded the performance of other variant pathogenicity prediction tools in differentiating benign and pathogenic de novo mutations in candidate developmental disorder genes, and in reproducing prior knowledge in Clinvar. These results suggest that PrimateAI is an important step forward for variant-classification tools that may lessen the reliance of clinical reporting on prior knowledge. In addition, deep generative models have shown promise for predicting the effects of genetic variants and are especially intriguing given their ability to evaluate the joint influence of multiple genetic variants and/or complex indels on protein function, a capability that is largely absent from most pathogenicity prediction tools. Deep generative models are a type of deep neural network that can learn to replicate data distributions and produce examples not previously observed by the model. For example, a deep generative model trained on images of birds could learn to generate novel bird images.

Another variant type, copy number variant (CNV), is the variant that exhibits differences in the number of copies in specific DNA segments, specifically manifested as duplication or deletion of a particular size of DNA fragments. A popular CNV caller, PennCNV, uses the HMM algorithm to detect CNVs from intensity data generated by high-resolution single nucleotide polymorphisms (SNP) arrays. (The Hidden Markov Model [HMM] is a statistical model used to describe systems with changing unobservable states over time).

The parameters of HMM models were first optimized by training using the Baum-Welch algorithm on large CNV regions from a large set of training samples. The optimized HMM then modelled the observed intensity data as a mixture of normal distributions, incorporated with the Log R Ratio (LRR) and B Allele Frequency (BAF) values for each SNP in the genome to predicted copy number states (e.g., 0, 1, 2, or more copies) at each genomic location. Next, the detected CNVs were validated using the posterior probabilities of each copy number state calculated by the Bayesian algorithm with the use of pedigree information to obtain reliable CNVs. The same framework was further extended and adapted for calling CNVs from whole genome sequencing (WGS) data in PennCNV-Seq. Another DL-based tool, DeepCNV, aims for CNV validation instead of CNV calling. It attempts to replace human visual examination in order to reduce the false positive rate of CNVs, centering around the CNVs called by PennCNV. DeepCNV is constructed by a hybrid deep neural network architecture consisting of a deep convolutional neural network (CNN) and a deep fully connected neural network (DNN). It can deal with both image data and summary statistics output from PennCNV, using CNN and DNN algorithms respectively. This tool has completely changed the ability of CNV studies and can trim the raw CNV calls into reliable CNV sets with high effectiveness and efficiency.

With current high-throughput technology, various tools have emerged for identifying CNVs from next generation sequencing (NGS) data using AI models. Based on a machine-learning approach, CN-Learn accurately detects high-confidence CNVs by aggregating multiple CNV-detection methods (CANOES, CODEX, CLAMMS, and XHMM) from exome sequencing data. Caller-specific and genomic features such as guanosine/cytosine (GC) content, CNV concordance, and CNV size were obtained from multiple CNV callers and further used as the training dataset for a Random Forest classifier, eventually used to distinguish true or false positive calls for the identified CNVs. Similarly, CNV-JACG was developed with a random forest model for judging the accuracy of CNVs and genotyping using paired-end WGS data. CNV-JACG was trained on 21 distinct features characterizing true CNV regions, including 13 features characterizing the breakpoints of CNVs, 6 features of the region encompassed by the CNV, and 2 features related to the variants called within the CNV region. After training, the model learns to determine true and false CNVs and make predictions on the input dataset, calling real CNVs.

CNVs have been reported to have a high impact on congenital surgical diseases. For example, it has been reported that around 3%–25% of congenital heart disease

(CHD) cases harbor rare pathogenic CNVs that can produce proteins that did not function properly. To access the contribution of de novo CNVs in the pathogenesis of sporadic CHD, investigators applied PennCNV and XHMM (exome hidden Markov model) for the detection of high-confident de novo CNVs from the genotyping array and whole exome sequencing (WES) data respectively. CNVs detected in silico were then validated experimentally using digital droplet PCR. Ultimately, a significant increase in CNV burden in CHD cases compared with healthy controls was detected.

The Tetralogy of Fallot (TOF) is the most common subtype of CHD, characterized by pulmonary stenosis, ventricular septal defect, overriding aorta and hypertrophy of the right ventricle. A WGS study on 146 Chinese non-syndromic TOF parent-offspring trios for the identification of high-confidence CNVs (>50 bp) from the WGS data. The study identified 16 de novo CNVs in 14 TOF patients, accounting for 9.6% in the Chinese TOF cohort, which is higher than that in the general population.

CNV analysis on Hirschsprung disease (HSCR) identified a novel candidate gene, NRG3, with an increased burden of intronic CNVs (both deletions and duplications) in patients. Furthermore, the CNV analysis also revealed the differential genetic architecture in relation to CNVs, such that syndromic HSCR was associated with longer CNVs whereas isolated HSCR were found to have an increased burden of shorter CNVs.

Biliary atresia (BA) is a rare paediatric hepatobiliary disorder with multifactorial aetiology. It is characterized by progressive fibro-inflammatory obstruction of the bile duct. The exact cause of BA is still unknown, but it is thought to be caused by both genetic and environmental factors. One study detected 29 BA-private CNVs from SNP array data of BA patients and controls using PennCNV, Birdseye and iPattern. By exploring the interconnectivity of CNVs, SNPs and genetic networks in BA patients, a significant enrichment in the immune inflammatory pathway for genes associated with these BA-associated CNVs was detected.

Generally, the critical process of genomic analysis includes variant detection and variant annotation. Variants could be annotated with multiple variant features, like their associated gene symbol, protein consequence of nucleotide change, and allele frequency, among which deleterious prediction is the important term. With the predicted deleterious score, prioritization of potentially damaging causative variants, could facilitate the clinical interpretation of variants and thus contributing significantly to the study of congenital diseases.

Classification of non-coding variants

The computational identification and prediction of non-coding pathogenic variation is an open challenge in human genomics. Recent findings suggest that AI algorithms will substantially improve the ability to understand non-coding genetic variation. Splicing defects in genes are responsible for at least 10% of rare pathogenic genetic variation, but they can be difficult to identify because of the complexity of intronic and exonic splicing enhancers, silencers, insulators, and other long range and combinatorial DNA interactions that influence gene splicing. SpliceAI, a 32-layer deep neural network, is able to predict both canonical and non-canonical splicing directly from exon–intron junction sequence data. Remarkably, SpliceAI was able to use long-range sequence information to boost prediction accuracy from 57%, using a short window size (80 nucleotides) typical for many prior splicing prediction tools, to 95% when a 10 kb window size was ingested by the AI algorithm, and was able to identify candidate cryptic splicing variants underlying neurodevelopmental disorders.

Deep learning-based approaches have also substantially improved the ability to detect regulatory elements and to predict the influence of genetic variation on those elements. DeepSEA, a multitask hierarchically structured CNN trained on large-scale functional genomics data, was able to learn sequence dependencies at multiple scales and simultaneously produce predictions of DNase hypersensitive sites, transcription factor binding sites, histone marks, and the influence of genetic variation on those regulatory elements, with a level of accuracy superior to those of other tools for prioritizing non-coding functional variants. As with SpliceAI, the ability of DeepSEA to ingest DNA sequences of 1 kb, which is substantially larger than the input to typical motif-based search tools, was critical to this improved performance. Extensions of DeepSEA have been applied to whole-genome sequencing data from families with autism spectrum disorder to reveal several candidate non-coding mutations. Further extension to the ExPecto algorithm demonstrated its ability to predict gene expression levels directly from DNA sequence information. Further investigation of these new deep-learning based frameworks for the analysis of noncoding sequence data is likely to provide new insights into the regulatory code of the human genome.

Phenotype-to-genotype mapping

Human genomes contain numerous genetic variants that are either previously described as pathogenic or predicted to be pathogenic, regardless of the individual's health status. Therefore, the molecular diagnosis of disease often requires both the identification of candidate pathogenic variants and a determination of the correspondence between the diseased individual's phenotype and those expected to result from each candidate pathogenic variant. AI algorithms can significantly enhance the mapping of phenotype to genotype, especially through the extraction of higher-level diagnostic concepts that are embedded in medical images and EHRs.

Image to genetic diagnosis

The human phenotype ontology lists 1007 distinct terms defining different abnormalities of the face. These abnormalities are associated with 4,526 diseases and 2,142 genes. These abnormalities can be identified individually and synthesized into a clinical diagnosis. The clinical diagnosis may then inform targeted gene sequencing or phenotype-informed analysis of more comprehensive genetic data. Often the human-provided clinical diagnosis and molecular diagnoses overlap but do not match precisely because of the phenotypic similarity of genetically distinct syndromes. DeepGestalt, a CNN-based facial image analysis algorithm, dramatically outperforms human dysmorphologists in this task and is precise enough to distinguish between molecular diagnoses that are mapped to the same clinical diagnosis, for example, distinct molecular forms of Noonan syndrome. (Noonan syndrome is a genetic disorder that may present with mildly unusual facial features, short height, congenital heart disease, bleeding problems, and skeletal malformations. Facial features include widely spaced eyes, light-colored eyes, low-set ears, a short neck, and a small lower jaw. Heart problems may include pulmonary valve stenosis. The sternum may either protrude or be sunken, while the spine may be abnormally curved. Intelligence is often normal. Complications of NS can include leukemia).

When combined with genomic data, PEDIA, a genome interpretation system incorporating DeepGestalt, was able to use phenotypic features extracted from facial photographs to accurately prioritize candidate pathogenic variants for 105 different monogenic disorders across 679 individuals. Deployment of DeepGestalt as a face-scanning app has the potential to both democratize and revolutionize the identification of genetic syndromes. Genetic syndromes that are identified through facial analysis can be readily confirmed with DNA testing, but adequate material for somatic mutation testing is not always available in some instances of cancer. However, knowledge of the genomic underpinnings of a tumour are critical to treatment planning. AI can bridge the gap between image-derived phenotypes and their probable genetic source. A 'survival CNN', which is a combination of a CNN with Cox proportional hazards-based outcomes (a type of statistical survival analysis), was able to learn the histological features of brain tumors that were associated with survival and correlated with somatic mutation status. Importantly, this algorithm was not trained to predict genomic aberrations directly. Inspection of the CNN concepts used to make the survival predictions identified novel histological features that are important for prognosis determination. Like the faces of individuals with phenotypically overlapping genetic syndromes, these results suggest that the genomic aberrations underpinning an individual's tumour could potentially be predicted directly from tumour histology images. More generally, AI-based computer vision systems appear to be capable of predicting the genomic aberrations that are likely to be present in an individual's genome on the basis of the complex phenotypes embedded in relevant clinical images.

Electronic health record (EHR) and genetic diagnosis

Disease phenotypes can be complex and multimodal, captured not only by medical imaging, but also by biochemical and other tests that may be ordered at different times and perhaps by different physicians during the course of a differential diagnosis. These results are documented in an EHR where physicians synthesize these findings to provide diagnoses and inform clinical decision-making. Although human specialists can accomplish this task accurately within their area of expertise, AI-based algorithms can recognize patterns in EHRs. In a study involving more than 500,000 patients, an AI-based natural language processing (NLP) approach was used to extract clinically relevant features from EHR data. A hierarchical statistical model, tiered on the basis of anatomic divisions in a manner meant to mimic the clinical reasoning of a composite of experienced physicians, was trained on the NLP output to generate a diagnostic system. Overall, this system was able to differentiate between 55 common paediatric diagnoses with 92% accuracy.

When linked with genomic data, an AI-based diagnostic agent coupled with a genome interpretation system can rapidly produce genetic diagnoses. For example, an NLP system was designed to extract phenotypic descriptions automatically from EHR data of paediatric patients with rare diseases, and to rank matches to the expected phenotypic features of candidate pathogenic variants in the patients' genomes. In 101 children with 105 genetic diseases, automated retrospective genomic diagnoses agreed with expert human interpretation at 97% recall and 99% precision. The system was also able to provide automated genomic diagnoses prospectively for three of seven seriously ill ICU infants. A simpler phenotypic risk score approach, applied to an adult population with EHR and genomic data, was able to identify previously unrecognized monogenic conditions in 18 individuals from a population of 21,701. These results suggest that AI-based phenotype-to-genotype mapping approaches could significantly improve the diagnostic yield of genetic testing and the identification of individuals with unrecognized genetic disorders.

Genotype-to-phenotype prediction

The purpose of clinical genetics is to provide diagnoses and forecasts of future disease risk. Relatively simple statistical approaches to polygenic risk prediction allow for personally and clinically useful stratification of risk for some common complex diseases. One application of machine learning to genomic prediction of height was able to provide relatively accurate predictions within expected bounds, suggesting that AI-based methods can be used to improve upon statistical techniques. However, the true utility of AI-based approaches in genotype-to-phenotype prediction will probably come from the integration of a variety of health data types and risk factors into comprehensive predictors of disease risk.

Common diseases are a result of a complex interplay between inherited genetic risk factors, environmental exposures, and behaviours. Genetic risk alone provides a baseline estimate of lifetime risk for disease, but genetic risk combined with other risk factors allows for a narrowing of that probability space into a short-term projection of disease risk. For example, several non-genetic risk factors are associated with breast cancer risk, including mammographic density, age at first birth, age at menarche, and age at menopause. Combining these non-genetic risk factors with genetic data significantly improves the accuracy of breast cancer risk models and can inform risk-based mammographic screening strategies. Similarly, significant improvement in risk stratification can be achieved by integrating conventional and genetic risk factors for coronary artery disease. Genetic risk score models are more useful than simple pathogenicity assertions in cases where a common disease is the result of a combination of weak effects from multiple loci. However, current models integrate genetic and non-genetic risk factors in simple additive models that probably do not capture the complex causal relationships between these heterogenous risk factors. AI algorithms, given an appropriate volume of data, excel at dissecting this complexity. Unravelling the complex interplay between genetic data, EHR data, digital health monitoring devices, and other sources of health information with AI-based algorithms is a compelling prospect for the future.

With the introduction of these advanced AI-based, especially DL-based, detection and prediction tools, many disease-causing variants have been identified and prioritized from big genomic data, dramatically enhancing understanding of the aetiology of numerous congenital surgical diseases and promoting the uptake of this new evidence into clinical practice.

Prioritizing deleterious mutations in the coding region

Combined Annotation-Dependent Depletion (CADD) is the most widely used annotation tool to predict the deleteriousness of short variants (SNVs and indels) in genetic studies of both monogenic and complex diseases. It applies a machine learning model to aggregate diverse annotations, including evolutionary conservation metrics from other annotated tools (phastCons scores, GERP, and phyloP), regulatory information and functional prediction, into a single, comprehensive measure, including evolutionary conservation, regulatory information, functional prediction score for each variant. Using the SVM algorithm, the model was trained on a set of known pathogenic and benign variants, learning to discriminate between these two classes based on the input annotations with high precision and accuracy for all kinds of variants such as missense, splice, and frameshift variants.

In contrast, another tool rare exome variant ensemble learner (REVEL), was designed only to predict the pathogenicity of missense variants. Similar to CADD, REVEL is an ensemble method integrated with 13 other prediction tools: MutPred, FATHMM, VEST, PolyPhen, SIFT, PROVEAN, MutationAssessor, MutationTaster, LRT, GERP, SiPhy, phyloP, and phastCons. It is trained by Random Forest using a dataset of known pathogenic and rare neutral missense variants to predict the potential effect of the query variants. REVEL had better performance on pathogenicity prediction of missense variants than other ensemble methods such as MetaSVM, MetaLR, KGGSeq, Condel, CADD, DANN, and Eigen and thus has been widely adopted for predicting in silico damaging effect as supporting evidence of pathogenicity.

AI-based variant annotation has been instrumental in the genetic analysis of rare congenital surgical diseases. In a WGS study of a Chinese cohort with TOF, Tang et al. (2022) extracted potential rare damaging variants by the damaging Phred-scaled CADD scores, thereby identifying 6 TOF patients with ultra-rare damaging variants in 3 known TOF genes (KDR, FLT4 and NOTCH1). It also pointed out novel biological pathways and developmental hotspots relevant to the dysregulation of cardiac development in TOF through enrichment analysis. Another study called variants using GATK and defined likely pathogenic nonsynonymous variants with a scaled CADD score ≥ 20, highlighting the increased burden of NOTCH1 mutations in TOF. Likewise, a trio-based whole exome sequencing (WES) study on identified rare, deleterious de novo or biallelic variants in liver-expressed ciliary genes in 31.5% (28/89) of the biliary atresia (BA) patients with the help of the CADD, SIFT and PolyPhen2. They found that these rare deleterious variants in liver-expressed ciliary genes were associated with a significant two-fold increased risk of BA, underlying the potential disease mechanism of BA led by the malformation and dysfunction of cilia.

Current advances and challenges in variant interpretation

While AI-based tools have made significant contributions to the detection and prioritization of disease-causing variants, a persistent challenge in genomic research lies in variant interpretation. In 2015 the American College of Medical Genetics and Genomics and the Association for Molecular Pathology (ACMG/AMP) published an authoritative guideline to standardize variant interpretation, which categorizes variants into five classes ranging from benign to pathogenic. Subsequently, multiple platforms were developed for automated variant interpretation based on the ACMG/AMP criteria, such as VarSome, VSClinical, and AION from Nostos genomics. However, although these platforms have facilitated the effective and efficient prioritization of pathogenic or likely pathogenic variants along with their supporting evidence, they still face challenges in interpreting variants of uncertain significance (VUS).

Conclusions and Future directions

AI makes it possible to integrate and model vast amounts of genomic data quickly and accurately, facilitating the identification, annotation and prioritization of genetic mutations that contribute to disease development. However, large amounts of diverse data are required to train the AI models. Overall, AI is a powerful tool that has revolutionized disease-specific genomic analysis by providing speedy and precise insights into the complex relationship between genetics and disease development. Ultimately, these findings that traditional methods might have missed will lead to earlier diagnosis and better prognoses for patients with complex congenital disorders.

AI systems have surpassed the performance of state-of-the-art methods and have gained FDA clearance for a variety of clinical diagnostics, especially imaging-based diagnostics. The availability of large datasets for training, for example, large collections of annotated medical images or large functional genomics datasets, in conjunction with advances in AI algorithms and in the GPU systems used to train them, is driving this surge of productivity. Currently, the most promising applications of AI in clinical genomics appear to be the AI extraction of deep phenotypic information from images, EHRs, and other medical devices to inform downstream genetic analysis. However, deep-learning algorithms have also shown great promise in a variety of clinical genomics tasks such as variant calling, genome annotation, and functional impact prediction. It is possible that more generalized AI tools will become the standard in these areas, especially for clinical genomics tasks where inference from complex data (that is, variant calling) is a frequently recurring task. These applications have benefited from advances in CNNs and RNNs which appear to be particularly well suited for the analysis of genomic data. However, the utility of AI algorithms as the ultimate clinical decision support tool in predicting common complex human phenotypes has not been convincingly demonstrated. The rise of biobank-scale efforts with longitudinal health data collection, such as the UK Biobank and All of Us Research Program, will potentially provide the training datasets necessary to make this goal a reality. Given the reliance of AI on large-scale training datasets, it is likely that the scalable collection of phenotype data, and not genomic data, will be the more difficult barrier to overcome in realizing this ambition. Modern DNA sequencing technology allows for the generation of genomic data uniformly and at scale, but the collection of phenotype data requires numerous data collection modes, and tends to be slow, expensive, and highly variable across collection sites. Finally, the interpretability and identification of machine bias are essential to broad acceptance of AI technology in any clinical diagnostic modality.

Chapter 26. How AI will improve drug discovery

AI has proven invaluable in the field of drug discovery by expediting the search for potent therapeutic compounds, and subsequently, accelerating the drug development process. For example, AI can predict the pharmacokinetic and pharmacodynamic properties of novel compounds, pinpoint potential drug targets, and simulate clinical trials, substantially reducing both time and costs associated with drug development (Vamathevan, J, et al., 2019).

The use of artificial intelligence in medicinal chemistry has gained significant attention in recent years as a potential means of revolutionizing the pharmaceutical industry. Drug discovery, the process of identifying and developing new medications, is a complex and time-consuming endeavour that traditionally relies on labour-intensive techniques, such as trial-and-error experimentation and high-throughput screening. However, AI techniques such as machine learning (ML) and natural language processing offer the potential to accelerate and improve this process by enabling more efficient and accurate analysis of large amounts of data. The successful use of deep learning (DL) to predict the efficacy of drug compounds with high accuracy has been described. AI-based methods have also been able to predict the toxicity of drug candidates. Different algorithms based on AI, including supervised and unsupervised learning methods, reinforcement, and evolutionary or rule-based algorithms, can potentially contribute to solving the problems listed above that are associated with traditional ways of developing new medications. The AI methods for new drug discovery are typically based on the analysis of large amounts of data that can be exploited in different ways. Additionally, AI-based algorithms can also be employed to identify new targets for drug development, such as the specific proteins or genetic pathways involved in diseases (Blanco-González A, et al., 2023)

The role of ML in predicting drug efficacy and toxicity

One of the key applications of AI in medicinal chemistry is the prediction of the efficacy and toxicity of potential drug compounds. Based on the analysis of a large amount of information, ML algorithms can identify patterns and trends that may not be apparent to human researchers. This can enable the identity of new bioactive compounds with minimum side effects in a much faster process than traditional methods: a DL algorithm has recently been trained using a dataset of known drug compounds, along with their corresponding biological activity. The algorithm was then able to predict the activity of novel compounds with high accuracy. Significant contributions to prevent the toxicity of potential drug compounds, employing intensive training using large databases of known toxic and non-toxic compounds for ML, have also been described.

Another important application of AI in drug discovery is the identification of drug–drug interactions that take place when several drugs are combined for the same or different diseases in the same patient, resulting in altered effects or adverse reactions. This issue can be identified by AI-based approaches by analysing large datasets of known drug interactions and recognizing the patterns and trends. This has been addressed recently by an ML algorithm used to accurately predict the interactions of novel drug pairs. The role of AI to identify possible drug–drug interactions in the context of personalized medicine is also relevant, enabling the development of custom-made treatment plans that minimize the risk of adverse reactions. Personalized medicine aims to tailor treatment to the individual characteristics of each patient, including their genetic profile and response to medications.

The impact of AI on the drug discovery process and potential cost savings

Another key application of AI in drug discovery is the design of novel compounds with specific properties and activities. For example, a deep learning algorithm has recently been trained on a dataset of known drug compounds and their corresponding properties, to propose new therapeutic molecules with desirable characteristics such as solubility and activity, demonstrating the potential of these methods for the rapid and efficient design of new drug candidates.

DeepMind made a significant contribution to the field of AI research with the development of AlphaFold, a software platform for advancing the understanding of biology. The algorithm uses protein sequence data and AI to predict the proteins' corresponding three-dimensional structures.

ML techniques and molecular dynamics (MD) simulations are being used in the field of de novo drug design to improve efficiency and accuracy. The technique of combining these methodologies is being explored to take advantage of the synergies between them. The use of interpretable machine learning (IML) and DL methods is also contributing to this effort.

Case studies of successful AI-aided drug discovery efforts

The potential of AI in the context of drug discovery has been demonstrated in several case studies: the successful use of AI to identify novel compounds for the treatment of cancer has been reported. In this study the investigators trained a DL algorithm on a large dataset of known cancer-related compounds and their corresponding biological activity. The use of ML to identify small-molecule inhibitors of the protein MEK has been described. MEK is a possible target for the treatment of cancer, but the development of effective inhibitors has been challenging. The ML algorithm was able to identify novel inhibitors for this protein. Another example is the identification of novel inhibitors of beta-secretase (BACE1), a protein involved in the development of Alzheimer's disease by using an ML algorithm. AI has also been successfully applied in the discovery of new antibiotics. A pioneering ML approach has identified powerful types of antibiotics from a pool of more than 100 million molecules, including one that works against a wide range of bacteria, including tuberculosis.

The role of collaboration between AI researchers and pharmaceutical scientists

This collaboration can help improve the accuracy and efficiency of clinical trials, as AI algorithms can be used to analyse the data collected during these trials to identify trends and the potential adverse effects of the drugs being tested. This can help pharmaceutical companies to make informed decisions about which drug candidates to pursue and can speed up the overall drug development process. By working together, they can help to identify new targets for drug development and improve the effectiveness of existing treatments, ultimately benefiting patients and improving their quality of life.

Challenges and limitations of using AI in drug discovery

Current AI-based approaches are not a substitute for traditional experimental methods, and they cannot replace the expertise and experience of human researchers. AI can only provide predictions based on the data available, and the results must then be validated and interpreted by human researchers.

Conclusions and summary

AI has the potential to revolutionize the drug discovery process, offering improved efficiency and accuracy, accelerated drug development, and the capacity for the development of more effective and personalized treatments. However, the successful application of AI in drug discovery is dependent on the availability of high-quality data, the addressing of ethical concerns, and the recognition of the limitations of AI-based approaches.

Chapter 27. Portable and wearable sensors

Application of ML in noninvasive biosensors

A noninvasive biosensor is a sensing system that generally utilizes body fluids that can be easily obtained, including exhaled breath, saliva, tears, sweat, urine, and interstitial fluid, for detection of the target analyte; the sensor can be integrated into wearable and portable devices. These easily access body fluids to provide sources of various biomarkers that can enable the diagnosis and monitoring of multiple diseases (Kadian et al. 2023). In addition, the development of non-invasive biosensors offers the capability of continuous monitoring of multiple physiologic parameters. In this context, ML through computer programs can enhance the performance of biosensors with experience. For example, the electrical and optical signals collected from the biosensors can be used as an input to the ML models. Data processing steps such as data cleaning, feature extraction, and hyper parameter tuning can be performed. Different ML models play unique roles in classification and pattern recognition to enhance sensing performance and assist in decision-making.

Portable biosensors

A portable biosensor is a device that offers the detection of target analytes outside the laboratory environment. Recent advances in portable biosensors mainly involve the testing of easily accessible body fluids, including urine, exhaled gas, and saliva; as such, these devices are pertinent to long-time tracking and continuous health monitoring. Two types of portable biosensors are commonly used: lateral flow assays and microfluidic-based biosensors. Lateral flow assay-based biosensors often involve paper-based strips, which consist of a nitrocellulose membrane, sample application pad, adsorption pad, and conjugate pad. In this approach, when the liquid test sample containing the target analyte flows over the different parts of the paper-based strip, the pre-immobilized reagents present on the strip indicate different characteristics. These devices contain several attractive features, including ease-of-use, low-cost, rapid detection, scalability, and exceptional portability; these biosensors have been widely accepted in food safety and healthcare applications. Portable biosensors have been integrated with ML to enhance data interpretation. For example, investigators prepared an ML-based smartphone app using binary (LS-

SVM) as well as multi-class (Random Forest) classifiers for paper strip-based colorimetric detection of peroxide. The binary and multi-class classifiers were supplied with the mean Hue-Saturation-Value (HSV), Red-Green-Blue (RGB), and LAB values of the paper-based strip image under different illumination settings in the presence and absence of grey-world color constancy algorithm. Another group demonstrated a deep learning-enabled economical paper-based vertical flow assay for C-reactive protein detection. They used an ML-based framework to measure an optimal configuration of immunoreaction spots in order to understand the target biomolecule concentration. Other investigators utilized a high-throughput colorimetric sensor to analyse the total organic carbon content of a water sample with the help of a CNN model developed using ML. The ML model mapped a relationship between the total organic carbon value and the colorimetric sensor data. Investigators prepared an intelligent paper-based colorimetric sensor that can automatically perform a test with a precision of over 86% without user interference. The new system was created using morphological operation, global thresholding, channel separation, and object recognition. Researchers have demonstrated a smartphone-enabled colorimetric detection of saliva alcohol concentrations, employing ML algorithms and optimal colour space. The smartphone camera captured the colour generated on the test strip with different concentrations of alcohol; analysis was performed via three different ML algorithms, including LDA, SVM, and ANN.

Many microfluidic-based biosensors utilize a lab-on-a-chip approach, which reduces the utilization of reagents and processing time; this approach offers the possibility of analysis using small-volume samples. Since microfluidic approaches utilize the movement of liquids at the microscale level with high spatiotemporal precision and throughput, these approaches generate large multidimensional datasets. Therefore, machine intelligence has been employed as a deep analytical tool to learn from microfluidics-generated data and enhance biosensor performance. Researchers reported that the peptide-based biofilm/bacteria interface induced a bacteria-particle aggregation pattern through supervised machine learning. Since every peptide acts differently with the bacterial species, it leads to different amounts of aggregation; this phenomenon alters the viscosity and surface tension of the fluid moving via the paper pores. The resulting variations in flow velocity created a different fingerprinting profile for each bacterial species; this phenomenon was captured through a smartphone. To classify and differentiate five bacterial species, *Pseudomonas aeruginosa, Escherichia coli, Staphylococcus aureus, Enterococcus faecium,* and *Salmonella typhimurium*, an advanced SVM model was used; this approach was found to be 93.3% accurate. Mercan et al. (2021) developed a portable colorimetric paper-based microfluidics device to quantify the glucose concentration in artificial saliva with an ML-based smartphone application. The change in the images of the colorimetric paper-based microfluidics device was captured with smartphones under discrete illumination situations, which were further processed for feature extraction and employed to train ML classifiers; the results of the strategy in the colorimetric analysis demonstrated a classification accuracy as high as 98.24%. Another group demonstrated a flexible microfluidic device that sticks to human skin and analyzes sweat during exercise. The colorimetric microfluidic device was integrated with a smartphone to capture and analyze the images for the detection of chloride ions, glucose, and lactate in sweat during a monitored cycling exercise.

Wearable biosensors

Wearable biosensors are sensing systems that can gather biofluids from the body surface to detect the concentration of various biological markers. Based on the interface with the human body, these non-invasive sensing systems are classified into three groups: accessories-based, on-body clothing, and textile-based biosensors. Accessories-based wearable biosensors describe sensing devices that loosely link to the body. For instance, eyeglasses can be integrated with metabolite sensors that are located on the nose-bridge sticker pads, which can monitor sweat metabolites Textile-based wearable biosensors refer to the sensors that are combined with wearable items such as clothing, which can be utilized to monitor analyte levels. Similarly, on-body wearable biosensors involve sensors that stick to the human body, such as contact lenses and skin patches. These devices can detect the target biomolecule in sweat and interstitial fluid. With advances in ML and artificial intelligence-enabled sensing technology, wearable sensors are being developed that can collect physiological signals from the host and share the data wirelessly for processing and storage; ML models can be utilized to assist in diagnosis. For instance, one group proposed an ML model to predict the Unified Parkinson's Disease Rating Scale using a wearable sensing device. In this study, a wrist-watch-type wearable gadget containing a gyroscope and accelerometer was used to gather the tremor signals of 85 Parkinson's disease patients. Nineteen features were extracted from the obtained angular velocity, acceleration, calculated displacement, and angle signal values; a pairwise correlation scheme was employed to decrease the number of feature dimensions. Using the preferred features, a k-nearest-neighbor (kNN), discriminant analysis (DA), support vector machine (SVM), decision tree (DT), and random forest (RF) model were investigated for computerized scoring of the disease severity. They observed that the performance of the ML model in scoring symptom severity was similar to that of neurologist-provided scoring in clinical practice. Others developed a non-invasive wearable seizure detection system using deep neural networks. In this approach, a deep neural network-based long-short-term memory model was developed by training the model over a modest amount of seizure data collected through a wristband device. Transfer learning was used for the classification of non-EEG physiological signals, including heart rate, blood volume pulse, accelerometry, electrodermal activity, and temperature. To evaluate the efficacy of the seizure detection system, the wearable sensing band was used over several days with an embedded neurostimulator for recording the iEEG data. The algorithm performed well during motor and non-motor seizures when tested in-hospital.

Wearable devices based on electrochemical detection

Electrochemical wearable sensors are generally based on the modified electrodes on the flexible substrates, which react chemically with the target biomolecules once the analyte contacts with the electrodes. Due to the change of electrons during chemical reactions, the concentration of analytes could be translated into electrical signals such as voltage or current. One group proposed a flexible sensing array integrated into multi-parametric sensing functions, for monitoring K+, Na+, glucose, lactate, and body temperature. Another group proposed a graphene-hybrid wearable patch for monitoring of blood glucose levels while calibrating the glucose signal in real time by the simultaneous measurement of pH, temperature, and humidity. The device compared well with a commercial glucose monitoring kit. Electrochemical wearable sensors have many uses as they are a pain-free method for directly analysing interstitial fluid (ISF). Various commercial devices have been developed for real-time monitor of glucose level. Examples are Guardian REAL-Time by

Medtronic and FreeStyple Libre by Abbot. Other than glucose levels, other analytes in ISF have also been successfully measured, including lactate, urea, alcohol, levodopa, pH, various ions and oxygen concentrations. Electrochemical sensors integrated with contact lenses are commonly used for measuring intraocular glucose concentration.

Wearable devices based on optical detection

Optical detection has also gained many interests for wearable sensors due to its low cost and relatively simple system construction compared with electrochemical detection. The commonest optical wearable sensors are based on colorimetric detection. When combined with the smartphone, the changes of colour can be quantified via the digital camera and processed using built-in apps. Investigators used an integrated colorimetric sweat sensing patch capable of measuring the sweat rate, pH, chloride, glucose, and lactate levels. The sweat was routed into the microfluidic channel via serpentine channels with corresponding reservoirs for the assays of various analytes. The build-in app in the smartphone was used to determine the red/green/blue (RGB) values of chromogens. The wearable optical sensors can also be used for measuring pulse oximetry. Using the ultra-flexible, and thin organic LEDs, the pulse oximeters could be minimized and worn on the finger, which is suitable for all-day monitoring.

Wearable dialysis devices

Dialysis is the main treatment for ESRD. Wearable dialysis devices can measure the real-time analysis of equipment alarms, dialysis parameters, and patient-related data with a real-time feedback response. One group combined AI and regenerative medicine technology to develop wearable dialysis devices. These devices can conduct continuous dialysis, remove toxins effectively and have little effect on hemodynamics. The devices have been tested in 15 ESRD patients. The results showed that dialysis was effective without any adverse reactions. The devices were authorized as a breakthrough device by the USA Food and Drug Administration. Another interesting approach is the wearable artificial kidney, a 5-kg wearable, miniaturized device with a sorbent-based haemodialysis system that is worn on the waist like a toolkit belt and is currently under development at the University of Washington, USA. An exploratory clinical trial with 10 patients received therapy with a wearable artificial kidney for 24 hours. However, the trial was stopped after the inclusion of the 7th subject because of device-related technical problems, including an excessive presence of carbon dioxide bubbles in the dialysate circuit, which exceeded its degassing capacity, tubing kinks and variable pump function that resulted in fluctuating blood and dialysate flow rates. Another innovation is the implantable Renal Assist Device (iRAD) that uses micromachining techniques to fabricate a biohybrid system able to mimic renal morphology and function. This artificial kidney is a bionic device that incorporates a silicon nanopore membrane and a bioreactor of live kidney cells that will concentrate the ultrafiltrate into urine. The bundle is enclosed in a body-friendly box and connected to a patient's circulatory system and bladder. Despite having been used with success in animal models, it is still under development to scale it up for the clinical environment.

Recently, experts found MXene sorbents for removal of urea from dialysate, which open a new opportunity in designing a miniaturized dialysate regeneration system for a wearable artificial kidney. Meng et al. (2018) showed that two-dimensional titanium carbide (MXene) with the composition of Ti3C2Tx, where Tx represents surface termination groups such as −OH, −O–, and −F, can adsorb urea, reaching 99% removal efficiency from aqueous solution and 94% from dialysate at the initial urea concentration of 30 mg/dL, with the maximum urea adsorption capacity of 10.4 mg/g at room temperature.

Conclusions, challenges, and future recommendations

The advances in the area of noninvasive biosensors have laid the groundwork for real-time and onsite analyte testing. The incorporation of ML with portable and wearable biosensing devices adds value by managing large amounts of biosensing data and converting it into understandable information. For example, ML-enabled wearable devices can predict the probability of injury and cardiac arrhythmia as well as the hydration level of an athlete. Since the demand for accurate, multifunctional, and precise sensors is increasing, ML-enabled biosensors appear to fulfill many needs of the healthcare market.

Interpretative output is not only necessary for acceptance in clinical practice but is also important for unveiling the knowledge discovered by AI systems and for detecting biases that may result in undesirable behavior. AI systems must be carefully applied to differentiate between these types of bias. When medical AI systems are not inspected for non-causal bias, they can act as propagators of disparity. For example, DeepGestalt, the previously described AI system for facial dysmorphology analysis, displayed poor accuracy for the identification of Down syndrome in individuals of African versus European ancestry (36.8% versus 80%, respectively). Retraining the model with examples of Down syndrome in individuals of African ancestry improved the diagnosis of Down syndrome in individuals of African ancestry to 94.7%. Genetic risk prediction is also prone to unequal performance in different population groups because of underrepresentation in the training data.

In some cases, however, the bias is embedded in ostensibly representative training data. For example, gender bias is common in written documents and can be rapidly incorporated into NLP systems. Extensions to these models were required to 'debias' word embeddings. In clinical applications, EHR data may be representative overall, but the contents may include biases that result from the delivery of care or physician bias. For example, recent immigrants in Canada are more likely to receive aggressive care and die in intensive care units than are other residents. Furthermore, the substructure of genomic data is correlated with population structure, which can lead to the appearance of non-causal trait associations. However, tools that will help to address machine bias are being developed, and careful attention to these issues could not only help to resolve machine bias issues but could eventually lead to diagnostic systems that are free from human bias.

Regulatory issues

A growing number of AI algorithms have been approved by the FDA. These algorithms raise a number of regulatory and ethical challenges around the sourcing and privacy of the data used to train the algorithms, the transparency and generalizability of the underlying algorithms themselves, the regulatory process for refreshing these algorithms as further data become available, and the liability associated with prediction errors. Some of these issues can and should be addressed by open sharing of AI models in detail (including source codes, model weights, and meta graphs) with the scientific and medical community in order to improve transparency. Other issues will need to be addressed by the development of: (i) best practices for the interpretability of predictions to protect patient autonomy and shared decision-making; (ii) fairness standards to minimize disparities induced by machine bias; and (iii) ad hoc guidance to allow for continuous improvement of the algorithms.

AI interpretability

AI is often criticized for being a 'black box': a system that produces an output without any explanation or justification. While this may be acceptable in low-risk situations, clinical decision-making is not a low-risk situation. 'What?' may sufficiently encompass the question of interest in a general object-detection task, but 'why?' is an inherent part of the question in most clinical diagnostic tasks, because it is often crucial to subsequent clinical decision-making or at least necessary for acceptance of the prediction by both physicians and patients. An ideal AI-based clinical diagnostic system should produce accurate predictions and provide human-interpretable explanations of those predictions. A common approach to answering 'why?' in computer vision applications is to generate a visual overlay of the portions of an image that contribute most strongly to an output prediction. This strategy works well for image-based and other CNN-based clinical diagnostic tasks. In fact, many AI-based clinical diagnostic methods include some form of interpretive analysis.

When complex interdependencies form the basis of a prediction, however, accurate interpretation of AI output becomes more challenging. Interpretable machine-learning methods are an active area of computer science research, but most interpretable AI approaches involve the production of a simplified and potentially inaccurate approximation of the more complex AI system. Recently, a move towards more interactive models of interpretability through 'dialogue' with the AI system has been proposed. This approach allows the human user to ask questions of the AI system in order to explore how its output predictions would change if inputs were modified. This approach could also facilitate a dialogue between physician and patient, with the aid of the AI interpretation system, to help them to understand the clinical diagnosis and, in some instances, the risk factors that could be modified to change the predicted outcome. Thus, further improvements to interpretable AI systems should not only substantially enhance the acceptability of AI predictions but also enhance the transparency of health communication between physicians and patients.

Data and machine bias

Interpretative output is not only necessary for acceptance in clinical practice but is also important for unveiling the knowledge discovered by AI systems and for detecting biases that may result in undesirable outcomes. There is substructure embedded in genomic and health data. Some substructure is due to truly differing causal relationships between alleged risk factors and health outcomes, whereas other substructure can be attributed to external factors such as socioeconomic status, cultural practices, unequal representation, and other non-causal factors that relate to the delivery and accessibility of medicine and clinical tests rather than to their efficacy. AI systems must be carefully applied to differentiate between these types of bias. When medical AI systems are not inspected for non-causal bias, they can act as propagators of disparity. Genetic risk prediction is also prone to unequal performance in different population groups because of underrepresentation in the training data.

However, not all machine bias can be resolved by addressing underrepresentation in training data. In some cases, the bias is embedded in ostensibly representative training data. For example, gender bias is common in written documents and can be rapidly incorporated into NLP systems. Extensions to these models were required to 'debias' word embeddings. In clinical applications, EHR data may be representative overall, but the contents may include biases that result from the delivery of care or physician bias. Tools that will help to address machine bias are being developed, and careful attention to these issues could not only help to resolve machine bias issues but could eventually lead to diagnostic systems that are free from human bias.

Conclusions and future directions

AI systems have surpassed the performance of state-of-the-art methods and have gained FDA clearance for a variety of clinical diagnostics, especially imaging-based diagnostics. The availability of large datasets for training, for example, large collections of annotated medical images or large functional genomics datasets, in conjunction with advances in AI algorithms and in the GPU systems used to train them, is driving this surge of productivity. Currently, the most promising applications of AI in clinical genomics appear to be the AI extraction of deep phenotypic information from images, EHRs, and other medical devices to inform downstream genetic analysis. However, deep-learning algorithms have also shown tremendous promise in a variety of clinical genomics tasks such as variant calling, genome annotation, and functional impact prediction. It is possible that more generalized AI tools will become the standard in these areas, especially for clinical genomics tasks where inference from complex data (that is, variant calling) is a frequently recurring task. These applications have benefited from advances in CNNs and RNNs which appear to be particularly well suited for the analysis of genomic data. Yet, the utility of AI algorithms as the ultimate clinical decision support tool in predicting common complex human phenotypes has not been convincingly demonstrated. The rise of biobank-scale efforts with longitudinal health data collection, such as the UK Biobank and All of Us Research Program, will potentially provide the training datasets necessary to make this goal a reality. Given the reliance of AI on large-scale training datasets, it is likely that the scalable collection of phenotype data, and not genomic data, will be the more difficult barrier to overcome in realizing this ambition. Modern DNA sequencing technology allows for the generation of genomic data uniformly and at scale, but the collection of phenotype data requires numerous data collection modes, and tends to be slow, expensive, and highly variable across collection sites. Finally, the interpretability and identification of machine bias are essential to broad acceptance of AI technology in any clinical diagnostic modality.

Chapter 29. The future of AI

From the early days of X-ray imaging in the 1890s to more recent advances in CT, MRI and PET scanning, medical imaging continues to be a pillar of medical management. Current advances in imaging hardware — in terms of quality, sensitivity and resolution — enable the discrimination of minute differences in tissue densities. Such differences are, in some cases, difficult to recognize by a trained eye and even by some traditional AI methods used in the clinic. These methods are thus not fully on par with the sophistication of imaging instruments, yet they serve as another motivation to pursue this paradigm shift towards more powerful AI tools. Moreover, and in contrast to traditional methods based on predefined features, deep learning algorithms scale with data, that is, as more data are generated every day and with ongoing research efforts, relative improvements in performance are expected.

In contrast to traditional AI algorithms locked within proprietary commercial packages, the most popular deep learning software platforms available today are open-source. This has fostered, and continues to foster, experimentation on a massive scale. In terms of data, AI efforts are expected to shift from processed medical images to raw acquisition data. Raw data are almost always down sampled and optimized for human viewers. This simplification and loss of information are both avoidable when the analyses are run by machines but are associated with caveats including reduced interpretability and impeded human validation. As more data are generated, more signal is available for training. However, more noise is also present. With difficulties in curating and labelling data, a major push towards unsupervised learning techniques to fully utilize the vast archives of unlabelled data is foreseen.

Future prospects

The medical field in AI is expanding to disease severity assessment and prognosis prediction. Although most AI research in pathology is still focused on cancer detection and the grading of tumours, pathological diagnosis is not simply a morphological diagnosis, but is a complex process of evaluation and judgment of various types of clinical data that deal with various organs and diseases. A large amount of data, including genetic data, clinical data, and digital images, is needed to develop AI that covers the range of clinical situations. There are a number of public medical databases, including TCGA, and a number of studies have been performed based on those databases. They provide a good starting point in researching and developing medical AI, but much more high-quality data is required. Detailed annotations on a large number of pathology images, created and validated by several experienced pathologists, are necessary to develop a pathology-image-analyzing AI that is comparable to that of human pathologists.

Eventually, there will be a medical AI application of the prognostic prediction model, combining clinical data, genetic data, and morphology. Also, a new grading system applicable to several tumours can be created by an AI model that has learned from the patient's prognosis combined with a number of variables including morphology, treatment modality, and tumour markers. This will also help to overcome the poor reproducibility and the variety of current grading and staging results among pathologists, leading to better clinical outcomes for patients.

Chapter 30. Conclusions

Artificial intelligence is alive and well and is already integrated into aspects of human activity: an example is the virtual assistant, such as Siri, now available on iphones.

The internet was a huge event in accessing information to millions, if not billions, of people on any topic as long as they had a computer with a search engine and wifi access.

AI will be bigger than the internet because it will solve problems that humans cannot solve. Many improvements still need to be made and the appropriate use of AI by regulatory authorities is essential.

References

Abertawe H, et al. A Novel CNN-Based CAD System for Early Assessment of Transplanted Kidney Dysfunction. Sci Rep. 2019 Apr 11;9(1):5948. doi: 10.1038/s41598-019-42431-3. PMID: 30976081; PMCID: PMC6459833.

Abràmoff et al. Pivotal trial of an autonomous AI-based diagnostic system for detection of diabetic retinopathy in primary care offices. Yearbook of Paediatric Endocrinology 2019. DOI:10.1530/ey.16.12.1

Agrebi S and Larbi A. Use of artificial intelligence in infectious diseases. Artificial Intelligence in Precision Health. 2020:415–38. doi: 10.1016/B978-0-12-817133-2.00018-5. Epub 2020 Mar 13. PMCID: PMC7153335.

Ahn JS, et al. Artificial Intelligence in Breast Cancer Diagnosis and Personalized Medicine. J Breast Cancer. 2023 Oct;26(5):405-435. doi: 10.4048/jbc.2023.26.e45. PMID: 37926067; PMCID: PMC10625863.

Almansour NA et al. Neural network and support vector machine for the prediction of chronic kidney disease: A comparative study. Comput Biol Med. 2019 Jun; 109:101-111. doi: 10.1016/j.compbiomed.2019.04.017. Epub 2019 Apr 25. PMID: 31054385.

Antonelli M, Johnston EW, Dikaios N, et al. Machine learning classifiers can predict Gleason pattern 4 prostate cancer with greater accuracy than experienced radiologists. Eur Radiol. 2019;29:4754–4764. doi: 10.1007/s00330-019-06244-2.

Arnaout R, et al. An ensemble of neural networks provides expert-level prenatal detection of complex congenital heart disease. Nat Med. 2021 May;27(5):882-891. doi: 10.1038/s41591-021-01342-5. Epub 2021 May 14. PMID: 33990806; PMCID: PMC8380434.

Aslam N, Khan IU, Bashamakh A, Alghool FA, Aboulnour M, Alsuwayan NM, Alturaif RK, Brahimi S, Aljameel SS, Al Ghamdi K. Multiple Sclerosis Diagnosis Using Machine Learning and Deep Learning: Challenges and Opportunities. Sensors (Basel). 2022 Oct 16;22(20):7856. doi: 10.3390/s22207856. PMID: 36298206; PMCID: PMC9609137.

Attia Z.I., Noseworthy P.A., Lopez-Jimenez F., Asirvatham S.J., Deshmukh A.J., Gersh B.J., Carter R.E., Yao X., Rabinstein A.A., Erickson B.J., et al. An artificial intelligence-enabled ECG algorithm for the identification of patients with atrial fibrillation during sinus rhythm: A retrospective analysis of outcome prediction. Lancet. 2019;394:861–867. doi: 10.1016/S0140-6736(19)31721-0.

Avendi MR, Kheradvar A, Jafarkhani H. A combined deep-learning and deformable-model approach to fully automatic segmentation of the left ventricle in cardiac MRI. Med Image Anal. 2016, 30:108-119. doi: 10.1016/j.media.2016.01.005. Epub 2016 Feb 6. PMID: 26917105.

Axelsson GT, et al. The Proteomic Profile of Interstitial Lung Abnormalities. Am J Respir Crit Care Med. 2022 Aug 1;206(3):337-346. doi: 10.1164/rccm.202110-2296OC. PMID: 35438610; PMCID: PMC9890263.

Bashat, B et al. (2018). COMP-18. Machine learning differentiation between plexiform neurofibromas and malignant nerve sheath tumors in patients with neurofibromatosis type 1 (NF1) based on MRI. neuro-oncology. 20. vi67-vi67. 10.1093/neuonc/noy148.273.

Bermejo-Peláez D, et al. Classification of Interstitial Lung Abnormality Patterns with an Ensemble of Deep Convolutional Neural Networks. Sci Rep. 2020 Jan 15;10(1):338. doi: 10.1038/s41598-019-56989-5. PMID: 31941918; PMCID: PMC6962320.

Blanco-González A, Cabezón A, Seco-González A, Conde-Torres D, Antelo-Riveiro P, Piñeiro Á, Garcia-Fandino R. The Role of AI in Drug Discovery: Challenges, Opportunities, and Strategies. Pharmaceuticals (Basel). 2023 Jun 18;16(6):891. doi: 10.3390/ph16060891. PMID: 37375838; PMCID: PMC10302890.

Bogunovic H, et al (a). Machine Learning of the Progression of Intermediate Age-Related Macular Degeneration Based on OCT Imaging. Invest Ophthalmol Vis Sci. 2017;58(6):BIO141-BIO150. doi: 10.1167/iovs.17-21789. PMID: 28658477.

Bogunovic H, et al (b). Prediction of Anti-VEGF Treatment Requirements in Neovascular AMD Using a Machine Learning Approach. Invest Ophthalmol Vis Sci. 2017;58(7):3240-3248. doi: 10.1167/iovs.16-21053. PMID: 28660277.

Briggs FB, et al. Supervised machine learning and logistic regression identifies novel epistatic risk factors with PTPN22 for rheumatoid arthritis. Genes Immun. 2010

Apr;11(3):199-208. doi: 10.1038/gene.2009.110. Epub 2010 Jan 21. PMID: 20090771; PMCID: PMC3118040.

Brinker TJ, Hekler A, Enk AH et al. Deep learning outperformed 136 of 157 dermatologists in a head-to-head dermoscopic melanoma image classification task. Eur J Cancer 2019; 113:47–54.

Brinker TJ, Hekler A, Enk AH, et al. A convolutional neural net-work trained with dermoscopic images performed on par with145 dermatologists in a clinical melanoma image classification task. Eur J Cancer 2019; 111:148–54.

Calivà, F, et al. Studying osteoarthritis with artificial intelligence applied to magnetic resonance imaging. Nat Rev Rheumatol 18, 112–121 (2022). https://doi.org/10.1038/s41584-021-00719-7.

Castle JR, et al. Assessment of a Decision Support System for Adults with Type 1 Diabetes on Multiple Daily Insulin Injections. Diabetes Technol Ther. 2022 Dec;24(12):892-897. doi: 10.1089/dia.2022.0252. Epub 2022 Sep 5. PMID: 35920839; PMCID: PMC9700374.

Castle, JR, et al. Assessment of a Decision Support System for Adults with Type 1 Diabetes on Multiple Daily Insulin Injections. Diabetes Technology & Therapeutics 2022 24:12, 892-897

Chaki, J et al. Machine learning and artificial intelligence based Diabetes Mellitus detection and self-management: A systematic review. Journal of King Saud University - Computer and Information Sciences, 2022, 34, 3204-3225, ISSN 1319-1578, https://doi.org/10.1016/j.jksuci.2020.06.013.

Chang HY, Jung CK, Woo JI, Lee S, Cho J, Kim SW, Kwak TY. Artificial Intelligence in Pathology. J Pathol Transl Med. 2019 Jan;53(1):1-12. doi: 10.4132/jptm.2018.12.16. Epub 2018 Dec 28. PMID: 30599506; PMCID: PMC6344799.

Chen W, et al. 2021). "Deep Learning Methods for Heart Sounds Classification: A Systematic Review". Entropy. 23 (6):

Chiu HY, Chao HS, Chen YM. Application of Artificial Intelligence in Lung Cancer. Cancers (Basel). 2022 Mar 8;14(6):1370. doi: 10.3390/cancers14061370. PMID: 35326521; PMCID: PMC8946647.

Cho HH, Lee SH, Kim J, Park H. Classification of the glioma grading using radiomics analysis. PeerJ. 2018 Nov 22;6:e5982. doi: 10.7717/peerj.5982. PMID: 30498643; PMCID: PMC6252243.

Christou CD and Tsoulfas G. Challenges and opportunities in the application of artificial intelligence in gastroenterology and hepatology. World J Gastroenterol. 2021 Oct 7;27(37):6191-6223. doi: 10.3748/wjg.v27.i37.6191. PMID: 34712027; PMCID: PMC8515803.

Cohen-Shelly M, et al. Electrocardiogram screening for aortic valve stenosis using artificial intelligence. Eur Heart J. 2021;42(30):2885–96.

Dias, R., Torkamani, A. Artificial intelligence in clinical and genomic diagnostics. Genome Med 11, 70 (2019). https://doi.org/10.1186/s13073-019-0689-8.

Djavan B, Remzi M, Zlotta A, Seitz C, Snow P, Marberger M. Novel artificial neural network for early detection of prostate cancer. J Clin Oncol. 2002;20:921–929. doi:10.1200/JCO.2002.20.4.921.

Duarte JV, et al. Multivariate pattern analysis reveals subtle brain anomalies relevant to the cognitive phenotype in neurofibromatosis type 1. Hum Brain Mapp. 2014 Jan;35(1):89-106. doi: 10.1002/hbm.22161. Epub 2012 Sep 11. PMID: 22965669; PMCID: PMC6869472.

Ellahham S. Artificial Intelligence: The Future for Diabetes Care. Am J Med. 2020 Aug;133(8):895-900. doi: 10.1016/j.amjmed.2020.03.033. Epub 2020 Apr 20. PMID: 32325045.

Eriksen A, et al. Use of GPT-4 to Diagnose Complex Clinical Cases. New England Journal of Medicine AI 2023;1, 1. DOI: 10.1056/AIp2300031.

European Society of Radiology (ESR). What the radiologist should know about artificial intelligence - an ESR white paper. Insights Imaging. 2019 Apr 4;10(1):44. doi: 10.1186/s13244-019-0738-2. PMID: 30949865; PMCID: PMC6449411.

Fehr D, t al. Automatic classification of prostate cancer Gleason scores from multiparametric magnetic resonance images. Proc Natl Acad Sci U S A 2015;112:E6265–6273. doi: 10.1073/pnas.1505935112.

Fernandes AC Souto MEVC. Benefits, Limits, and Risks of GPT-4 as an AI Chatbot for Medicine. N Engl J Med. 2023 Jun 22;388(25):2399-2400. doi: 10.1056/NEJMc2305286. PMID: 37342940

Finne P, et al. Predicting the outcome of prostate biopsy in screen-positive men by a multilayer perceptron network. Urology. 2000;56:418–422. doi:10.1016/S0090-4295(00) 00672-5 11.

Flynn, B.I., Javan, E.M., Lin, E. et al. Deep learning based phenotyping of medical images improves power for gene discovery of complex disease. npj Digit. Med. 6, 155 (2023). https://doi.org/10.1038/s41746-023-00903-x.

Galloway CD et al. Development and Validation of a Deep-Learning Model to Screen for Hyperkalemia From the Electrocardiogram. JAMA Cardiol. 2019 May 1;4(5):428-436. doi: 10.1001/jamacardio.2019.0640. PMID: 30942845; PMCID: PMC6537816.

Gandhi Z, et al. Artificial Intelligence and Lung Cancer: Impact on Improving Patient Outcomes. Cancers (Basel). 2023 Oct 31;15(21):5236. doi: 10.3390/cancers15215236. PMID: 37958411; PMCID: PMC10650618.

Ge P, et al. Predictive models for prostate cancer based on logistic regression and artificial neural network. 2015 IEEE International Conference on Mechatronics and Automation (ICMA). 2015;1472–1477. 12.

Green WJ, Bal G, Hulman G, et al. KI-67 and DLX2 predict increased risk of metastasis formation in prostate cancer – a targeted molecular approach. Br J Cancer. 2016;115:236–242. doi: 10.1038/bjc.2016.169.

Gulshan V, et al. Development and Validation of a Deep Learning Algorithm for Detection of Diabetic Retinopathy in Retinal Fundus Photographs. JAMA. 2016 13;316:2402-2410. doi: 10.1001/jama.2016.17216. PMID: 27898976.

Guo, P et al. (2014). Gene expression profile based classification models of psoriasis. Genomics 103, 48 – 55.

Gustafson E, et al. A Machine Learning Algorithm for Identifying Atopic Dermatitis in Adults from Electronic Health Records. IEEE Int Conf Healthc Inform. 2017 Aug; 2017:83-90. doi: 10.1109/ICHI.2017.31. Epub 2017 Sep 14. PMID: 29104964; PMCID: PMC5664951.

Han, SS et al. Augmented Intelligence Dermatology: Deep Neural Networks Empower Medical Professionals in Diagnosing Skin Cancer and Predicting Treatment Options for 134 Skin Disorders Journal of Investigative Dermatology (2020) 140, 1753e1761; doi:10.1016/j.jid.2020.01.019.

Handa T., et al. Novel Artificial Intelligence-Based Technology for Chest Computed Tomography Analysis of Idiopathic Pulmonary Fibrosis. Ann. Am. Thorac. Soc. 2022;19:399–406. doi: 10.1513/AnnalsATS.202101-044OC.

Hashimoto DA, et al. Artificial Intelligence in Surgery: Promises and Perils. Ann Surg. 2018 Jul;268(1):70-76. doi: 10.1097/SLA.0000000000002693. PMID: 29389679; PMCID: PMC5995666.

Ho CY, et al. Image segmentation of plexiform neurofibromas from a deep neural network using multiple b-value diffusion data. Sci Rep. 2020 Oct 20;10(1):17857. doi: 10.1038/s41598-020-74920-1. PMID: 33082502; PMCID: PMC7575542.

Hogarty, D.T.et al. Artificial Intelligence in Dermatology—Where We Are and the Way to the Future: A Review. Am J Clin Dermatol 21, 41–47 (2020). https://doi.org/10.1007/s40257-019-00462-6

Honavar SG. Artificial intelligence in ophthalmology - Machines think! Indian J Ophthalmol. 2022, 70:1075-1079. doi: 10.4103/ijo.IJO_644_22. PMID: 35325987; PMCID: PMC9240552

Horimasu Y., et al. A Machine-Learning Based Approach to Quantify Fine Crackles in the Diagnosis of Interstitial Pneumonia: A Proof-of-Concept Study. Medicine. 2021;100:e24738.

Hosny A, Parmar C, Coroller TP, Grossmann P, Zeleznik R, Kumar A, et al. (2018) Deep learning for lung cancer prognostication: A retrospective multi-cohort radiomics study. PLoS Med 15(11): e1002711. https://doi.org/10.1371/journal.pmed.1002711

https://doi.org/10.1016/j.compbiomed.2019.103488.

https://doi.org/10.1016/j.talo.2023.100267.

Hughes MS, Addala A, Buckingham B. Digital Technology for Diabetes. N Engl J Med. 2023 Nov 30;389(22):2076-2086. doi: 10.1056/NEJMra2215899. PMID: 38048189.

Humbert-Droz M, et al. Development of a Natural Language Processing System for Extracting Rheumatoid Arthritis Outcomes From Clinical Notes Using the National Rheumatology Informatics System for Effectiveness Registry. Arthritis Care Res (Hoboken). 2023 Mar;75(3):608-615. doi: 10.1002/acr.24869. Epub 2022 Oct 31. PMID: 35157365.

Ismail, L., Materwala, H., Tayefi, M. et al. Type 2 Diabetes with Artificial Intelligence Machine Learning: Methods and Evaluation. Arch Computat Methods Eng 29, 313–333 (2022). https://doi.org/10.1007/s11831-021-09582-x.

Jamshidi N, et al. The radiogenomic risk score stratifies outcomes in a renal cell cancer phase 2 clinical trial. Eur Radiol. 2016 Aug;26(8):2798-807. doi: 10.1007/s00330-015-4082-8. Epub 2015 Nov 11. PMID: 26560727.

Jeong S, et al. Integrated Magneto-Electrochemical Sensor for Exosome Analysis. ACS Nano. 2016 Feb 23;10(2):1802-9. doi: 10.1021/acsnano.5b07584. Epub 2016 Jan 28. PMID: 26808216; PMCID: PMC4802494.

Joseph, GB, et al. AI MSK clinical applications: cartilage and osteoarthritis. Skeletal Radiol 51, 331–343 (2022). https://doi.org/10.1007/s00256-021-03909-2.

Kadian, S, et al. Recent advancements in machine learning enabled portable and wearable biosensors,Talanta Open,Volume 8,2023,100267,ISSN 2666-8319,

Kannan S, et al. Segmentation of Glomeruli Within Trichrome Images Using Deep Learning. Kidney Int Rep. 2019 Apr 15;4(7):955-962. doi: 10.1016/j.ekir.2019.04.008. PMID: 31317118; PMCID: PMC6612039.

Kazemi Y and Mirroshandel SA. A novel method for predicting kidney stone type using ensemble learning. Artif Intell Med. 2018 Jan;84:117-126. doi: 10.1016/j.artmed.2017.12.001. Epub 2017 Dec 11. PMID: 29241659.

Kigka VI, et al. Detection of Asymptomatic Carotid Artery Stenosis through Machine Learning. Annu Int Conf IEEE Eng Med Biol Soc. 2022 Jul;2022:1041-1044. doi: 10.1109/EMBC48229.2022.9870927. PMID: 36085692.

Kim Y, et al. Targeted proteomics identifies liquid-biopsy signatures for extracapsular prostate cancer. Nat Commun. 2016;7:11906.

Komura D., Ishikawa S. Machine Learning Methods for Histopathological Image Analysis. Comput. Struct. Biotechnol. J. 2018;16:34–42.
doi: 10.1016/j.csbj.2018.01.001.

Kras, Celi and Miller. Accelerating ophthalmic artificial intelligence research: the role of an open access data Repository. Curr Opin Ophthalmol 2020;31:337–50.doi:10.1097/ICU.0000000000000678pmid:http://www.ncbi.nlm.nih.gov/pubmed/32740059

Kröner PT, et al. Artificial intelligence in gastroenterology: A state-of-the-art review. World J Gastroenterol. 2021 Oct 28;27(40):6794-6824. doi: 10.3748/wjg.v27.i40.6794. PMID: 34790008; PMCID: PMC8567482.

Kwon JM, et al. Deep learning-based algorithm for detecting aortic stenosis using electrocardiography. J Am Heart Assoc. 2020;9(7): e014717.

Lareyre F, et al. Applications of artificial intelligence for patients with peripheral artery disease. J Vasc Surg. 2023 Feb;77(2):650-658.e1. doi: 10.1016/j.jvs.2022.07.160. Epub 2022 Jul 31. PMID: 35921995.

Lawrentschuk N, et al. Predicting prostate biopsy outcome: artificial neural networks and polychotomous regression are equivalent models. Int Urol Nephrol. 2011;43:23–30. doi:10.1007/s11255-010-9750-7.

Lee HC, et al. Derivation and Validation of Machine Learning Approaches to Predict Acute Kidney Injury after Cardiac Surgery. J Clin Med. 2018 Oct 3;7(10):322. doi: 10.3390/jcm7100322. PMID: 30282956; PMCID: PMC6210196.

Lee, E, et al. Artificial Intelligence for Mental Health Care: Clinical Applications, Barriers, Facilitators, and Artificial Wisdom. Biological Psychiatry: Cognitive Neuroscience and Neuroimaging. 6 (9): 856–
864. doi:10.1016/j.bpsc.2021.02.001. PMC 8349367. PMID 33571718.

Leung, R.K., et al. Using a multi-staged strategy based on machine learning and mathematical modeling to predict genotype-phenotype risk patterns in diabetic kidney disease: a prospective case–control cohort analysis. BMC Nephrol 14, 162 (2013). https://doi.org/10.1186/1471-2369-14-162.

Li Z, et al. Artificial Intelligence in Dermatology Image Analysis: Current Developments and Future Trends. J Clin Med. 2022 Nov 18;11(22):6826. doi: 10.3390/jcm11226826. PMID: 36431301; PMCID: PMC9693628.

Li Z., et al. Artificial Neural Network Identified the Significant Genes to Distinguish Idiopathic Pulmonary Fibrosis. Sci. Rep. 2023;13:1225. doi: 10.1038/s41598-023-28536-w.

Lin Q, Tam PK, Tang CS. Artificial intelligence-based approaches for the detection and prioritization of genomic mutations in congenital surgical diseases. Front Pediatr. 2023 Aug 1;11:1203289. doi: 10.3389/fped.2023.1203289. PMID: 37593442; PMCID: PMC10429173.

Lin, CS et al. Artificial intelligence may speed heart attack diagnosis and treatment. Presented at the American Heart Association's Annual Meeting Scientific Sessions 2023.

Liu F, et al. Fully Automated Diagnosis of Anterior Cruciate Ligament Tears on Knee MR Images by Using Deep Learning. Radiology: Artificial Intelligence. 2019; 1: 180091.

Liu Y, et al. Prediction of ESRD in IgA Nephropathy Patients from an Asian Cohort: A Random Forest Model. Kidney Blood Press Res. 2018;43(6):1852-1864. doi: 10.1159/000495818. Epub 2018 Dec 7. PMID: 30537719.

Liu Y,. et al. Prediction of ESRD in IgA Nephropathy Patients from an Asian Cohort: A Random Forest Model. Kidney Blood Press Res. 2018;43:1852-64.

Lofaro, D et al. Prediction of Chronic Allograft Nephropathy Using Classification Trees, Transplantation Proceedings, 42, 1130 – 1133, 2010. ISSN 0041-1345, https://doi.org/10.1016/j.transproceed.2010.03.062.

Long, E, et al. Monitoring and Morphologic Classification of Pediatric Cataract Using Slit-Lamp-Adapted Photography. Trans. Vis. Sci. Tech. 2017;6(6):2. https://doi.org/10.1167/tvst.6.6.2.

Low, M. et al. Automating vitiligo skin lesion segmentation using convolutional neural networks. 2020 IEEE 17th International Symposium on Biomedical Imaging (ISBI), 2020.

Lu, W, et al. Applications of Artificial Intelligence in Ophthalmology: General Overview, Journal of Ophthalmology, vol. 2018, Article ID 5278196, 15 pages, 2018. https://doi.org/10.1155/2018/5278196

Lui YW, et al. Artificial Intelligence in Neuroradiology: Current Status and Future Directions. AJNR Am J Neuroradiol. 2020 Aug;41(8):E52-E59. doi: 10.3174/ajnr.A6681. Epub 2020 Jul 30. PMID: 32732276; PMCID: PMC7658873.

M. Schinkel, K. Paranjape, R.S. Nannan Panday, N. Skyttberg, P.W.B. Nanayakkara. Clinical applications of artificial intelligence in sepsis: A narrative review. Computers in Biology and Medicine, 115, 2019,103488,ISSN 0010-4825,

Mayr C.Het al. Integrative Analysis of Cell State Changes in Lung Fibrosis with Peripheral Protein Biomarkers. EMBO Mol. Med. 2021;13:e12871. doi: 10.15252/emmm.202012871.

Melina A, et al. Artificial Intelligence for the Objective Evaluation of Acne Investigator Global Assessment. J Drugs Dermatol. 2018 Sep 1;17(9):1006-1009. PMID: 30235389.

Meng, F., Seredych, M., Chen, C., Gura, V., Mikahlovsky, S., Sandeman, S., Ingavle, G., Ozulumba, T., Miao, L., Anasori, B., & Gogotsi, Y. (2018). MXene Sorbents for Removal of Urea from Dialysate: A Step toward the Wearable Artificial Kidney. ACS Nano, 12(10), 10518-10528. https://doi.org/10.1021/acsnano.8b06494.

Mercan, OB, Kılıç, and Şen, M. Machine learning-based colorimetric determination of glucose in artificial saliva with different reagents using a smartphone coupled μPAD

Mohamadlou H, et al. Prediction of Acute Kidney Injury With a Machine Learning Algorithm Using Electronic Health Record Data. Can J Kidney Health Dis. 2018 Jun

8;5:2054358118776326. doi: 10.1177/2054358118776326. PMID: 30094049; PMCID: PMC6080076.

Mohsin S, , et al. (2023) The Role of Artificial Intelligence in Prediction, Risk Stratification, and Personalized Treatment Planning for Congenital Heart Diseases. Cureus 15(8): e44374. DOI 10.7759/cureus.44374.

Morgan, J; Vagal, A; Wu, CC. AI imaging in Practice: Introducing the Special Issue. Radiology. Published Online: Mar 23 2022 https://doi.org/10.1148/ryai.220039.

Myasoedova E, et al. Pharmacogenetics of Methotrexate in Rheumatoid Arthritis Consortium. Toward Individualized Prediction of Response to Methotrexate in Early Rheumatoid Arthritis: A Pharmacogenomics-Driven Machine Learning Approach. Arthritis Care Res (Hoboken). 2022 Jun;74(6):879-888. doi: 10.1002/acr.24834. Epub 2022 Apr 6. PMID: 34902228.

Naguib RN, et al. Neural network analysis of combined conventional and experimental prognostic markers in prostate cancer: a pilot study. Br J Cancer. 1998;78:246–250. doi:10.1038/bjc.1998.472.

Najjar R. Redefining Radiology: A Review of Artificial Intelligence Integration in Medical Imaging. Diagnostics. 2023; 13(17):2760. https://doi.org/10.3390/diagnostics13172760.

Narula S., Shameer K., Salem Omar A.M., Dudley J.T., Sengupta P.P. Machine-Learning Algorithms to Automate Morphological and Functional Assessments in 2D Echocardiography. J. Am. Coll. Cardiol. 2016; 68:2287–2295. doi: 10.1016/j.jacc.2016.08.062.

Neeraj K, et al. Convolutional neural networks for prostate cancer recurrence prediction. Proc SPIE. 2017.

Onishchenko, D et al (2022). Screening for idiopathic pulmonary fibrosis using comorbidity signatures in electronic health records. Nature Medicine. 28. 1-10. 10.1038/s41591-022-02010-y.

Pawar S.P. and Talbar S.N. Two-Stage Hybrid Approach of Deep Learning Networks for Interstitial Lung Disease Classification. BioMed Res. Int. 2022:7340902. doi: 10.1155/2022/7340902.

Pilia N, et al. ECG-based Estimation of Potassium and Calcium Concentrations: Proof of Concept with Simulated Data. Annu Int Conf IEEE Eng Med Biol Soc. 2019 Jul; 2019:2610-2613. doi: 10.1109/EMBC.2019.8857634. PMID: 31946431.

Poon, H. Multimodal generative AI for precision medicine. NEJM AI December 2023. doi: 10.1056/AI-S2300233

Pyrros, A., Borstelmann, S.M., Mantravadi, R. et al. Opportunistic detection of type 2 diabetes using deep learning from frontal chest radiographs. Nat Commun 14, 4039 (2023). https://doi.org/10.1038/s41467-023-39631-x

Raffort, J, et al. (2020). Artificial intelligence in abdominal aortic aneurysm, Journal of Vascular Surgery,72, 321-333.e1. ISSN 0741-5214. https://doi.org/10.1016/j.jvs.2019.12.026.

Ray A, et al. Artificial intelligence and Psychiatry: An overview. Asian J Psychiatr. 2022 Apr;70:103021. doi: 10.1016/j.ajp.2022.103021. Epub 2022 Feb 12. PMID: 35219978; PMCID: PMC9760544.

Remzi M,, et al. An artificial neural network to predict the outcome of repeat prostate biopsies. Urology. 2003;62:456–460. doi:10.1016/S0090-4295(03)00409-6.

Retson TA, et al. Reader Perceptions and Impact of AI on CT Assessment of Air Trapping. Radiol Artif Intell. 2021 Nov 10;4(2):e210160. doi: 10.1148/ryai.2021210160. PMID: 35391767; PMCID: PMC8980862.

Roblot V, et al. Artificial intelligence to diagnose meniscus tears on MRI. Diagnostic and Interventional Imaging. 2019; 100: 243–249.

Liu F, et al. Deep Learning Approach for Evaluating Knee MR Images: Achieving High Diagnostic Performance for Cartilage Lesion Detection. Radiology. 2018; 289: 160–169.

Schnürle, S. et al. On using Support Vector Machines for the Detection and Quantification of Hand Eczema. 9th International Conference on Agents and Artificial Intelligence (2017). DOI:10.5220/0006125000750084

Sens. Actuators B Chem., 329 (2021), 10.1016/j.snb.2020.129037

Sharma K, et al. Automatic Segmentation of Kidneys using Deep Learning for Total Kidney Volume Quantification in Autosomal Dominant Polycystic Kidney Disease.

Sci Rep. 2017 May 17;7(1):2049. doi: 10.1038/s41598-017-01779-0. PMID: 28515418; PMCID: PMC5435691.

Shrivastava VK et al, (2015). First review on psoriasis severity risk stratification: An engineering perspective. Computers in biology and medicine, 63, 52-63.

Smyser CD, Dosenbach NU, Smyser TA, Snyder AZ, Rogers CE, Inder TE, Schlaggar BL, Neil JJ. Prediction of brain maturity in infants using machine-learning algorithms. Neuroimage. 2016 Aug 1;136:1-9. doi: 10.1016/j.neuroimage.2016.05.029. Epub 2016 May 11. PMID: 27179605; PMCID: PMC4914443.

Soun, J.E.; Chow, D.S.; Nagamine, M.; Takhtawala, R.S.; Filippi, C.G.; Yu, W.; Chang, P.D. Artificial Intelligence and Acute Stroke Imaging. AJNR Am. J. Neuroradiol. 2021, 42, 2–11

Stephan C, et al. Multicenter evaluation of an artificial neural network to increase the prostate cancer detection rate and reduce unnecessary biopsies. Clin Chem. 2002;48:1279–1287. doi:10.1093/clinchem/48.8.1279.

Stojadinovic M, Stojadinovic M, Pantic D. Decision tree analysis for prostate cancer prediction. Srp Arh Celok Lek. 2018;147:39.

Ström P, et al. Artificial intelligence for diagnosis and grading of prostate cancer in biopsies: a population-based, diagnostic study. Lancet Oncol. 2020 Feb;21(2):222-232. doi: 10.1016/S1470-2045(19)30738-7. Epub 2020 Jan 8. Erratum in: Lancet Oncol. 2020 Feb;21(2):e70. PMID: 31926806.

Sun, X. et al. Artificial intelligence in cardiovascular diseases: diagnostic and therapeutic perspectives. Eur J Med Res 28, 242 (2023). https://doi.org/10.1186/s40001-023-01065-y.

Tallam, H et al. Fully Automated Abdominal CT Biomarkers for Type 2 Diabetes Using Deep Learning. Radiology 2022 304:1, 85-95.

Tang CQ, et al. (2018) Comparison of machine learning method and logistic regression model in prediction of acute kidney injury in severely burned patients. Zhonghua Shao Shang Za Zhi. 2018 Jun 20;34(6):343-348. Chinese. doi: 10.3760/cma.j.issn.1009-2587.2018.06.006. PMID: 29961290. (In Chinese).

Tang CSM, et al. Sequencing of a Chinese tetralogy of Fallot cohort reveals clustering mutations in myogenic heart progenitors. JCI Insight. 2022 Jan 25;7(2):e152198. doi: 10.1172/jci.insight.152198. PMID: 34905512; PMCID: PMC8855809.

Toivonen J, et al. Radiomics and machine learning of multisequence multiparametric prostate MRI: towards improved non-invasive prostate cancer characterization. PLoS One. 2019;14:e0217702. doi: 10.1371/journal.pone.0217702.

Tomašev N, et al. A clinically applicable approach to continuous prediction of future acute kidney injury. Nature. 2019 Aug;572 (7767):116-119. doi: 10.1038/s41586-019-1390-1. Epub 2019 Jul 31. PMID: 31367026; PMCID: PMC6722431.

Tyler NS, et al. An artificial intelligence decision support system for the management of type 1 diabetes. Nat Metab. 2020 Jul;2(7):612-619. doi: 10.1038/s42255-020-0212-y. Epub 2020 Jun 1. PMID: 32694787; PMCID: PMC7384292.

Vamathevan, J, et al. Applications of machine learning in drug discovery and development. Nat. Rev. Drug Discov. 2019, 18, 463–477.

Vamathevan, J, et al. Applications of machine learning in drug discovery and development. Nat. Rev. Drug Discov. 2019, 18, 463–477.

Vamathevan, J.; Clark, D.; Czodrowski, P.; Dunham, I.; Ferran, E.; Lee, G.; Li, B.; Madabhushi, A.; Shah, P.; Spitzer, M.; et al. Applications of machine learning in drug discovery and development. Nat. Rev. Drug Discov. 2019, 18, 463–477.

Van Booven, DJ, et al (2021) A Systematic Review of Artificial Intelligence in Prostate Cancer, Research and Reports in Urology, 31-39, DOI: 10.2147/RRU.S268596

van Gastel MDA, et al. Automatic Measurement of Kidney and Liver Volumes from MR Images of Patients Affected by Autosomal Dominant Polycystic Kidney Disease. J Am Soc Nephrol. 2019 Aug;30(8):1514-1522. doi: 10.1681/ASN.2018090902. Epub 2019 Jul 3. PMID: 31270136; PMCID: PMC6683702.

Wang H, et al.2021). Application of Artificial Intelligence in Acute Coronary Syndrome: A Brief Literature Review. Advances in Therapy. 38 (10): 5078–5086. doi:10.1007/s12325-021-01908-2. PMID 34528221. S2CID 237522871.

Wang Q, et al. Prediction and Diagnosis of Venous Thromboembolism Using Artificial Intelligence Approaches: A Systematic Review and Meta-Analysis. Clin Appl Thromb Hemost. 2021 Jan-Dec;27:10760296211021162. doi: 10.1177/10760296211021162. PMID: 34184560; PMCID: PMC8246532.

Wang, P, et al. Automatic classification of breast cancer histopathological images based on deep feature fusion and enhanced routing. Biomedical Signal Processing and Control, 65, 2021,102341, ISSN 1746-8094. https://doi.org/10.1016/j.bspc.2020.102341.

Wei CJ, et al. Computed Tomography-Based Differentiation of Benign and Malignant Craniofacial Lesions in Neurofibromatosis Type I Patients: A Machine Learning Approach. Front Oncol. 2020 Jul 31;10:1192. doi: 10.3389/fonc.2020.01192. PMID: 32850344; PMCID: PMC7411852.

Xiao J, et al. Comparison and development of machine learning tools in the prediction of chronic kidney disease progression. J Transl Med. 2019 Apr 11;17(1):119. doi: 10.1186/s12967-019-1860-0. PMID: 30971285; PMCID: PMC6458616.

Yang F., et al. Pneumoconiosis Computer Aided Diagnosis System Based on X-Rays and Deep Learning. BMC Med. Imaging. 2021;21:189. doi: 10.1186/s12880-021-00723-z.

Yao T, et al. A Deep Learning Pipeline for Assessing Ventricular Volumes from a Cardiac MRI Registry of Patients with Single Ventricle Physiology. Radiol Artif Intell. 2024; 6(1):e230132. doi: 10.1148/ryai.230132. PMID: 38166332.

Yedavalli, V.S.; Tong, E.; Martin, D.; Yeom, K.W.; Forkert, N.D. Artificial intelligence in stroke imaging: Current and future perspectives. Clin. Imaging 2021, 69, 246–254.

Yeo L, et al. Expression of chemokines CXCL4 and CXCL7 by synovial macrophages defines an early stage of rheumatoid arthritis. Ann Rheum Dis. 2016 Apr;75(4):763-71. doi: 10.1136/annrheumdis-2014-206921. Epub 2015 Apr 9. PMID: 25858640; PMCID: PMC4819606.

Yin WJ, et al. Preprocedural Prediction Model for Contrast-Induced Nephropathy Patients. J Am Heart Assoc. 2017 Feb 3;6(2): e004498. doi: 10.1161/JAHA.116.004498. PMID: 28159819; PMCID: PMC5523753.

Yoosuf N, et al. Early prediction of clinical response to anti-TNF treatment using multi-omics and machine learning in rheumatoid arthritis. Rheumatology (Oxford). 2022 Apr 11;61(4):1680-1689. doi: 10.1093/rheumatology/keab521. PMID: 34175943; PMCID: PMC8996791.

Yuan, Q et al. Int J Med Sci. 2020; 17(7): 970–984. Published online 2020 Apr 6. doi: 10.7150/ijms.42078. PMCID: PMC7163364. PMID: 32308551.

Zacharias HU, et al. A Novel Metabolic Signature To Predict the Requirement of Dialysis or Renal Transplantation in Patients with Chronic Kidney Disease. J Proteome Res. 2019 Apr 5;18(4):1796-1805. doi: 10.1021/acs.jproteome.8b00983. Epub 2019 Mar 12. PMID: 30817158.

Zugang, Y, et al. Application of artificial intelligence in diagnosis and treatment of colorectal cancer: A novel prospect. Frontiers in Medicine 10, 2023. https://www.frontiersin.org/articles/10.3389/fmed.2023.1128084. DOI=10.3389/fmed.2023.1128084.

Abbreviations used

2TBN, two-timeslice Bayesian network

3SFCA, three-step floating catchment area

ABCA4, ATP-binding cassette transporter gene sub-family A

ACO, ant colony optimization

ACPA, anti-cyclic citrullinated peptide antibody

AD, Alzheimer's disease

ADC, apparent diffusion coefficient

ADHD, adult attention deficit hyperactivity disorder

ADPKD, autosomal dominant polycystic kidney disease

ADR, adenoma detection rate

ADR, adenoma detection rate

ADRD, attention-aware dense net with residual deconvolution

AGI, artificial general intelligence

AI, artificial intelligence

AI-ECG, AI-enhanced electrocardiogram

AION, ischemic optic neuropathy

AIP, autoimmune pancreatitis

AIQCT, artificial-intelligence-based quantitative CT image analysis software

AIRS, artificial immune recognition system

AKI, acute kidney injury

ALBI, albumin-bilirubin

ALD, alcoholic liver disease

ALK, anaplastic lymphoma kinase

ALVD, asymptomatic left ventricular dysfunction

AMD, age-related macular degeneration

AMI, acute myocardial infarction

AMR, adenoma miss rate

ANN, artificial neural network

APO, artificial plant optimization

AREDS, age-related eye disease studies

ARIMA, autoregressive integrated moving average

AS, aortic stenosis

ASD, autism spectrum disorder

ATP, adenosine triphosphate

AUC, area under the receiver operating characteristic curve

AUROC, area under the receiver operating characteristic curve

AUROC: Area under the receiver operating characteristic curve.

BACE1, beta-secretase

BAF, B allele frequency

BCC, basal cell carcinoma from smartphone-captured

BCLC, Barcelona-Clinic-Liver-Cancer (staging system)

bDMARD, biologic disease-modifying antirheumatic drug

BE, Barrett's esophagus

BMI, body mass index

bp, base pairs

BP, blood pressure

CAD, computer-aided detection

CADD, combined annotation-dependent depletion approach

CADe, computer-aided detection

CAKUT, congenital abnormalities of the kidney and urinary tract

CAP, credit assignment path

CARD, comprehensive antibiotic resistance database

CART, classification and regression tree

CCA, cholangiocarcinoma

CD, Crohn's disease

CDAI, clinical disease activity index

CDE, common data element

CDN, content delivery network or content distribution network

CDS, Clinical Decision Support System

CeD, celiac disease

CETZ, contrast enema transition zone

Chat GPT, Chat Generative Pre-trained Transformer

ChatGPT, Chat Generative Pre-trained Transformer

CHD, congenital heart disease

CIN, contrast-induced nephropathy

CIN, contrast-induced nephropathy

CKD, chronic kidney disease

CKD, chronic kidney disease

CKD, chronic kidney disease

CKD-MBD, chronic kidney disease mineral and bone metabolism disorders

CML, continuous machine learning

CMRI, cardiovascular magnetic resonance imaging

CNF, conjunctive normal form

CNN, convolutional neural network

CNV, copy number variant

CPU, central processing unit

CR = complete remission

CRC, colo-rectal cancer

CRP, C-reactive protein

csDMARDS, conventional synthetic disease-modifying antirheumatic drugs

CT, computed tomography

CTC, connectionist temporal classification

CTP, Child–Turcotte–Pugh

CVD, cardiovascular disease

CXR, chest x-ray

Cycle GANS-consistent adversarial networks

DA, discriminant analysis

DALY, disability-adjusted life year

DAS, disease activity score

DAS, disease activity score

DBN, dynamic Bayesian network

dbNSFP, database for nonsynonymous SNPs' functional predictions

DBT, digital breast tomosynthesis;

DC, dilated cardiomyopathy

DCIS, ductal carcinoma in situ

DCIS, ductal carcinoma in situ

DCNN, deep convoluted neural network

DEG, differentially expressed gene

DFC, deep feature classification

DFC, deep feature classification

DIA, digital imaging analysis

DICE, diverse counterfactual explanations

DICOM, digital imaging and communications in medicine

DIHM, digital in-line holographic microscopy

DKD, diabetic kidney disease

DL, deep learning

DL, deep learning

DL, description logic

DNN, deep neural network

DPLL, Davis–Putnam–Logemann–Loveland

DR, diabetic retinopathy

DRE, digital rectal examination

DRI, donor risk index

DSC, Sørensen–Dice coefficient

DSL, digital subscriber line

DSM-5, The Diagnostic and Statistical Manual of Mental Disorders, Fifth Edition

DT, decision tree

DVT, deep vein thrombosis

DWI, diffusion weighted imaging

EA, evolutionary algorithm

EDA, estimation of distribution algorithm

EDA, exploratory data analysis

EDV, end-diastolic volume

EEC, early esophageal adenocarcinoma

EEG, electroencephalogram

EF, ejection fraction

EFS, ensemble feature selection

EGF, epidermal growth factor

EGFR, epidermal growth factor receptor

EHR, electronic health record

ELISA, enzyme-linked immunosorbent assay

ELM, extreme learning machine

EMT, extended mind thesis

EPO, erythropoietin

ER, estrogen receptor

ESR, erythrocyte sedimentation rate

ESR, European Society of Radiology

ESR, European Society of Radiology

ESRD, end-stage renal disease

ESRD, end-stage renal disease

ESV, end-systolic volume

EUS, endoscopic ultrasound

FCN, fully convolutional neural network

FDA, Food and Drug Administration (USA)

FDR, false discovery rate

FDR, Fischer discriminant ratio

FFN, feedforward neural network

FISH, fluorescence in situ hybridization

FLD, fatty liver disease

FOL, first-order logic

GA, genetic algorithm

GAD, Genetic Association Database

GATK, genome analysis toolkit

GB, gradient boosting

GBM, glioblastoma low-grade glioma

GBS, Glasgow-Blatchford score

GC, gastric cancer

G-CSF, granulocyte colony-stimulating factor

GEO, Gene Expression Omnibus

GEO, gene expression omnibus

GEP, gene expression programming

GIB, gastrointestinal bleeding

GIM, gastric intestinal metaplasia

GMDH, group method of data handling

GM-LARS, generalized linear model-based least angle regression

GO, gene ontology

GOFAI, good old-fashioned AI

GP, genetic programming

GPU, graphics processing unit

GRNN, generalized regression neural network

GRO, growth-regulated oncogene

GSEA, gene set enrichment analysis

GTEx, genotype-tissue expression

HASTE, Half-Fourier Acquisition Single-shot Turbo spin Echo imaging.

HBV, hepatitis B

HCC, hepatocellular carcinoma

HCC, hepatocellular carcinoma

HCM, hypertrophic cardiomyopathy

HCV, hepatitis C

HDCP, high-definition care platform

H&E, hematoxilin and eosin

HEMLBC, H&E manual liquid-based cytology

HER, electronic heath record

HER2, human epidermal growth factor receptor 2

HGDM, human gene mutation database

HIV, human immunodeficiency virus

HMM, hidden Markov model

hPSC, human pluripotent stem cell

HRCT, high resolution computed tomography

HSCR, Hirschsprung disease

HTM, hierarchical temporal memory

I/O, input/output

IBD, identity-by-descent

IBD, inflammatory bowel disease

IBD, inflammatory bowel disease

IBD, inflammatory bowel disease

IC, interval cancer

ICC, intraclass correlation coefficient

ICC, intraclass correlation coefficients

ICD, International Classification of Disease

ICU, intensive care unit

IFN, interferon

IGAN, IgA nephropathy

IHC, immunohistochemistry

IHC, immunohistochemistry

IL, interleukin

ILD, interstitial lung disease

ILP, inductive logic programming

IML, interpretable machine learning

IOP, intra-ocular pressure

IoT, internet of things

IPF, idiopathic pulmonary fibrosis

iRAD, implantable renal assist device

IS, interstitial fluid

ISH, in situ hybridization

ISIC, skin imaging collaboration

ISR, information support robot

JAGG, Judging the Accuracy of CNVs and Genotyping

JDPCA, joint diagonalization principal component analysis

JPEG, joint photographic experts group

KEGG, Kyoto Encyclopedia of Genes and Genomes

kNN, k-nearest neighbor

KR, KR^2 and KR&R, knowledge representation and reasoning

LCS, learning classifier system

LGG, low grade glioma

LIDAR, light imaging, detection, and ranging

LLaVA-Med, an open source multimodal language model that can be used for visual question answering and has limited support for object detection.

LLM, large language model

LLM, large language model

LMM, Large Multimodal Model

LN, lymph node

LN, lymph node

LNM, lymph node metastasis

LOA, limits of agreement (LOA)

LR, logistic regression

LRR, Log R Ratio

LSTM, long short-term memory

LVF, left ventricular failure

LVH, left ventricular hypertrophy

MARVEL, multiscale analysis of regulatory variants on the epigenomic landscape

MAS, multi-agent system

MCC, Merkel cell carcinoma

MD, molecular dynamics

MEA, means-ends analysis

Med-PaLM M, a LLM specialized to the medical domain and can take images, as well as text prompts, as inputs. This allows it to be used for a wider variety of tasks than an LLM alone.

MELD, model for end-stage liver disease

MEM, micro-electro-mechanical system

MF, mycosis fungoides

MI, mutual information

MILD, Multicentric Italian Lung Detection (trial)

ML, machine learning

MIP, macrophage inflammatory protein

MIT, Massachusetts Institute of Technology

MLA, manifold learning algorithms

MLP, multilayer perceptron

MLP, multi-layer perceptron

MLR, machine-learned ranking

MMG, mammography

MOI, microscopic ocular images

MP3, motion picture experts group

MPI, myocardial perfusion imaging

MPNST, malignant peripheral nerve sheath tumor

MPRA, massively parallel reporter assay

MPT, multiphoton tomography

MR, mitral regurgitation

MRCP, magnetic resonance cholangiopancreatography

MVI, microvascular invasion

NAFLD, non-alcoholic fatty liver disease

NAION, non-arteritic anterior ischemic optic neuropathy

NASH, non-alcoholic steatohepatitis

NBI, narrow band imaging

NGS, next generation sequencing

NGS, next-generation sequencing

NHS, National Health Service (UK)

NLI, natural language interpretation

NLP, natural language processing

NLU, natural language understanding

NLUI, natural-language user interface

NP, nondeterministic polynomial time

NPDR, nonproliferative diabetic retinopathy

NSCLC, non-small cell lung cancer

NSCLC, non-small cell lung cancer

OAG, open-angle glaucoma

OCR, optical character recognition

OCT, optical coherence tomography

OCT, optical coherence tomography

OCTA, optical coherence tomography angiography

ODR, optic cup-to-disc ratio

ODx, oncotype diagnosis

OLT, orthotopic liver transplantation

OMIM, Online Mendelian Inheritance in man

ONH, optic nerve head

OSIC, Open Source Imaging Consortium

PACS, picture archiving and communication system

PAD, peripheral arterial disease

PARTZ, plain abdominal radiograph transition zone

PCA, principal component analysis

PCN, pancreas cystic neoplasms

PCR, polymerase chain reaction

PD = progressive disease

PDAC, pancreatic ductal adenocarcinoma

PD-L1, programmed death ligand 1

PDR, proliferative diabetic retinopathy

PET, positron emission tomography

PgR, progesterone receptor

PheWAS, phenome-wide association study

PMBGA, probabilistic model-building genetic algorithm

PN, plexiform neurofibroma

POC, point-of-care

PPI, protein–protein interactive

PR, partial response

PR, progesterone receptor

pRAS, psoriasis risk assessment system

PRISM, Preferred Reporting Items for Systematic Review and Metaanalysis

PSA, prostate specific antigen

PSSP, patient-specific survival prediction

PTH, parathyroid hormone

RBC, red blood cell

RBF, radial basis function

RBF, radial basis function

RBM, restricted Boltzmann machine

RCC, renal cell carcinoma

REVEL, rare exome variant ensemble learner

RF, random forest

RFA, radiofrequency ablation

RGB, red, green and blue

RMSE, root mean squared error

RNA, ribonucleic acid

RNFL retina nerve fiber layer

RNN, recurrent neural network

RO, random optimization

ROC, receiver operating characteristic curve

ROC, receiver operating characteristic curve

ROI, region of interest

RoS, risk of sepsis score

RPA, robotic process automation

RPF, recursive partitioning forest

RSNA, Radiology Society of North America

RVF, Rift Valley fever

RVSD, right ventricular systolic dysfunction

SA, simulated annealing

SARIMA, seasonal autoregressive integrated moving average

SARIMA-NNAR, seasonal autoregressive integrated moving average neural network auto-regression

SC, soft computing

SCC, squamous cell carcinoma

SD = stable disease

SD-OCT, spectrum domain OCT

SI, swarm intelligence

SIANN, shift invariant or space invariant artificial neural networks

SL, supervised learning

SLN, sentinel lymph node

SLNB, sentinel lymph node biopsy

SLNB, sentinel lymph node biopsy

SNP, single nucleotide polymorphism

SNV, single-nucleotide variation

SO, stochastic optimization

SOAR, security orchestration, automation and response

SOC, security operations center

SOFA, sequential organ failure assessment

SROC, summary receiver operating characteristic

SSL, semi-supervised learning

STEMI, ST-elevation myocardial infarction

SVM, support vector machine

SVR, sustained virological response

TCAG, The Cancer Genome Atlas

TFI, tubule formation indicator

TGF, transforming growth factor

TGN, thioguanine nucleotide

TGN, thioguanine nucleotide

TIL, tumor-infiltrating lymphocyte

TKV, total kidney volume

TMA, tissue microarray

TNBC, triple-negative breast cancer

TNF, tumor necrosis factor

TNM, tumor node metastasis

TOF, Tetralogy of Fallot

TRUS, transrectal ultrasound

tsDMARDS, targeted synthetic DMARDs

UC, ulcerative colitis

US, ultrasound.

VCE, video capsule endoscopy

VEGF, vascular endothelial growth factor

VF, visual field

VQSR, variant quality score recalibration

VQSR, variant quality score recalibration

VUS, variants of uncertain significance

VUS, variants of uncertain significance

WES, whole exome sequencing

WGS, whole genome sequencing

WGS, whole genome sequencing

WLI, white light imaging

WSI, whole-slide image.

XAI, explainable AI

XHMM, exome hidden Markov model

Made in United States
Orlando, FL
04 November 2026

90201577R00231